Current Concepts in Parenteral Nutrition

Current Concepts in Parenteral Nutrition

edited by

J. M. Greep
P. B. Soeters
R. I. C. Wesdorp
C. W. R. Phaf
J. E. Fischer

1977

Martinus Nijhoff Medical Division
The Hague

ISBN-13:978-94-010-1072-6 e-ISBN-13:978-94-010-1070-2
DOI: 10.1007/978-94-010-1070-2

Contents

2 Specific aspects of management

List of contributors

Ronald M. Abel, M.D., Assistant Professor of Surgery, Director of Hyperalimentation Unit, The New York Hospital-Cornell Medical Center, New York, USA

F. W. Ahnefeld, Professor of Anaesthesiology, University of Ulm, W.Germany

Thomas L. Anderson, M.D., Department of Pediatrics, Columbia College of Physicians and Surgeons, Columbia-Presbyterian Medical Center, New York City, New York, USA

Bruce R. Bistrian, M.D., Ph.D., Cancer Research Institute, New England Deaconess Hospital; Harvard Medical School, Boston, Massachusetts, USA

George L. Blackburn, M.D., Ph.D., Cancer Research Institute, New England Deaconess Hospital; Harvard Medical School, Boston, Massachusetts, USA

K. D. Bury, M.D., ScM., FRCS (C), FACS, University of Toronto, Department of Surgery, Wellesley Hospital, Toronto, Ontario, Canada

P. E. Carlo, Ph.D., Consultant to the Drug Industry, Paris, France

R. Colley, Nurse, Clinician Hyperalimentation Unit, Massachusetts General Hospital, Boston, USA

Edward M. Copeland, M.D., Associate Professor of Surgery, The University of Texas Medical School at Houston, USA

R. Dölp, University of Ulm, Department of Anaesthesiology, Ulm, W.Germany

Stanley J. Dudrick, M.D., Chairman Department of Surgery, The University of Texas Medical School at Houston, USA

Josef E. Fischer, M.D., Associate Professor of Surgery, Harvard Medical School, Chief of Hyperalimentation Unit, Massachusetts General Hospital, Boston, USA (editor)

Jean-Pierre Flatt, Ph.D., Cancer Research Institute, New England Deaconess Hospital; Harvard Medical School, Boston, Massachusetts, USA

J. M. Greep, Professor of Surgery, Medical Faculty, University of Limburg, Maastricht, The Netherlands (editor)

M. Halmágyi, University of Mainz, Professor of Anaesthesiology, Mainz, W.Germany

E. L. M. Hardy, Pharmacist, Department of Clinical Pharmacy, St. Annadal Hospital, Maastricht, The Netherlands

William C. Heird, M.D., Department of Pediatrics, Columbia University, College of Physicians and Surgeons, Columbia-Presbyterian Medical Center, New York City, New York, USA

L. Heller, Prof. Dr., Zentrum der Frauenheilkunde und Geburtshilfe, Frankfurt a/Main, W.Germany

K. N. Jeejeebhoy, M.D., Professor of Medicine, University of Toronto, Canada

Friedrichkarl Jekat, Prof. Dr., Fachbereich Ernährungswissenschaften Universität Giessen

Direktor, Chemische Untersuchungsanstalt Oberhausen, Bochum, W.Germany

H. A. Lee, B.Sc., M.B., B.S., FRCP, Professor of Metabolic Medicine, Department of Nephrology, University of Southampton, Wessex Regional Renal Unit, St. Mary's Hospital, Portsmouth, Hampshire, UK

James M. Long, M.D., Attending Surgeon, Hermann Hospital, Houston, Texas, USA

Bruce V. MacFadyen, Jr., M.D., Assistant Professor of Surgery, The University of Texas Medical School at Houston, USA

Baltej S. Maini, M.D., Cancer Research Institute, New England Deaconess Hospital; Harvard Medical School, Boston, Massachusetts, USA

John D. B. Miller, M.D., FRCS, Ed., Cancer Research Institute, New England Deaconess Hospital; Harvard Medical School, Boston, Massachusetts, USA

H. N. Munro, M.D., Physiological Chemistry Laboratories Department of Nutrition and Food Science Massachusetts Institute of Technology Cambridge, Mass., USA

C. W. R. Phaf, Hospital pharmacist, Chief Department of Clinical Pharmacy, St. Anna dal Hospital, Maastricht, The Netherlands (editor)

Hugh Rienhoff, B.A., Cancer Research Institute, New England Deaconess Hospital; Har vard Medical School, Boston, Massachusetts, USA

Peter B. Soeters, Chief Resident, Ziekenhuis St. Annadal, Maastricht, The Netherlands (editor)

R. I. C. Wesdorp, Department of Surgery, Ziekenhuis St. Annadal, Maastricht, The Netherlands (editor)

Douglas W. Wilmore, M.D., United States Army Institute of Surgical Research Brooke Army Medical Center, Fort Sam Houston, Texas, USA

Robert W. Winters, M.D., Department of Pediatrics, Columbia University, College of Physicians and Surgeons, Columbia-Presbyterian Medical Center, New York City, New York, USA

Arvid Wretlind, Department of Human Nutrition, Medical Faculty, Karolinska institutet, Stockholm, Sweden

Introduction

J. E. Fischer, M.D.

Professor Greep, ladies and gentlemen. It is a great pleasure for me and the participants to be present at this International Meeting of Parenteral Nutrition. This meeting would not have been possible five years ago. At that time we were still arguing about central vs. peripheral routes, efficacy of the technique, and still getting accustomed to our ability to support patients nutritionally. Within the last five years these discussions, which seem almost futile in retrospect, have been put aside. Both techniques, we know how, work quite well and have their own indications.

Having become comfortable with the technique, it is now time to enter the second phase of parenteral nutrition, and that is the differentiation of the technique for the benefit of different patients. Over the next two days we will be discussing several problems which at the present time are central to the entire subject of parenteral nutrition. Is a fat calorie the same as a carbohydrate calorie? What is the effect on protein metabolism of the fat calorie as opposed to the carbohydrate calorie? Are they equivalent? Are there situations in which one is superior to the other? Perhaps we will find out tomorrow in the panel.

It has long been clear that patients with hepatic and renal failure do not tolerate nitrogen in the usual sense. Using the now available crystalline amino acids, can we now determine which amino acids are best for these patients and can we devise optimal protein and caloric intakes, based on carefully done studies now within our grasp? This afternoon we shall hear a little more about these two disease conditions.

Although the different needs in these conditions are obvious, the differences between the requirements of the usual patients and pediatric, burn patients, and the regrowing depleted patients, are more subtle. Are the requirements for these patients different, and if so, how? How may we best optimize their care?

We shall also hear over the next two days about patients with cancer and the possibilities that part of the ravages of that disease are due to nutritional deficiencies. Can we help patients with cancers survive radical surgery, aggressive chemotherapy, and supervoltage radiation by the addition of adequate nutrition? Perhaps.

Parenteral nutrition has been one of the most significant advances in patient care, certainly in the last decade, and perhaps in this century. Through its benefits, many patients are surviving that ordinarily would not have. It is altogether fitting and appropriate the inaugural conference of the new department of surgery at the University of Limburg Medical School, under the direction of Professor Greep, itself, a significant departure in medical education, be held on parenteral nutrition. Professor Greep is widely known as a surgical innovator and a man of wide vision. On a more personal note, several of the young men you will see over the next two days are people who I have a personal stake in. I assure you you will be hearing a lot more from the new department of surgery in Maastricht, from Professor Greep, and from some of the people in his department.

1

General principles of parenteral nutrition

Applications and hazards of intravenous hyperalimentation

Stanley J. Dudrick, M.D., James M. Long, M.D.

Among the primary functions of the gastrointestinal tract are ingestion, digestion and absorption of food and assimilation of resulting substrates into the body cell mass. Any one or more of a variety of pathologic processes may significantly compromise any or all of these vital functions, and homeostasis and nutritional integrity might well become dependent upon parenteral administration of essential biochemical substrates for extended periods of time. The successful clinical application of intravenous hyperalimentation has allowed total parenteral nutrition to be a reality for the first time (1). By this technique, it is now possible to provide the quantity and quality of essential nutrients necessary to maintain positive nitrogen balance and to achieve weight stability or gain in adults and normal growth and development in infants under a wide variety of conditions usually associated with a catabolic response. Having the capacity to feed patients adequately by vein has given the physician an option to bypass a malfunctioning alimentary tract for as long as necessary to allow return of normal or maximal function, while simultaneously maintaining or improving the nutritional status of the patient. Moreover, a period or relative gastrointestinal tract rest, which total parenteral nutrition makes possible, allows time for the diseased or disordered segment of the system to be spared from secretory and mechanical stimulation and its usual functions while it is being repaired or restored. Furthermore, the feasibility of administering all required nutrient substrates by parenteral means has provided basic and clinical investigators with a valuable and novel model for studying the physiologic and pathophysiologic processes and reactions of the gastrointestinal tract and other body systems and for achieving absolute control of substrate input for metabolic studies.

Restoration and maintenance of nutritional and metabolic homeostasis must be concomitant goals throughout all phases of diagnosis, therapy, recovery, convalescence and rehabilitation of patients (2). This is best accomplished by conscientious attention to dietary regimens, tailored to the specific requirements and conditions in individual patients, and delivered to the gastrointestinal tract by mouth, by a variety of enteral feeding tubes or by surgical ostomies whenever possible and practical. However, when use of the alimentary tract for delivering nutrients is inadequate, ill-advised or impossible for extended periods of time, nourishment must be supplemented or accomplished entirely by parenteral routes. The basic indications for application of total parenteral nutrition clinically are for support and management of patients who cannot eat, who will not eat, who should not eat or who cannot eat enough.

Applications when adequate enteral intake is impossible

The many specific conditions in which use of the alimentary tract for nourishing a patient optimally may be impossible can be classified into the following categories: a) mechanical obstruction; b) reflex or postoperative ileus; c) acute inflammatory, catabolic or malabsorptive processes; d) short-gut syndrome.

Enteral nutrition is impaired by obstruction of the alimentary tract by any lesion or disorder that either totally or partially impedes the natural flow of nutrients through the lumen. Conditions that gradually produce obstruction of the alimentary tract often cause a progressive and insidious form of malnutrition which may be easily corrected by total parenteral nutrition. However, sudden onset of acute obstruction of the alimentary tract usually requires prompt operative intervention before a meaningful program of nutritional rehabilitation can be undertaken. The most frequent and significant complications following definitive operations for lesions that have gradually obstructed the upper gastrointestinal tract are related directly to the nutritional deficits incurred before operation. Every patient who is to undergo a surgical procedure for a non-acute obstructing lesion of the alimentary tract should be given serious consideration as a candidate for preoperative parenteral feeding. Thereby, not only can the incidence of postoperative anastomotic failure be reduced, but the patient will better tolerate the effects of the catabolic response to the operation and avoid many of the other complications that often prolong morbidity or increase mortality. If an anastomotic leak occurs, it can frequently be managed satisfactorily by a conservative regimen of simple drainage, bowel rest and total parenteral nutrition, thus avoiding another major operation in most cases.

Complete obstruction of the small or large bowel is usually treated best by immediate operation. Occasionally, when the question of complete versus partial obstruction is unanswered, especially when the primary etiology is regional enteritis, granulomatous colitis, ulcerative colitis or diverticulitis, patients can be partially replenished with vital biochemical substrates until the diagnosis is established and definitive therapy is undertaken. Operation should not be delayed when the clinical condition of the patient suggests imminent danger. On the other hand, every opportunity should be taken to supply the depleted cellular milieu with essential nutrients from which life-sustaining proteins can be synthesized.

Total parenteral nutrition in children has been particularly applicable to situations in which extensive operative resection or reconstruction of gastro-intestinal continuity has been necessary during the neonatal period, as well as to conditions that render the alimentary tract temporarily ineffective as a means of sustaining normal nutrition. Despite the gravity of the insult imposed by lesions of the alimentary tract, infants have been successfully supported during preoperative, operative and postoperative management of complex congenital anomalies. Moreover, intravenous hyperalimentation allows growth and development of the infant, permitting specific organs to mature, heal or recover sufficiently to achieve normal function or to adapt to resected or altered components of the alimentary tract. The problem of managing severely premature or immature neonates is just as great as managing an infant who has the short-gut syndrome. In both instances, the infant's inability to maintain normal enteral nutrition is aggravated by limited organ function. Total parenteral nutrition can support normal growth and development of the infant until the alimentary tract is functional and self-sufficient.

Prolonged adynamic ileus may result from myriad metabolic, traumatic, reflex, or inflammatory disorders. In all of these conditions, the association of starvation with the catabolic process, determined in large measure by the etiology of the ileus, establishes a sequence of events that can lead to steady deterioration and death, if the process is not interrupted. If a patient is unable to resume oral intake within seven to ten days after an operation, parenteral nutrition should be instituted. However, total parenteral nutrition is never a substitute for adequate surgical or medical therapy, and abscesses must be drained, obstructions relieved, foreign bodies removed, infections controlled and fluid and electrolyte balance achieved for optimal patient management to be realized.

Enteral feeding is not only frequently impossible but may be contra-indicated in a patient who has acute pancreatitis. Bowel rest appears to be one of the most important therapeutic measures in managing this disorder because of the reduced stimulation of digestive hormones and enzymes. But, total bowel rest imposes *de facto* a state of starvation upon a patient who already has increased demands for nutrients. The application of total parenteral nutrition has obviated this therapeutic dilemma. Moreover, pancreatic fistulas have closed spontaneously while the patient was maintained on this regimen (3).

In patients who have sustained major full-thickness burns or other complicated trauma in whom nutrient requirements cannot be met by enteral feeding, as many as 5000 to 7000 calories a day have been provided totally by vein or by using a combination of oral, tube and intravenous feedings. Using combination techniques, over 200 grams of protein equivalent have been given to selected patients with multiple injuries.

Massive loss of small bowel, for whatever reason, leaves the patient in a situation in which normal oral nutritional sustenance is impossible. Following massive resections, the residual bowel is incapable of immediately performing the secretory and absorptive functions formerly accomplished by the entire intestine. Applying the technique of total parenteral nutrition for several months in such patients has been lifesaving (4).

Applications when adequate enteral intake is inadvisable

During the early phases of granulomatous enterocolitis, mucosal involvement passes through a phase which may be compared to a first-degree burn, that is, minimal inflammation without significant loss of tissue and with the possibility of complete recovery. Another group of patients with granulomatous enterocolitis has a bowel injury roughly comparable to a second-degree burn, that is, serious epithelial damage from which recovery is possible if the residual viable basilar cells are adequately protected from further injury. The institution of a regimen of bowel rest and total parenteral nutrition has significant application in both of these circumstances. In some patients, however, the inflammatory response is so severe that spontaneous complete recovery of the bowel is unlikely or impossible, a condition analogous to a third-degree burn. Under these circumstances, operation is usually required.

In a series of 52 consecutive patients with inflammatory bowel disease treated with intravenous hyperalimentation, patients with granulomatous enterocolitis responded more favorably than those with chronic or acute ulcerative colitis (4, 5, 6). The responses to bowel rest and total parenteral nutrition delineated three categories to which the burn analogy could again be applied: a) those patients in whom the disease became quiescent in a few weeks and normal oral intake was reinstituted, a situation comparable to first-degree burns; b) those in whom the disease became inactive after several weeks of intravenous hyperalimentation, a group analogous to second-degree burns; and c) those in whom the disease process did not respond and in whom some form of operative procedure was required, similar to third-degree burns. The second group could actually be subdivided into two categories analogous to superficial areas which usually heal completely, and more deeply diseased areas which do not heal and often become the foci of abscesses, fistulas, or obstructions, as a result of superimposed infection and mechanical or chemical trauma.

In our clinical study, 53.8% of the patients responded to bowel rest and total parenteral nutrition by sufficient healing of the involved tissues to allow resumption of normal oral feeding. During the period of intravenous hyperalimentation, which averaged 36.3 days for each patient in this group, the epithelium apparently healed in a manner similar to that of a first-degree burn. The second group consisted of 13 patients (25%) in whom remission of the disease was achieved, but operation was required because of a complication associated with some other manifestation of the disease process; they were analogous to second-degree burn patients. Eleven of the patients (21.2%) had a favorable response to the regimen of bowel rest and total parenteral nutrition but did not show any objective evidence of improvement of the underlying disease process. Although all of these patients eventually required operation, many of them did not have evidence of cicatrix formation and obstruction. However, the damage to the bowel was sufficiently advanced that even with the prolonged elimination of intraluminal food from and reduction of digestive juices in the diseased bowel segments, appreciable mucosal regeneration had not occurred. These patients were analogous to third-degree burn patients.

In all categories of inflammatory bowel disease treated by a program of total parenteral nutrition, significant improvement of the overall nutritional status of the patient was observed regardless of the response of the disease. Even when operation was ultimately required, the patient was much better able to tolerate the surgical trauma and to achieve prompt and complete recovery and rehabilitation. We conclude, therefore, that total parenteral nutrition is indicated in patients who have granulomatous enterocolitis in each of the following conditions: a) prolonged periods of active disease associated with significant catabolism; b) preoperative and postoperative periods of patients requiring operation; c) intestinal obstruction; d) short-bowel syndrome resulting from massive intestinal resection; e) indolent wounds and fistulas; f) periods of bowel rest during acute exacerbation of the disease.

Prior to the clinical application of intravenous hyperalimentation, the management of internal and external intestinal fistulas was accompanied by significant morbidity and very high mortality rates. Virtually all patients with such complications suffered from some degree of nutritional depletion, which was further aggravated by the presence of a fistula. Although the nutritional deficits were obvious, a uniformly successful technique for the repair of such deficits was not available. The level of the fistula within the alimentary tract usually determined whether or not some form of enteral alimentation could be accomplished. A fistula from the upper intestinal tract, such as the duodenum or jejunum, could not be managed successfully in most instances with enteral feedings. Fistulas from the distal portions of the alimentary tract, particularly the colon, were more likely to close while on oral feeding. For these reasons, prompt operation was the classical treatment for all upper gastrointestinal tract fistulas; the operative risk was high, and failure was common. Application of the technique of bowel rest and total parenteral nutrition has eliminated the urgency for early high-risk operations and has yielded much more satisfactory results (7).

Our series now includes more than 100 consecutive patients with enterocutaneous or enteroenteral fistulas, and we have accomplished a spontaneous closure rate of 70.5% of those fistulas. The overall mortality rate in this group has been 6.45%, which is in contrast to previously reported mortality rates of 40 to 65% in similar series. Of the 21.8% of our patients who required operation, the mortality rate was only 6.67%. The 7.7% of fistulas which never did close were all in patients who died.

Several specific conditions can inhibit spontaneous closure of internal and external fistulas despite an adequate program of bowel rest and total parenteral nutrition. Distal bowel obstruction, the presence of a foreign body, epithelialization of the fistula tract, the presence of an adjacent intra-abdominal abscess, and sometimes the effects of irradiation or of contiguous malignant disease will render nonoperative therapy inadequate. Recently, however, spontaneous closure has been achieved in some patients who had fistulas associated with irradiation damage or neoplasm. Total parenteral nutrition serves as an excellent means for preparing such patients for operation, but spontaneous fistula closure should not be expected or sought when such major obstacles are present.

Patients who have acute or chronic renal failure and in whom feeding via the alimentary tract is either impossible or inadequate have also been supported satisfactorily by vein with specially formulated solutions of L-amino acids, hypertonic dextrose, vitamins and minerals (8, 9). In addition to the usual catabolic state in such patients, a self-imposed state of semi-starvation often results from the associated anorexia. In other patients who have some degree of hepatic dysfunction, total parenteral feeding has been successful by using diets tailored to specific amino acid requirements which appear to exist under these conditions (10). Finally, patients with certain cardiac disorders have shown significant improvement both in myocardial function and nutritional status following relatively short periods of parenteral nutritional support (11).

Applications where adequate enteral intake is improbable

Table 1 lists a diverse group of disease states in which the maintenance of a balanced enteral dietary regimen is very unlikely, even though the alimentary tract may be potentially or partially functional. Some of these conditions appear more than once in the table because the disease process may have very different effects on enteral nutrition in particular patients. The interrelationships of these conditions to each other and to malnutrition in general need no further comment.

The nutritional status of patients receiving cancer chemotherapy warrants brief discussion. Many of these patients are already in a state of significant malnutrition secondary to a combination of the parasitic nature of the malignant process itself, the catabolism of previous surgical procedures or postoperative complications, and the anorexia associated with both. Chemotherapeutic agents themselves cause additional insult to the nutritional status of the patient by aggravating the catabolic process and often rendering the patient anorectic. In cancer patients receiving chemotherapy, radiation therapy, immunotherapy or a combination of these modalities, application of bowel rest and total parenteral nutrition has reduced the manifestations of alimentary tract toxicity and has allowed administration of as much as two to three times the usual chemotherapeutic dose without serious deleterious effects and with enhanced salutary results in many instances (12).

In many patients who have malignant diseases or other debilitating processes, immuno-incompetence, indicated by anergic responses to a battery of skin test antigens, has been reversed, and normal immunologic mechanisms have been restored, when sufficient nutritional support was provided via intravenous hyperalimentation (13, 14). Early results indicate that this effect improves the ability of the patient to resist infection and bolsters natural immunologic defense mechanisms against the neoplastic process. The potential of this technique as an adjunct to the various forms of cancer therapy has not yet been fully explored or exploited.

Table 1. Applications of total parenteral nutrition

To avoid or correct malnutrition when adequate enteral intake is:			
Impossible	Improbable	Inadvisable	Hazardous
1. Alimentary tract obstruction or ileus a. Oropharynx-neoplasm b. Esophagus-achalasia, neoplasm, stricture c. Stomach-benign or malignant ulcer or neoplasm, post-operative atony, gastroschisis d. Duodenum-ulcer, neoplasm, veil, atresia, duplication, choledochal cyst, annular pancreas, carcinoma of the head of the pancreas, superior mesenteric artery syndrome e. Small intestine-atresia, intussusception, neoplasm, polyp, regional enteritis, adhesions, bands, veils, gallstone ileus, foreign body, malrotation f. Colon-diverticulitis, volvulus, neoplasm, ulcerative colitis, granulomatous colitis	1. Malnourished geriatric patients 2. Chronic starvation-marasmus, kwashiorkor 3. Anorexia nervosa 4. Hyperemesis gravidarum 5. Severe mental depression 6. Chronic alcoholism 7. Chronic relapsing pancreatitis 8. Recurrent regional enteritis 9. Chronic granulomatous or ulcerative colitis 10. Radiation effects 11. Chemotherapy effects 12. Short-gut syndrome-after maximal adaptation 13. Myocardial insufficiency 14. Chronic respiratory tract disease 15. Bronchopleural fistula 16. Moderate catabolism-burns, trauma, multiple operations	1. Enterocutaneous and enteroenteral fistulas 2. Renal failure-acute or chronic 3. Acute hepatitis 4. Reversible liver failure 5. Partial intestinal obstruction 6. Acute pancreatitis 7. Acute regional enteritis 8. Acute granulomatous or ulcerative colitis Chronic respirator dependence 10. Severe alkaline reflux gastritis 11. Severe cachexia 12. Malabsorption syndromes 13. Extreme prematurity 14. Failure to thrive 15. Intractable diarrhea	1. Cerebrovascular accident 2. Mental obtundity 3. Reversible coma 4. Tetanus 5. Laryngeal incompetence 6. Tracheoesophageal fistula 7. Toxic megacolon 8. Meteorism 9. Occult gastrointestinal bleeding

2. Acute hemorrhagic pancreatitis
3. Short-gut syndrome-2 months postoperative
4. Radiation effects-entire GI tract
5. Chemotherapy effects-entire GI tract
6. Infectious gastroenteritis-cholera, salmonellosis, shigellosis
7. Intra-abdominal abscess and/ or peritonitis
8. Wound dehiscence
9. Protein-losing gastroenteropathy-sprue, Ménétrier's disease
10. Massive catabolism-major burns, multiple trauma
11. Other congenital anomalies-omphalocele, diaphragmatic hernia

In patients with such disorders as anorexia nervosa, hyperemesis gravidarum and senile dementia, total parenteral nutrition can be a valuable technique for restoring nutritional status when attempts to use the gastrointestinal tract are ineffective. Finally, maintenance of the anabolic state in patients who have major debilitating disorders or who require major operative procedures may decrease the incidence of complications, reduce the duration and cost of hospitalization and achieve more rapid and complete patient recovery and rehabilitation

Applications when adequate enteral intake is hazardous
Each of the conditions listed in Table 1 has an apparent association with malnutrition, but to use standard diets or even specialized enteral feeding techniques can be hazardous and potentially lethal. In almost all of these situations, oral or tube feedings are associated with an unacceptably high incidence of aspiration pneumonia. When properly carried out, total parenteral nutrition affords the safest and most judicious means of achieving satisfactory metabolic rehabilitation of such patients.

Hazards of total parenteral nutrition
The infectious and technical problems related to long-term central venous catheters are listed in Table 2. Of course, prevention of infection and sepsis is of utmost importance to the safety and efficacy of long-term total parenteral nutrition. If aseptic and antiseptic principles are conscientiously practiced during the insertion and subsequent maintenance of the indwelling central venous feeding catheter, the incidence of catheter-related sepsis is indeed very low (15, 16). Because hypertonic nutrient solutions are excellent culture media for many species of bacteria and fungi, meticulous asepsis must also be maintained during solution preparation, additive injection and long-term infusion. If fever should occur in a patient receiving total parenteral nutrition, the physician must immediately attempt to define its source in the ears, nose or throat, chest, urinary tract, gastrointestinal tract or wound. If the etiology of the fever cannot be determined readily, the nutrient solution and tubing must empirically and promptly be replaced, and specimens of the blood and the solution must be cultured for aerobic and anaerobic bacteria and for fungi. Should the fever persist after replacement of the solution and administration apparatus, the infusion must be terminated immediately. The indwelling subclavian vein catheter must be removed, and the distal tip of the catheter must be cultured for aerobic and anaerobic bacteria and for fungi. Depending upon the clinical situation, an-

other feeding catheter may be inserted into the opposite subclavian vein, or administration of isotonic dextrose solution may be started via peripheral vein to insure against postinfusion hypoglycemia. Septemic broad-spectrum antibiotic therapy or antifungal therapy is rarely required. However, if desired, or if the patient shows persistent signs of sepsis, an antimicrobial regimen may be instituted at this time and modified when specific sensitivity testing has been completed.

The existence of fever or evidence of sepsis prior to the institution of total parenteral nutrition does not necessarily contraindicate the use of the technique (17). In a traumatized, debilitated or critically ill patient, sepsis often accentuates the nutritional requirements. Specific antimicrobial therapy has already been instituted in most of such patients, and although seeding of the indwelling catheter by circulating microorganisms is a definite possibility, it has not proved to be an overwhelming clinical problem. In fact, resolution of

Table 2. Hazards of total parenteral nutrition related to central venous catheterization

Infectious	Technical
1. Insertion site contamination	Pneumothorax
a. Contamination during insertion	Tension pneumothorax
b. Contamination during routine care	Hemothorax
2. Catheter contamination	Hydrothorax
a. Improper technique inserting catheter	Hydromediastinum
	Cardiac tamponade
b. Administration of blood via feeding catheter	Brachial plexus injury
	Horner's syndrome
c. Use of catheter to measure central venous pressure	Phrenic nerve paralysis
	Carotid artery injury
d. Use of catheter to obtain blood samples	Subclavian artery injury
	Subclavian hematoma
e. Use of catheter to administer medications	Thrombosis, subclavian vein or superior vena cava
f. Contaminated solution during preparation or additives	Arteriovenous fistula
	Venobronchial fistula
g. Contaminated tubing via connections	Air embolism
	Catheter embolism
h. Three-way stopcocks in system	Thromboembolism
3. Secondary contamination	Catheter misplacement
a. Septicemia, bacterial or fungal	Cardiac perforation
b. Septic emboli	Endocarditis
c. Osteomyelitis of clavicle	Thoracic duct laceration
d. Septic arthritis	Innominate or subclavian vein laceration
e. Endocarditis	

systemic infections has occurred regularly during the periods of total parenteral nutrition. However, if the clinician suspects that the infectious course of the patient might be caused or aggravated by the superior vena caval catheter, it should be removed and cultured promptly.

Although development of thrombophlebitis is always possible with the use of long-term indwelling catheters and hypertonic solutions, superior vena caval thrombosis has not been observed clinically in more than 4000 patients. Apparently the high rate of blood flow in this large diameter vessel assures prompt dilution of the hypertonic fluid and prevents chemical phlebitis. Furthermore, attention to sterility has practically eliminated infectious thrombophlebitis. However, rare incidences of thrombosis have occurred in patients when the catheter tips were misdirected into or malpositioned in an external jugular, internal jugular, internal mammary or axillary vein. Other central venous catheter-related hazards such as an inadvertent air embolism and catheter embolism can be avoided easily by adherence to principles and techniques of safe central venous catheterization reported in previous publications (1, 18, 19). A thorough knowledge of anatomy, combined with common sense and strict adherence to the principles and techniques of percutaneous subclavian vein catherization should minimize the potential hazards of accidental pneumothorax, hydrothorax, hemothorax, hydromediastinum, subclavian artery puncture, bleeding, arteriovenous fistula, endocarditis, injury to the thoracic duct, venobronchial fistula, injury to the brachial plexus or sympathetic chain, osteomyelitis of the clavicle or even death.

Nonketotic hyperosmolar hyperglycemia can be precipitated acutely by infusion of the hypertonic nutrient solution too rapidly with resultant marked osmotic diuresis, serum and urine electrolyte aberrations, dehydration and central nervous system derangements. This syndrome can also occur insidiously when chronically impaired glucose utilization is not recognized, particularly in the patient with diabetes mellitus, sepsis, extensive burns, major trauma, or following intracranial operations. If blood and urine sugar concentrations are not conscientiously monitored in such patients, significant hyperglycemia and dehydration can ensue with accompanying weakness, listlessness and eventually coma. Basic treatment of nonketotic hyperosmolar hyperglycemia consists of judicious infusion of isotonic or half-strength solutions of saline or dextrose together with insulin, while simultaneously obtaining frequent measurements of fluid loss, central venous pressure, serum and urine electrolytes and blood glucose. Thorough assessment and understanding of the patient's underlying disease processes and metabolic status and proper use of established principles of the technique of intravenous hyperalimentation will obviate the vast majority of the potential metabolic hazards of total parenteral nutrition listed in Table 3 (20).

Other rare metabolic hazards which can arise during total parenteral nutrition are usually iatrogenic and include fluid overload, hypernatremia, hyponatremia, hypermagnesemia, trace element deficiencies, acne, and acalculous cholescystitis. Although these infrequent hazards can usually be avoided by adherence to the established principles and techniques of total parenteral nutrition, the clinician must be ever alert to the possibility of their occurrence.

Table 3. Potential metabolic hazards of total parenteral nutrition

Hazards	Possible explanations
I. Glucose metabolism:	
A. Hyperglycemia, glycosuria, osmotic diuresis, non-ketotic hyperosmolar dehydration and coma	Excessive total dose or rate of infusion of dextrose; inadequate endogenous insulin; glucocorticoids; sepsis
B. Ketoacidosis of diabetes mellitus	Inadequate endogenous insulin response; inadequate exogenous insulin therapy
C. Postinfusion (rebound) hypoglycemia	Persistence of endogenous insulin production secondary to prolonged stimulation of islet cells by high-carbohydrate infusion
II. Amino acid metabolism:	
A. Hyperchloremic metabolic acidosis	Excessive chloride and monohydrochloride content of crystalline amino acid solutions
B. Serum amino acid imbalance	Unphysiologic amino acid profile of the nutrient solution; different amino acid utilization with various disorders
C. Hyperammonemia	Excessive ammonia in protein hydrolysate solutions; deficiencies of arginine, ornithine, aspartic acid and/or glutamic acid in crystalline amino acid solutions; primary hepatic disorder
D. Prerenal azotemia	Excessive total dose or rate of infusion of protein hydrolysate or amino acid solution
III. Calcium and phosphorus metabolism:	
A. Hypophosphatemia	
1. Decreased erythrocyte 2,3-diphosphoglycerate	Inadequate phosphorus administration, redistribution of serum phosphorus into cells and/or bone
2. Increased affinity of hemoglobin for oxygen	
3. Aberrations of erythrocyte intermediary metabolites	

Table 3 continued.

B. Hypocalcemia	Inadequate calcium administration; reciprocal response to phosphorus repletion without simultaneous calcium infusion; hypoalbuminemia
C. Hypercalcemia	Excessive calcium administration with or without high doses of albumin; excessive vitamin D administration
D. Vitamin D deficiency; hypervitaminosis D	Inadequate or excessive vitamin D administration
IV. Essential fatty acid metabolism:	
Serum deficiencies of phospholipid linoleic and/or arachidonic acids, serum elevations of Δ-5,8,11-eicosatrienoic acid	Inadequate essential fatty acid administration; inadequate vitamin E administration
V. Miscellaneous:	
A. Hypokalemia	Inadequate potassium intake relative to increased requirements for protein anabolism; diuresis
B. Hyperkalemia	Excessive potassium administration especially in metabolic acidosis; renal decompensation
C. Hypomagnesemia	Inadequate magnesium administration relative to increased requirements for protein anabolism and glucose metabolism
D. Hypermagnesemia	Excessive magnesium administration; renal decompensation
E. Anemia	Iron deficiency; folic acid deficiency; vitamin B_{12} deficiency; copper deficiency; other deficiencies
F. Bleeding	Vitamin K deficiency
G. Hypervitaminosis A	Excessive vitamin A administration
H. Elevations in SGOT, SGPT, and serum alkaline phosphatase	Enzyme induction secondary to amino acid imbalance; excessive glycogen and/or fat deposition in the liver
I. Cholestatic hepatitis	Decreased water content of bile

CONCLUSIONS

The current technique of total parenteral nutrition (intravenous hyperalimentation) is relatively safe and efficacious, but will undoubtedly undergo change and modification as improved techniques and materials become available. With judicious application of the technique as a clinical therapeutic and investigative tool, new indications for general and specific total parenteral nutrition will likely expand and extend into every medical discipline. As relatively few of the potential applications for total parenteral nutrition have been thoroughly explored or exploited, the clinical and laboratory research possibilities appear to be virtually limitless. Thus, as increasing knowledge and experience are gained, applications of total parenteral nutrition will inevitably be expanded and will become more specific, and the hazards will no doubt decrease.

REFERENCES

1. Dudrick, S. J., Wilmore, D. W., Vars, H. M., Rhoads, J. E., Can intravenous feeding as the sole means of nutrition support growth in the child and restore weight loss in an adult? An affirmative answer. *Ann. Surg. 169:* 974-984 (1969).
2. Artz, C. P., Hardy, J. D., eds., *Management of Surgical Complications*. Philadelphia: W. B. Saunders, 834 pp (1975).
3. Dudrick, S. J., Wilmore, D. W., Steiger, E., Mackie, J. A., Fitts, W. T., Spontaneous closure of traumatic pancreatoduodenal fistulas with total intravenous nutrition. *J. Trauma. 10*: 542-553 (1970).
4. Bockus, H. L., ed., *Gastroenterology*, Vol. 2. Philadelphia: W. B. Saunders, 1171 pp. (1975).
5. Anderson, D. L., Boyce, H. W., Use of parenteral nutrition in treatment of advanced regional enteritis. *Dig. Dis. 18*: 633 (1973).
6. Clearfield, H. R., Dinoso, V. P., eds., *Gastrointestinal Emergencies*. New York: Grune and Stratton. 305 pp. (1976).
7. MacFadyen, B. V., Jr., Dudrick, S. J., Ruberg, R. L., The management of gastro-intestinal fistulas with parenteral hyperalimentation. *Surgery 74*: 100-105 (1973).
8. Dudrick, S. J., Steiger, E., Long, J. M., Renal failure in surgical patients. Treatment with intravenous essential amino acids and hypertonic glucose. *Surgery 68*: 180-186 (1970).
9. Abel, R. M., Beck, C. H., Jr., Abbott, W. M., Ryan, J. A., Jr., Barnett, G. O., Fischer, J. E., Improved survival from acute renal failure after treatment with intravénous essential L-amino acids and glucose. *N. Engl. J. Med. 288*: 695-699 (1973).
10. Fischer, J. E., *Total Parenteral Nutrition*. Boston: Little, Brown. 454 pp. (1976).
11. Abel, R. M., Fischer, J. E., Buckley, M. J., Austen, W. G., Hyperalimentation in cardiac surgery. *J. Thorac. Cardiovasc. Surg. 67*: 294-300 (1974).
12. Copeland, E. M., MacFadyen, B. V., Jr., Lanzotti, V. J., Dudrick, S. J., Intravenous hyperalimentation as an adjunct to cancer chemotherapy. *Am. J. Surg. 129*: 167-173 (1975).
13. Law, D. K., Dudrick, S. J., Abdou, N. I., Immunocompetence of patients with protein-calorie malnutrition. *Ann. Intern. Med. 79*: 545-550 (1973).
14. Copeland, E. M., MacFadyen, B. V., Jr., Dudrick, S. J., Effect of intravenous hyperalimentation on established delayed hypersensitivity in the cancer patient. *Ann. Surg. 184*: 60-64 (1976).
15. Copeland, E. M., MacFadyen, B. V., Jr., Dudrick, S. J., Prevention of microbial catheter contamination in patients receiving parenteral hyperalimentation. *South Med. J. 67*: 303-306 (1974).
16. Ryan, J. A., Abel, R. M., Abbott, W. M., Hopkins, C. C., Chesney, T. McC., Colley, R., Phillips, K., Fischer, J. E., Catheter complications in total parenteral nutrition. *N. Eng. J. Med. 290*: 6757-71 (1974).
17. Copeland, E. M., MacFadyen, B. V., Jr., McGown, C., Dudrick, S. J., The use of hyperalimentation in patients with potential sepsis. *Surg., Gynecol., Obstet. 138*: 377-380 (1974).

18. Ballinger, W. F., Collins, J. A., Drucker, W. R., Dudrick, S. J., Zeppa, R., eds., *Manual of Surgical Nutrition*. Philadelphia: W. B. Saunders. 527 pp. (1975).
19. Nyhus, L. M., ed., *Surgery Annual*. New York: Appleton-Century-Crofts. 418 pp. (1973).
20. Dudrick, S. J., MacFadyen, B. V., Jr., Van Buren, C. T., Ruberg, R. L., Maynard, A. T., Parenteral hyperalimentation: metabolic problems and solutions. *Ann. Surg.* *176*: 259-264 (1972).

Criteria for management of metabolic imbalance

C. W. R. Phaf and E. L. M. Hardy

I INTRODUCTION

In one paper on a subject as extensive as parenteral nutrition, we can only give outlines, highlights and problems. We will confront you with the available and the missing data.

In essence we will present the problems which have to be dealt with and will – we hope – in part be dealt with during this symposium.

As always we have to start from a number of certainties and uncertainties or perhaps better: probabilities and improbabilities. In nutrition we have to deal with the same problem as in pharmacotherapy: there is a discrepancy between the way we want the drug to behave and the behavior of the drug in each *specific case*. So let us be modest in our expectations.

This applies particularly to parenteral nutrition because we are dealing here with patients under very complex conditions who are often intoxicated with several kinds of drugs.

II PATIENT DATA TO BE USED AS CRITERIA FOR MANAGEMENT

Clinical situations such as starvation, cachexia, pre-operative weakness (especially in elderly patients), aggressive surgery with subsequent post-operative problems, traumata and intoxications may call for management.

Such clinical situations cause physiological situations, such as stress and hormonal imbalance.

Catabolic mechanisms will predominate over the anabolic mechanisms, causing protein degradation, protein loss and energy loss. The first proteins subject to degradation under such conditions are the functional proteins (1). This complicates matters considerably.

III CORRECTIVE MEASURES REQUIRED BY THE PATIENT AND CRITERIA FOR THE CHOICE OF PREPARATIONS

When the catabolic mechanisms predominate over the anabolic mechanisms the patient needs:

1. correction of hormonal imbalance:	insulin
2. correction of hypoalbuminemia:	human albumin
3. correction of nitrogen balance:	a. amino acids in an optimal pattern
	b. energy sources
	c. several vitamins
	d. several ions
4. correction of energy deficit:	energy sources.

Prior to the measures mentioned here, it is necessary to combat post-operative narcotic intoxication (causing liver and central nervous system impairment) and to correct hypoxia (4). Moreover several general measures must be taken such as neuroplegia and control of body temperature.

As to the factors necessary for stimulation of protein synthesis: all of these factors have to be balanced proportionally and must be provided at the right moment.

1. Correction of hormonal imbalance

In a post-operative stage the catabolic scale of the hormonal balance is forced downwards by an "overweight" of glucagon activity in particular. Insulin seems to be indicated to break the vicious circle (table 1). In post-traumatic situations however stress due to the effects of catecholamines and glucocorticosteroids causes varying degrees of inhibition of insulin activity and glucose tolerance.

This makes it very difficult to establish the proper doses of glucose and insulin for the different stages. In later stages glucose can be administered in increasing amounts (5).

As will be explained, in early post-traumatic stages the use of sorbitol instead of glucose seems to be preferable.

Among other reasons this provides a better situation for the proper use of insulin. High doses of insulin of up to 200 U daily are used to inhibit proteolysis. It is difficult to provide rules for such dosages (5).

As serious problems may arise from hyperglycemia as well as hypoglycemia, frequent determinations of the plasma glucose levels are necessary. Insulin is indicated when the plasma glucose level rises above 200 mg/100 ml; in general insulin is immediately indispensable when the plasma glucose level exceeds 300 mg/ml. An initial dose of 8-12 U daily can later be adapted to the patient's needs.

Since pure insulin preparations are available, and provided such pure preparations are used, the chance that insulin antibodies will be formed can no longer be considered a reason to avoid the use of insulin. One should be aware that after prolonged insulin administration the endogenous insulin response is depressed for some time.

Table 1. Insulin for correction of hormonal imbalance

Problems:	decreasing inhibition of insulin effect and increasing glucose tolerance serious danger of hypoglycemia or hyperglycemia
Management:	careful dosage (initial dose 8-12 U daily) frequent plasma glucose determinations (at least 4-6 times a day).

2. *Correction of hypoalbuminemia*

In the early post-traumatic or post-surgical phase catabolic effects (and eventual blood loss) tend to cause a hypoalbuminemia. Proper parenteral nutrition can obviously bring about quick restoration of the albumin level.

Nevertheless it is self-evident that administration of human albumin is the therapy of choice for hypoalbuminemia (table 2). It is unnecessary to use adequate parenteral nutrition to achieve goals that can be reached directly and better by providing the end products (2, 41).

Table 2. Human albumin for correction of hypoalbuminemia

Management:	correction of albumin level with human albumin.

3. *Correction of nitrogen balance*

3.a. Amino acids in an optimal pattern

The expression "essential" as used in relation to amino acids means that the body is not able to synthesize the product under consideration. It is understood now that a strict division between "essential" and "non-essential" (or a-specific) is untenable in practice.

Since several "non-essential" amino acids are deficient under certain problematical conditions, the expression "semi-essential" is used. These distinctions evidently depend on the tentative state of our knowledge (see table 3).

Table 3. Amino acids required for correction of nitrogen balance

Amino acids L-configuration	'essential' = e 'semi-essential' = s 'non-essential' = n	Required (adult)
Isoleucine	e	+
Leucine	e	+
Lysine	e	+
Methionine	e	+
Phenylalanine	e	+
Threonine	e	+
Tryptophan	e	+
Valine	e	+
Histidine	s	+
Arginine	s	+
Glycine	s	+
Alanine	s	+
Proline	s	+
Glutamic acid	s	+
Tyrosine	n	+
Cysteine/Cystine	n	–
Aspartic acid	n	–
Serine	n	–
Ornithine aspartate	n	–

Several amino acids formerly considered "non-essential" are nowadays evidently essential in for instance newborn babies or uremic patients.

Moreover in parenteral nutrition, when all reaction components must be directly available, some "non-essential" amino acids appear to be deficient.

Partial or total absence of such amino acids will be a limiting factor, a risk that is not acceptable (see table 4). For this reason we have made a practical differentiation in the second column of table 3. In current practice with ever-changing circumstances and conditions it is impossible to make a distinction between theoretically indispensable, in practice necessary, required or useful components.

Several criteria and parameters have been used to try to establish an optimal amino acid pattern for parenteral use (see table 5). As a means of comparison and as raw material for preparations, (several) natural products known to be useful in oral feeding are often used.

As such we find among others casein, chicken egg, potato protein-chicken egg mixtures and human milk. For such natural products a FAO/WHO group used the so-called E/T ratio to call attention to the fact that the proportion

Table 4

Methionine	is a component in protein structure, a catalyst for protein synthesis, a source of cystein and a methyl donor. After trauma it is often the first amino acid to be limited (43, 52).
Histidine	is essential for children and uremic patients. Histidine stimulates protein synthesis; when it is lacking hematopoiesis is inhibited (2, 15, 34, 44, 53, 54, 55).
Arginine	has a limited synthesis capacity, so deficiency can occur after a short time. Arginine can bind NH_3 molecules. Excess might have an inhibiting effect (60).
Glycine	is necessary for hemosynthesis and for detoxication processes, among others. It is 'essential' for uremic patients. Excess as a single non-essential nitrogen source might cause a certain degree of imbalance (especially in newborn babies) (52).
Alanine and *Proline*	are able to correct a negative nitrogen balance and may even create a very good positive balance. Both amino acids are not readily synthesized. Absence of proline causes an inadequate nitrogen balance (23, 35).
Glutamic acid	administered to an adequate glycine-alanine-proline mixture (the optimal proportions are: glycine:alanine:proline = 8:3:1) can even create an optimal balance. Excess lowers the pH, which may cause metabolic problems and trombophlebitis (23, 35, 52).
Tyrosine	can partly replace phenylalanine. In newborn babies synthesis from phenylalanine is inadequate. Tyrosine is 'essential' in uremic patients (36, 44, 48).
Cysteine	can partly replace methionine from which it can be synthesized in limited amounts. It is inadequately synthesized in newborn babies and remains a limiting factor during the period of growth (56, 57).
Aspartic acid	in excessive amounts, like glutamic acid, may cause undesirable side-effects (see under glutamic acid) (60).
Serine	is easily synthesized out of glycine (60).

of the non-essential amino acids is often comparatively low. In connection with this reference is often made to the so-called "proteins of biologically high standard". Since we do not know the meaning of this expression in terms of parenteral nutrition under a variety of conditions, it does not make things very much clearer.

On the grounds that amino acids are all absorbed smoothly and without delay, the criteria for oral feeding were used for parenteral nutrition as well.

Since other criteria were not available we were glad to be able to use the results of the good investigations of Rose. We have to realize that more fundamental data have only recently become available.

Table 5. Criteria and parameters for choice of amino acid patterns (2)

Oral requirements
Plasma amino acid composition
Potassium and phosphate plasma levels and balance
Plasma levels of several functional proteins, like:
transaminases
complement factors
cholinesterase
pre-albumin
albumin
transferrin
immunoglobulin
S.G.O.T. and S.G.P.T.
Wound healing and other conditions of the patient
Urea excretion
Nitrogen balance
Plasma levels of single amino acids to detect and correct limiting factors

This brings us to the question: are the amino acid patterns of mixtures for oral feeding useful as criteria for the composition of preparations for parenteral nutrition?

We want to point out some reasons why they are not.

1. Absorption of amino acids is often an intricate matter because of carriers and combinations of molecules, mutual stimulation or antagonism and dipeptides that are involved in absorption processes. This requires conditions that are not needed for parenteral purposes.

2. During the period of absorption (and this is not equal for all amino acids) the body would have time for the synthesis of several "non-essential" amino acids. Otherwise there could be a loss (to gluconeogenesis and/or renal excretion) of the indispensable components during the waiting period. This could be a reason why the patterns of "non-essential" amino acids for oral and parenteral requirements are generally found to differ.

In parenteral nutrition direct availability of all components (and in this respect energy sources are to be included) for protein synthesis is necessary.

3. The conditions under which parenteral nutrition is required call for direct satisfaction of needs (which stresses point 2). The composition of the solutions for parenteral nutrition must satisfy several practical conditions such as tolerance, a physiologically acceptable pH and osmolarity, solubility of components, etc.

4. Orally ingested amino acids, after absorption, primarily pass through the liver.

The plasma amino acid pattern does not accidently reflect a pattern of choice for solutions of parenteral nutrition. Most other parameters mentioned here can only provide additional information. Urea excretion reflects about 70-90% of the amino acid excretion. A nitrogen balance is a time-consuming procedure demanding controlled steady conditions before being useful.

The procedure (last mentioned in table 5) of using the plasma levels of single amino acids to detect and correct limiting factors seems to be the most exact method to tackle the problem, provided plasma levels are estimated in samples taken at the same time of the day (for instance in the morning, before breakfast) and under steady-state conditions. It has to be remarked here that such steady-state conditions never exist in the patients under consideration. This means that fundamental work with such patients can not easily be used for comparison purposes. Such fundamental work has been done for instance by Dolif and Jürgens, as well as several others, like Heg-

Table 6. Amino acid patterns for correction of nitrogen balance required and provided

Amino acids L-configuration	required daily g/g lysine (Dolif, Jürgens) (24)	required daily g Holt (24)		Hegsted (33)		(Rose) (49)	provided in 7 "normal" preparations* g/1000 ml (adult)
Isoleucine	0.89	0.55	-	0.55	-	(0.70)	1.4-3.9
Leucine	1.23	0.60	-	0.73	-	(1.10)	2.2-5.3
Lysine	1.0 (norm)	0.43	-	0.54	-	(0.80)	1.6-4.3 (HCl)
Methionine	1.11 (incl. cysteine)	0.27	-	0.70	-	(1.10)	1.9-2.4
Phenylalanine	1.11 (incl. tyrosine)	0.26	-	0.26	-	(1.10)	1.9-5.5
Threonine	0.56	0.35	-	0.38	-	(0.50)	1.0-3.0
Tryptophan	0.28	0.18	-	0.17	-	(0.25)	0.5-1.0
Valine	0.84	0.63	-	0.62	-	(0.80)	1.5-4.3
Histidine	0.5-1.0						0-1.0-2.4
Arginine	1.5-2.5						1.0-6.0
Glycine	(...-8.0 max.)						2.1-25.0
Alanine	2.0-3.0						0-3.0-17.1
Proline	2.0-3.0						0-1.7-8.1
Glutamic acid	3.5-5.0 (aspartic acid included)						0 or 9.0
Tyrosine	0.2-0.4						0-0.2-0.5
Cysteine/cystine							0 or 1.4
Aspartic acid							0 or 4.1
Serine							0-1.2-7.5
Ornithine aspartate							0-0.5-1.0

* These solutions are Aminofusin L600, Aminosteril KE, Aminosteril L600, Salviamin LX4, Travasol 4%, Trophysan L50, Vamin 7%.

sted and Svendseid who combined plasma level changes with nitrogen balances.

Dolif and Jürgens proposed a pattern for "essential" amino acids. Moreover they listed the quantities of other amino acids required in relation to the quantity of available lysine. We have combined these data in table 6.

Evidently within certain limits one can state that the amino acid pattern is more important than the amount (44, 52).

It will be clear from the facts mentioned above that hydrolysates of natural products are not to be used, because their amino acid pattern is not optimal.

Moreover the composition is not always constant, and such preparations may contain more than 20% peptides (52).

3.b. Energy sources

Energy is needed for two purposes:

- proper use of nitrogen sources
- and correction of energy deficit in general.

The following are used:

fats, ethanol, carbohydrates, polyalcohols providing carbohydrates, mixtures and amino acids (table 9).

For the proper use of nitrogen sources at least 120 Kcal (30 g carbohydrate source) per 6.25 g amino acid mixture are necessary (52). The choice of a proper carbohydrate source will be extensively discussed in section 4.

3.c. Several vitamins

Several vitamins might be essential for the utilization of the amino acid source and/or for the normal supply.

Because of the differences in the quantities given by several authors (9, 27, 58, 59) we will only list the names of vitamins used for this purpose (table 7).

Table 7. Several vitamins for correction of nitrogen balance

Thiamine	Biotin
Riboflavine	Ascorbic acid
Nicotinamide	Retinol
Pyridoxine	Ergocalciferol or cholecalciferol
Folic acid	
Cyanocobalamin	Phytomenadione
Pantothenic acid	Tocopherol

3.d. Several ions

For the correction of the nitrogen balance, several ions in a normal supply are indispensable.

The requirements for sodium, potassium, calcium, magnesium, phosphate, chlorine and iron are well-known.

Zinc seems to be essential in wound healing processes (30, 46) and as a trace element in the period of growth (47).

Several other trace elements might be essential, or at least might become limiting factors in long-term feeding.

For the same reasons as given under 3.c, we will give a list of ions without quantities (table 8) (9, 21, 27, 58, 59, 61).

Table 8. Several ions for correction of nitrogen balance

Na^{+}	Mn^{++}	Ni^{++}
K^{+}	Zn^{++}	Cl^{-}
Ca^{++}	Cu^{++}	H_2PO4^{-}
Mg^{++}	Cr^{+++}	F^{-}
Fe^{++}	$Mo_7O_{24}^{6-}$	I^{-}

4. Correction of energy deficit: energy sources

Table 9 contains a list of energy sources used for this purpose.

Table 9

Energy sources, used for correction of nitrogen balance for correction of energy deficit	
Fats	
Ethanol	
Carbohydrates	Glucose
	Fructose
Polyalcohols	Sorbitol
	Xylitol
Mixtures of carbohydrates and/or polyalcohols	
Amino acids	

Fats as an energy source

Fats contain a lot of energy (100 g = 1000-1100 Kcal) which might become available after total metabolism; however in early post-traumatic states, fats are not useful because up to 70-80% is lost in the first stages (2, 28).

They might even become noxious causing a negative nitrogen balance, with lipolysis being impaired because of inhibition of insulin. Moreover utilization of fats requires a lot of energy and fatty acids may compete with the already impaired glucose utilization. In addition, the infusion of fat emulsions involves the immunological defense capacity and might interfere with the determination of plasma levels of drugs or other parameters (1). Fats are contra-indicated during gravidity because they might cause an impairment of placental function and a tendency towards ketosis or trigger labor.

After one week "essential fatty acids" can become limiting factors (10, 45).

Thus in long-term feeding they have to be used. In such situations it might not be necessary to administer them parenterally, because it has been suggested that they are adequately absorbed percutaneously.

Ethanol as an energy source

Ethanol inhibits lactate utilization (38, 39), presents an unnecessary workload for the liver and can cause serious liver impairment. In post-operative situations in which liver functions are already impaired by the use of narcotics, this may cause a dangerous situation. Moreover ethanol may give rise to problems as a result of its effect on the central nervous system, which in pre-existing hypoxia might be very dangerous.

In view of the above-mentioned disadvantages we might conclude that ethanol should not be used as an energy source.

The maximum supply rate for healthy subjects is considered to be 0.1 g/kg BW/hr (51).

Carbohydrates and polyalcohols as energy source

After total metabolism, 100 g of such preparations can provide 400 Kcal. The daily dosages and the quantities that can be administered per kg bodyweight and per hour (/kg BW/hr) differ for different preparations.

As will be seen the effects under early post-traumatic conditions diverge markedly; moreover the adverse effects after high dosages vary considerably. All carbohydrates or polyalcohols normally used cause renal overflow to some extent when dosages which are too high are administered too quickly. To try and make a choice we will review the qualities, advantages and disadvantages of all available carbohydrate sources.

Glucose as an energy source

Glucose is quickly and effectively metabolized, provided insulin is available and glucose utilization is not inhibited; however in the early post-traumatic state insulin synthesis is inhibited and there is a poor glucose tolerance which together create a serious risk of hyperglycemia (6, 20, 26, 50).

In such situations after administration of 0.5 g/kg BW/hr, up to 21% of the glucose is lost through renal overflow (3, 32).

Moreover glucose solutions have a low pH with an evident buffer capacity which raises the risk of thrombophlebitis. Mixtures containing both glucose and amino acids may undergo the reaction of Maillard which makes the composition of such solutions doubtful after some time.

Fructose as an energy source

In the first phase of metabolism fructose is quickly utilized without the help of insulin (29).

The loss through renal overflow in early post-traumatic conditions is low (9% after administration of 0.5 g/kg BW/hr) (3).

The fact that fructose is quickly utilized presents some disadvantages:

When fructose is administered too quickly or when liver insufficiency exists, there is a serious danger of metabolic acidosis resulting from an excess of lactic acid and/or uric acid (6, 18, 29).

Furthermore there is the risk of a toxic accumulation of fructose-1-phosphate and a quick decrease in plasma phosphate levels (4, 19). Fructose solutions have a low pH, with an evident buffer capacity, which raises the risk of thrombophlebitis.

Solutions containing amino acids and fructose also undergo the reaction of Maillard.

Sorbitol as an energy source

In the first phases of metabolism insulin is not needed for the utilization of sorbitol and in a later stage sorbitol does not require an additional amount of insulin.

This quality makes sorbitol useful in early post-traumatic stages. After administration of amounts of up to 0.5 g/kg BW/hr renal excretion is about 12%. After administration of more than 0.5 g/kg BW/hr the renal overflow starts to increase (in healthy subjects) (17).

The good solubility and tolerability of sorbitol enable the use of high concentrations (in our hospital 40% solutions are used).

Sorbitol solutions do not affect the physiological pH.

Sorbitol is dehydrogenated by dehydrogenase to fructose.

This process takes place quietly and therefore sorbitol does not cause the problems which may occur after administration of fructose.

Sorbitol induces only slightly raised lactate levels (19).

In the first stage of metabolism of sorbitol an extra quantity of energy is released; moreover sorbitol might have a normalizing effect on fatty acid metabolism.

Xylitol as an energy source

Xylitol has major advantages similar to those of sorbitol, but the risk of lactate formation is higher than in the case of sorbitol (in healthy subjects) (17). Uric acid and oxalic acid may be formed in excess when high doses are used (25). It should however be stressed that dangerous situations were seen only after overdosages (1, 40).

Renal excretion exceeds 16% after administration of as little as 0.25 g/kg BW/hr (in healthy subjects) (17). It is very remarkable that in stress situations the utilization of xylitol in a dosage of up to 0.5 g/kg BW/hr is even better than the utilization of the same dosage of glucose (1, 3, 16, 31, 62).

Mixtures of carbohydrate-sources

Several mixtures have been tried in order to be able to administer higher total dosages than are possible using the single components.

Glucose - fructose - xylitol mixture (1:2:1)

This mixture has been found to be an adequate energy source (3, 7, 17). Side-effects such as renal overflow and lactate production might not be additive. 0.5 g/kg BW/hr can be used (3, 11, 12, 13, 14, 17, 32). Most other mixtures are known to have important disadvantages.

Sorbitol + xylitol — xylitol

uses the same enzyme for dehydrogenation as sorbitol and thus inhibits sorbitol utilization considerably (8).

Sorbitol or xylitol + ethanol

Inhibition of lactate utilization by ethanol makes this combination dangerous:
Ethanol delays xylitol metabolism (1)
Ethanol delays sorbitol metabolism (37)
Ethanol delays gluconeogenesis(22)

Glucose + fructose (1:1)

The disadvantages of fructose are sufficient reason to state that invertsugar should not be used.

Attention should be drawn to the possible development of glucose intolerance in the presence of fructose (19). However a combination of glucose and fructose is tolerated better than a concentrated glucose solution alone when administered as an energy source in total parenteral nutrition (42).

To make a proper choice from the useful carbohydrate sources, we present table 10 in which the most important criteria are taken into account.

Table 10

	Glucose	Fructose	Sorbitol	Xylitol	Glucose Fructose Xylitol Mixture
Utilization under post-traumatic conditions	0	+	++	++	++
Energy production in the first stage of metabolism (40)	+	+	++	++	++
Maximum usable supply rate in g/kg BW/hr	0.5	n.g.*	0.5	0.25	0.5
Renal overflow using the maximum usable supply rate (3, 17)	~21% in post-traumatic situations	n.g.*	~12%	~16%	~7%
Renal overflow using 0.5 g/kg BW/hr (3, 17)	~ 1% ~21% in post-traumatic situations	~2% ~9% in post-traumatic situations	~12%	~27%	~7%
Lactate production after usable dosages	+	++	0	+	+
Low pH, with high risk of thrombophlebitis	++	++	0	0	+
Maillard reaction in mixtures with amino acids (2)	++	++	–	–	+

* Not given

Amino acids as an energy source
Use of amino acids as an energy source has to be qualified as a waste or at least as improper because it is uneconomical. 160 g of amino acid can replace 100 g of carbohydrates (52).

Amino acids are much more expensive than carbohydrates or polyalcohols; moreover amino acids used as an energy source present an extra burden for the liver function (4).

From the arguments cited above it may be concluded that we tend to propose sorbitol as the energy source of choice, at least in the early post-traumatic stages. However it remains to be established whether interactions exist between sorbitol-dehydrogenation and liver-insufficiency.

IV MANAGEMENT AND RELATED PROBLEMS

Aspects of management is the subject of many papers in this symposium. Thus we will confine ourselves to some specific problems such as

- when is treatment indicated?
- should we prefer "loading" before surgical treatment or "refilling" after surgical treatment?
- are parenteral preparations always necessary or could the patient (under certain circumstances) be treated with oral preparations?
- how to make use of the data concerning the age and condition of the patient?

There remains the eternal problem in pharmacotherapy: the criteria for healthy adults (or at least healthy people) are used for patients with varying bodyweights or body surface, in all kinds of conditions and often treated with several medications.

If there is a difference in need, there is a difference in utilization and there should be a difference in dose.

Such differences could exist in quantity or even in the quality of the preparations that have to be used and also in the utilization of the components of the therapy.

So the proper rate of administration, length of treatment and daily and total quantities of the doses will have to be different for different people.

- Is it possible to find and use criteria and schemes for the treatment of individual patients or at least for the management of different categories of patients?
- Could such schemes be evaluated using existing preparations? If this is

not be possible, cost factors have to be taken into account as well.

By giving you this information and these problems we hope to have at least fluttered the dovecot.

It is necessary that parenteral nutrition be a team-effort involving several disciplines, such as physicians, pharmacists, nurses and others participating in the clinical team.

After the development of such a clinical team, we may be able to look at the problem from the positive, the anabolic, side.

ACKNOWLEDGEMENT

We wish to acknowledge the help and endurance of Ine Nederveen-van der Kragt, Marita Derwa and L. C. Edmunds.

REFERENCES

1. Ahnefeld, F. W., Bässler, K. H., et al., Die Eignung von Nicht-Glukose-Kohlenhydraten für die parenterale Ernährung. *Infusionstherapie 2*: 227-237 (1975).
2. Ahnefeld, F. W., Burri, C. et al., (ed.), General Discussions in: *Grundlagen der Postoperativen Ernährung*, Klinische Anaesthesiologie und Intensivtherapie, Band 6, Berlin, 1975.
3. Ahnefeld, F. W., Halmágyi, M. and Milewski, P., Glukose und Glukoseaustauschstoffe in der Infusionstherapie des operativen Bereiches. In: Ritzel, G. and Brubacher, G. (ed.), *Monosaccharides and Polyalcohols in Nutrition, Therapy and Dietetics*, Vienna, 1976, pp. 242-251.
4. Ahnefeld, F. W., Burri, C. et al., (ed.), General Discussions in: *Parenteral Nutrition, Klinische Anaesthesiologie und Intensivtherapie*, Band 7, (English edition), New York, 1976.
5. Allison, S. P., Metabolic aspects of intensive care. *Br. J. Hosp. Med.*, 860-872 (1974).
6. Allison, S. P., Carbohydrate and Fat Metabolism - Response to Injury. In: Lee, H. A. (ed.), *Parenteral Nutrition in Acute Metabolic Illness*, London, 1974, pp. 167-175.
7. Bässler, K. H. and Reimold, W. V., Lactatbildung aus Zuckern und Zuckeralkoholen in Erythrozyten. *Klin. Wschr. 43*: 169 (1965).
8. Bässler, K. H., Stein, G. and Belzer, W., Xylitstoffwechsel und Xylitresorption. *Biochem Z. 346*: 171 (1966).
9. Bässler, K. H., Berg, G., et al., Empfehlungen zur parenteralen Ernährung. *Med. u. Ernährung 11*: 201-205 (1970).
10. Bässler, K. H., Zur Zweckmässigkeit von Fettinfusionen im Rahmen der parenteralen Ernährung. *Infusionstherapie 3*: 198-200 (1976).
11. Berg, G., Bickel, H. and Matzkies, F., Bilanz- und Stoffwechselverhalten von Fructose, Xylit und Glucose, sowie deren Mischungen bei Gesunden während sechsstündiger parenteraler Ernährung. *Dtsch. med. Wschr. 98*: 602-610 (1973).
12. Berg, G., Matzkies, F. et al., Säure-Basen-Haushalt bei Dauerinfusionen von Xylit, Fructose, Glucose und Kohlenhydratmischungen. *Z. Ernährungs. Wiss.*, Suppl. 15, 47-54 (1973)
13. Berg, G., Matzkies, F. and Bickel, H., Dosierungsgrenzen bei der Infusion von Glucose, Sorbit, Fructose, Xylit und deren Mischungen. *Dtsch. med. Wschr.99*: 633 (1974).

14. Berg, G., Matzkies, F. et al., Wirkungen einer Kohlenhydratkombinationslösung auf den Stoffwechsel bei hochdosierter Kurzzeitinfusion. *Z. Ernähr. Wiss. 14*: 53-63 (1975).
15. Bergström, J., Fürst, P., et al., Improvement of nitrogen balance in a uremic patient by the addition of histidine to essential amino acid solutions given intravenously. *Life Sci 9*: 787 (1970).
16. Bickel, H., Bünte, H., et al., Die Verwertung parenteral verabreichter Kohlenhydrate in der postoperativen Phase. *Dtsch. med. Wschr. 98*: 809 (1973).
17. Bickel, H. and Halmágyi, M., Requirement and utilization of Carbohydrates and Alcohol. In: Ahnefeld, F. W., Burri, C., et al. (ed.), *Parenteral Nutrition, Klinische Anaesthesiologie und Intensivtherapie*, Band 7, (English edition), New York, 1976, pp. 66-79.
18. Bode, J. C., Zelder, O., et al., Depletion of Liver Adenosine Phosphates and Metabolic Effects of Intravenous Infusion of Fructose or Sorbitol in Man and in the Rat. *Europ. J. Clin. Invest. 3*: 436-441 (1973).
19. Carlo, P. E., Hormonal control of substrate utlization in Parenteral Nutrition. A model Proposal. Paper presented at the International Congress of the International Society of Parenteral Nutrition, Melbourne, Australia, March 4-7, 1974 (to be published).
20. Daly, J. M., Steiger, E., et al., Postoperative oral and intravenous nutrition. *Ann. Surg. 180*: 709-715 (1974).
21. Dick, W. and Seeling, W., Water and electrolyte requirements during Parenteral Nutrition. In: Ahnefeld, F. W., Burri, C., et al. (ed.), *Parenteral Nutrition, Klinische Anaesthesiologie und Intensivtherapie*, Band 7, (English edition), New York, 1976, pp. 99-112.
22. Dietze, G., Wicklmayr, M., et al., Glykogenolyse und Gluconeogenese der menschlichen Leber. *Verh. dt Ges. inn. Med. 79*: 914-917 (1973).
23. Dolif, D. and Jürgens, P., Die Bedeutung der nicht essentiellen Aminosäuren bei der parenteralen Ernährung. In: Berg, G. (ed.), *Advances in Parenteral Nutrition*, Proceedings of the Symposium of the International Society of Parenteral Nutrition, Prague, 1969. Stuttgart (Thieme Verlag).
24. Dolif, D. and Jürgens, P., Requirement and utilization of Amino-acids. In: Ahnefeld, F. W., Burri, C., et al. (ed.), *Parenteral Nutrition, Klinische Anaesthesiologie und Intensivtherapie*, Band 7, (English edition), New York, 1976, pp. 54-65.
25. Dölp, R. and Paulini, K., Oxalatbildung nach parenteraler Ernährung mit Aminosäuren und Xylit bei einem polytraumatisierten Patienten. In: Ritzel, G. and Brubacher, G. (ed.), *Monosaccharides and Polyalcohols in Nutrition, Therapy and Dietetics*, Vienna, 1976, pp. 228-233.
26. Dudrick, S. J., MacFadyen, B. V., et al., Parenteral hyperalimentation. Metabolic problems and solutions. *Ann. Surg. 176*: 259-264 (1972).
27. Dudrick, S. J. and Rhoads, J. E., New Horizons for intravenous feeding. *J.A.M.A. 215*: 939-949 (1973).
28. Eckart, J., Zur Verwertung von Fettemulsionen in der parenteralen Ernährung des Menschen, *Infusionstherapie 1*: 521-529 (1973/74).
29. Förster, H., Grundlagen für die Verwendung der drei Zuckeraustauschstoffen Fructose, Sorbit und Xylit. *Med. und Ernährung 1*: 7-16 (1972).
30. Hallböök, T. and Lanner, E., *Lancet II*: 780 (1972).
31. Halmágyi, M. and Israng, H. H., Auswahl der Kohlenhydrate zur intravenösen Anwendung in der intra- und postoperativen Phase. In: Lang, K., Frey, P. and Halmágyi, M., (ed.), *Kohlenhydrate in der dringlichen Infusionstherapie*, Berlin, 1968, pp. 25-29.
32. Halmágyi, M., Bilanzierte Substitutionstherapie durch Infusion bei schwerkranken, traumatisierten Patienten. *Infusionstherapie 1*: 473-476 (1973/74).
33. Hegsted, D. M., Variation in requirements of nutrients. – Amino acids. Presented at

the 47th Annual Meeting of the Federation of American Societies for Experimental Biology, Atlantic City, N.J., April 20, 1963.
34. Holt, L. E., György, P., et al., *Protein and Amino Acid Requirements in Eearly Life*, New York, 1960.
35. Jürgens, P. and Dolif, D., Die Bedeutung nichtessentieller Aminosäuren für den Stickstoffhaushalt des Menschen unter parenteraler Ernährung. *Klin. Wschr. 46*: 131 (1968).
36. Jürgens, P. and Dolif, D., Experimental results of parenteral nutrition with amino acids. In: Wilkinson, A. W., (ed.), *Parenteral Nutrition*, Edinburgh, pp. 47.
37. Kaden, M., Oadkley, N., and Field, J. B., The effect of ethanol on hepatic gluconeogenesis. *Diabetes 16*: 528 (1967).
38. Krebs, H. A., Freedland, R. A., et al., Inhibition of Hepatic Gluconeogenesis by Ethanol. *Biochem. 112*: 117-124 (1969).
39. Kreisberg, R. A., Siegal, A. M. and Owen, W. C., Hyperlacticacidemia in Man: Ethanol - Phenformin Synergism. *Diabetes 20*: Suppl. 1, 324 (1971).
40. Lang, K., Xylit, Stoffwechsel und klinische Verwendung. *Klin. Wschr. 49*: 233-245 (1971).
41. Meert, J. P., personal communication.
42. Meng, H. C., Wang, P. Y. and Lu, K. S., The use of fructose and glucose in total parenteral nutrition as an energy source. In: Ritzel, G. and Brubacher, G. (ed.) *Monosaccharides and Polyalcohols in Nutrition, Therapy and Dietetics*, Vienna, 1976, pp. 252-276.
43. Munro, H. N. and Allison, J. B., *Mammalian Protein Metabolism*, New York, 1964.
44. Munro, H. N., Basic concepts in the use of amino acids and protein hydrolysates for parenteral nutrition. *Drug Intell. Clin. Pharm. 6*: 216-225 (1972).
45. Paulsrud, J. R., et al., Essential fatty acid deficiency in infants induced by fat-free intravenous feeding. *Am. J. Clin. Nutr.*, 897-904, September 1972.
46. Pories, W. J., Henzel, J. H., et al., *Lancet 1*: 121 (1967).
47. Prasad, A. S., Miale, A., et al., *J. Lab. Clin. Med. 61*: 537 (1963).
48. Rose, W. C., et al., Comparative growth on diets containing ten and nineteen amino acids with further observations upon the role of glutaminic and aspartic acid. *J. Biol. Chem. 176*: 753 (1948).
49. Rose, W. C., Amino acid requirements of man. *Federation Prod. 8*: 364 (1949).
50. Sall, S., Brofman, B. and Stone, M. L., Nutritional support of patients with intravenous hyperalimentation. *Am. J. Obstet. Gynec. 114*: 500-606 (1972).
51. Schaub, P., Betzler, H., et al., Stoffwechselverhalten eines Gemisches aus Aethanol, Lävulose, und Xylit während mehrstündiger parenteraler Zufuhr bei Gesunden. *Therapiewoche 24*: 3594 (1974).
52. Semler, P. (ed.), *Parenterale Therapie mit Aminosäuren-Lösungen*, Symposium am 19. September 1973 im Rudolf-Virchow-Krankenhaus, Berlin. Edited by Fresenius Werke, Bad Homburg, 1974.
53. Snijderman, S. E., Prose, P. H. and Holt, L. E., Histidin, an essential amino acid for the infant, *Amer. J. Dis. Child. 98*: 459 (1959).
54. Snijderman, S. E., Holt, L. E., et al., Unessential nitrogen: a limiting factor for human growth. *J. Nutrit. 78*: 57 (1962).
55. Snijderman, S. E., The protein and amino acid requirements of the infant. In: *Anaesthesiologie und Wiederbelebung*, Band 72, Berlin, 1973, p. 21.
56. Sturman, J. A., Gaull, G., et al., Absence of cystathionase in human fetal liver. Is cystine essential? *Science N.Y. 169*: 74 (1970).
57. Womack, M. and Rose, W. C., Partial replacement of dietary methionine by cystine for purposes of growth. *J. Biol. Chem. 141*: 375 (1941).

58. Wretlind, A., Complete intravenous nutrition: theoretical and experimental background. *Nutr. Metabol. 14*, Suppl. 1-57 (1972).
59. Wretlind, A., Assessment of Patient Requirements. In: Lee, H. A. (ed.), *Parenteral Nutrition in Acute Metabolic Illness*, London, 1974, pp. 353-383.
60. Wretlind, A., Amino acids. In: Lee, H. A. (ed.), *Parenteral Nutrition in Acute Metabolic Illness*, London, 1974, pp. 53-76.
61. IJdenberg, F. N., Sporenelementen voor toevoegen aan voedingsinfusen. In: *Mededelingen van de Nederlandse Vereniging van Ziekenhuisapothekers* (Communications of the Dutch Hospital Pharmacists), 33, March 1976.
62. Zöllner, N. and Heuckenkamp, P. U., Vergleichende Untersuchungen über Plasmaspiegel, Ausscheidung und Verwertung von Glucose während mehrstündiger intravenöser Zufuhr bei Stoffwechselgesunden und Patienten mit asymptomatischem Diabetes. *Z. ges. exp. Med. 153*: 112 (1970).

Hormonal control of substrate utilization in parenteral nutrition

P. E. Carlo, Ph.D.

INTRODUCTION

Traditionally, an evaluation of the efficacy of parenteral nutrition is essentially based on clinical results on the one hand and on balance studies on the other whereby the output of the various constituents is compared quantitatively and occasionally qualitatively with their input. A positive or zero balance is generally the definitive criterion of effectiveness.

It is our opinion, however, that the value of parenteral nutrition is still based too much on the study of what goes in and what goes out, and not enough on what goes on. This is why, for some time now, we have tried to stress essentially two points.

The first point is that in each patient, the balanced preferential orientation toward catabolic or anabolic utilization of exogenously supplied amino acids, fats and carbohydrates is essentially controlled by the prevailing activities of the various hormones and enzymes that regulate these two fundamentally different types of utilization. Pathological situations modify these activities.

The second point is that the metabolic properties of carbohydrates and fats are not limited only to their ability to supply calories for either use or storage and to play a structural role; similarly, the metabolic properties of amino acids are not limited to their ability to enter into the synthesis of proteins, thus playing a structural role, and to be used for gluconeogenesis. These three fundamentally different nutritional substrates exert other specific effects. As their administration proceeds, each substrate may preserve, stimulate or inhibit the activities, the release and/or the synthesis of hormones and/or enzymes through what can be called a "*substrate effect*", the intensity of which is proportional to the substrate level.

It thus can be stated that normally these hormone and/or enzyme activities and levels are substrate-modulated and vice versa, all through complex feed-back mechanisms.

Under physiological conditions these feed-back mechanisms can be expected to function properly and maintain homeostasis. Conversely under pathological conditions it can be expected that a few or many of these mechanisms will be disturbed. Consequently it can also be expected that substrate effects and utilization will show disturbances characteristic of the pathological conditions considered in proportion to their severity.

These phenomena deserve and need to be studied to make further progress in parenteral nutrition, both in the choice of the constituents and their mode of administration. Unfortunately, it is not possible to cover the subject in some detail here and only an outline of our method of approach can be given together with some comments on recently made observations.

Nevertheless, this outline and the comments are based on extensive documentation.

STUDY APPROACH – The three stages

Ideally the study of parenteral nutritional therapy should involve at least three stages (1).

Stage one

This first stage should be the study of the metabolism and properties, i.e. the biochemical and physiological properties, of the various constituents of parenteral nutrition. Emphasis should be placed on interactions between the constituents and the various hormone and enzyme systems that control their metabolism and the substrate effects.

There is a large body of information available on the metabolism and properties of carbohydrates, fats and proteins. It should be pointed out, however, that relatively less information is available on fat metabolism.

A clear distinction must be made between the effects of a substrate which lead to the control of its metabolism through the mediation of one or more hormone(s) and those effects that, as far as we know today, apparently do not involve such mediation and seem to be exerted directly, possibly at the level of some enzymatic mechanism.

Obviously, regardless of the mechanism(s) involved, it is important to consider whether the end result is predominantely anabolic or catabolic in nature, not only from the point of view of an overall balance but *also from that of their metabolic balance in specific organs or tissues.*

Substrate effects mediated by hormones

The major hormones involved in glucose, fat and amino acid metabolism are *insulin (I), glucagon (G), catecholamines (CA), glucocorticoids (GC) and growth hormone (GH)*; the main properties of these hormones have been extensively described in the literature which will therefore only be quoted in exceptional cases.

It can be stated that *I* is primarily a storage hormone; the overall result of its action consists of the conservation of energy, glycogenesis, lipogenesis and the synthesis and/or maintenance of body structures.

Both *G*, which has been called the "fuel need hormone", and *CA* are essentially catabolic hormones that can mobilize energetic substrates at the expense of body reserves, through glycogenolysis and lipolysis, and proteins, through gluconeogenesis.

G in practically all respects is an insulin antagonist (2). *CA* in addition inhibit the release of insulin in response to various stimuli, such as glucose and amino acids, and decrease the *I* sensitivity of peripheral tissues while increasing energetic expenses and needs.

GC also participate mainly in catabolic activities and possess diabetogenic properties. It is believed that some of these actions are due to a "permissive" effect which they exert on other hormone activities.

GH action is rather complex and its effects fall between those of insulin and glucagon. The actions of *I* and *GH* can be regarded as both synergistic and antagonistic.

GH is the only lipolytic hormone that can have an anabolic effect under certain circumstances.

It must be noted that these last four hormones all have diabetogenic properties and that some have a reciprocal potentiating effect.

In considering the substrate effects of glucose, fats and amino acids on hormones and enzymes and vice versa it is important to stress that normally, for nutritional purposes, the administration of one substrate to the exclusion of any other (particularly amino acids) is generally not considered appropriate. Amino acids and carbohydrates are always administered together, fats may or may not be added.

The close interdependence between the metabolisms of these three substrates and between the hormonal mechanisms that regulate them must be kept in mind constantly. Experience demonstrates that an observation made with one substrate can be considerably modified when one or both of the other substrates is (are) added.

In addition, in view of the sequence of metabolic events caused by the supply of a substrate and/or the possible hormone level modifications associated with this supply, a particular substrate effect never occurs as an isolated phenomenon. When it is mentioned separately, it is to stress its relative importance.

The study of *substrate effects on hormones* reveals a positive (+), negative (−) or no (0) feed-back effect. Thus a) for glucose this effect is + on *I*, − on *G* and *GH*; b) for amino acids it is + or 0 on *I*, + on *G* and *GH*, the intensity of the effect varying with the nature of the amino acid; c) for lipids it is apparently 0 on *I* and *G* by i.v. route; d) for ketone bodies it is + on *I*.

It must be noted that if the presence of a substrate can stimulate or inhibit the activity and/or the release of certain hormones and/or enzymes, conversely its deficiency can often have exactly the opposite effect with the opposite metabolic consequences.

To obtain a better picture of the consequences of a substrate effect on the metabolism not only of the substrate initially considered but also eventually of other substrates present, the existence of *hormone-hormone feed-back regulation mechanisms* must be also considered.

One of the most important such feed-backs exists between *G* and *I*, and its functioning is carbohydrate-dependent (3). Under normal nutritional conditions, i.e. in the presence of normal glycogen stores, amino acids stimulate *G* and a compensating *I* release. *In the absence of liver glycogen, however, i.e. following starvation, I secretion is blocked while G secretion continues* (4).

In addition, it should be mentioned that: a) *G* secretion is stimulated by *epinephrine* (5) through a positive feed-back mechanism; b) *G* stimulates the liberation of *GH* (6, 7); c) *GC* increase the basal *G* level (8).

However, a positive feed-back effect can be exerted on a hormone activity by another hormone without modification of the level of the latter. This is what has been called a "permissive effect" as mentioned above. Thus, either GC are necessary for the action of lipolytic stimuli or they increase their effects at the fatty tissue as well as the liver level.

Substrate-substrate feed-back regulation of substrate metabolism

As already stressed, neither carbohydrates nor lipids nor amino acids should be administered alone for full metabolic benefit. The metabolisms of these substrates are so closely related that they generally exert a beneficial reciprocal influence on the utilization of the other(s).

Reciprocal influence on metabolism can be the result of the effects of a substrate on a particular hormone which in turn regulates the metabolism of one or two of the other major substrate(s). For example, *I* stimulation by glucose contributes to the uptake and utilization of amino acids for protein synthesis, which in turn contributes to increased glucose utilization; the effects of glucose on *I* and *G* secretion lead to increased lipogenesis and decreased lipolysis, thus influencing *FFA* metabolism.

Metabolic interaction among substrates and their utilization might not, however, always be positive.

An excessive lipid supply has been reported to produce signs of increased gluconeogenesis, therefore protein breakdown and amino acid catabolism which have a negative effect on their utilization.

In addition, *FFA* utilization by tissues is known to compete with glucose utilization and vice versa; this is the basis of the "glucose-free fatty acid cycle" principle postulated by Randle (9). This phenomenon can be considered to be the origin of the glucose intolerance associated with hyperlipacidemia.

Substrate effects not mediated by hormones

If with the exception of their depressant effect on *GH*, the metabolic effects of lipids can be exerted without affecting *I* and *G*, it appears that some of the metabolic effects of glucose (10) and the amino acids (10, 13) can also be mediated without an initial hormonal substrate effect, therefore by-passing reciprocal hormonal control. Proteolysis can thus be decreased and an overall protein sparing effect can be observed.

Metabolic significance of the *I*/*G* ratio

In view of the antagonistic properties of *I* and *G*, Unger (14) has suggested that the *I*/*G* ratio could be an important indicator of the predominantely "anabolic or catabolic state" of the organism. With partial or total nutritional restriction, a drop below the range of its physiological value should thus indicate predominance of catabolism and be proportional to the latter as well as to nitrogen losses and gluconeogenesis from endogenous proteins.

Reciprocally, administration of nutritional substrates should cause a rise in the *I*/*G* ratio to within or above physiological values through adequate substrate effects. This rise should be more or less proportional to the predominance of anabolic activity and nitrogen retention. Experience shows, however, that in the absence of an adequate amino acid supply, a physiological (or higher) *I*/*G* ratio caused by the supply of an energetic substrate which stimulates insulin and/or depresses glucagon release will not be associated with a return to a zero or positive nitrogen balance, i.e. without a return to essential lean body mass maintenance or repair. The patient will remain essentially catabolic from a nitrogen balance standpoint due to normal unavoidable protein turnover. This demonstrates that it is essential to distinguish between energy and nitrogen balances.

In view of the fact that both *I* and *G* mediated and non-mediated substrate effects participate in the control of anabolic activity:

1. some substrates can participate in anabolic activities and nitrogen sparing without directly influencing insulin and glucagon levels, and consequently the value of their ratio;
2. amino acids in the presence of sufficient glycogen reserves lead to a simultaneous increase in *I* and *G* levels; variations within or above the normal range of the *I*/*G* ratio, if any, may thus be minor in comparison with improvement in anabolic activity and nitrogen retention;
3. depending upon the conditions of substrate choice and administration, similar anabolic activity, as measured by overall nitrogen retention or sparing, can be observed in the presence of both a normal and a higher than normal *I*/*G* ratio (15, 16).

It can be concluded that:

a. a drop in the *I*/*G* ratio below what can most likely be considered as its physiological range can be taken as a sign of the predominance of catabolic over anabolic activity from the standpoint of both an energy balance and a nitrogen balance;

b. either a physiological or higher value of the *I*/*G* ratio appears to be a *necessary condition* for either a balanced anabolic versus catabolic or a predominantly anabolic state of the organism from the standpoint of the energy balance and a zero or positive nitrogen balance, but is not a *sufficient condition* as far as the induction of a zero or positive nitrogen balance is concerned. Amino acids must be administered in addition.

Finally, although *I* and *G* are released by the pancreas and are, therefore, carried together in the blood stream to various organs, it is important to determine whether the different organs which they reach are equally responsive but in opposite directions or not. Since *G* exerts only a weak effect on peripheral tissues, this would suggest that the absolute I concentration is most important at that level; conversely, its absolute concentration might be more important in the central organs such as the liver.

Many examples clearly illustrate that there can be large differences in organ sensitivity as far as the metabolic effects of *I* and *G* are concerned. They suggest also that the *I*/*G* ratio assumes its real metabolic significance only when individual organs are considered. Although variations in degree can be anticipated, it is reasonable to expect, and many observations point in this direction, that such differences in sensitivity not only can extend to many other tissues and organs but also concern other hormones. *These points are considered to be fundamental.*

Stage two

This *second stage* should deal with the study of the nature, origin and intensity of the *metabolic disturbances* characterizing the pathological conditions for which parenteral nutritional therapy is to be considered and which can have repercussions on the metabolism of nutritional substrates.

Patient classification

Efficacy and tolerance of parenteral nutrition cannot be evaluated without first adopting a patient classification based mainly on the above-mentioned metabolic disturbances essentially at the hormone level. Various degrees of overlapping can be anticipated between two or more of the situations summarized below.

1. TYPE ONE SITUATION – This is the immediate or initial post-traumatic or post-surgical phase which generally combines acute starvation and stress; the metabolic disturbances of which the negative nitrogen balance is an overall manifestation, are proportional to the intensity of this stress. These disturbances are associated with variations in *hormone level* which can be summarized as follows:

In general, the *I level* shows a drop during surgery, followed by a significant rise with a maximum on the first to second post-operative day; then a progressive drop can be observed.

An increase in the *G level* appears to be a constant factor during the post-operative phase although occasionally no increase is observed during surgery. The increase can be particularly marked on the first day, still significantly increased on the second, third and fourth day and may not decrease until the seventh day. Sepsis and other complications also cause a *G* increase proportional to their severity.

CA levels increase significantly during stress situations, particularly when acute.

GC levels, especially with progressive stress situations, show a marked elevation which may last much longer than the elevation of other catabolic hormones. In surgical patients, levels can still be significantly increased on the 8th post-operative day.

GH levels show a rapid rise on the day of surgery but further development varies according to the author.

The simultaneous effects of the increase in the *G*, *CA*, *GC* and *GH* levels without a compensating *I* increase induce an *unrestrained energetic substrate mobilization* beyond immediate utilization capacity; this is illustrated by *hyperglycemia and hyperlipacidemia.*

Hormone substrate and hormone-hormone feed-back disturbances can also be observed. They include inhibition of the negative feed-back between hyperglycemia and glucagonemia (17), between hyperglycemia and *GH* for many hours (18, 19) and between *FFA* and *GH*; the positive feed-backs between hyperglycemia and *I* (19) and between *G* and *I* (19) are also inhibited.

All the above-mentioned disturbances increase the activity of those hormones which carry a diabetogenic component. It should not be surprising, therefore, to observe endogenous substrate utilization disturbances not unlike those of diabetes (1) where elevated *FFA* seems to play an important role (9).

In view of this characteristic hormonal profile the ratio $\frac{I}{G+CA+GC}$ has been suggested as being more representative of the overall anabolic versus catabolic activities (1, 20) than the I/G ratio.

2. TYPE TWO SITUATION – This is the secondary post-traumatic or post-surgical phase which in the absence of complications will progressively replace type one within three to five days as the stress stimuli decrease, i.e. *CA* and *GC* stimulation.

Major metabolic features and disturbances will generally speaking closely resemble those of simple starvation. Predominant *FFA* utilization as energy source, a decrease in glucose-metabolizing enzymes such as hexokinase, elevated *C* and decreased *I* levels are again diabetogenic factors and contribute to diabetic-like glucose intolerance and *I* resistance. Nitrogen losses decrease progressively together with other cell constituent losses to stabilize at minimum negative values.

In view of the above-mentioned hormone profile, it appears that now the I/G ratio is more suitable as *a metabolic model* of the anabolic versus catabolic activities.

3. TYPE THREE SITUATION – This situation can develop under two essentially different circumstances:

a. when the *type one* situation has been particularly intense and prolonged due to the severity of the trauma of surgery and/or if the *type two* situation has been allowed to progress too far without proper nutritional measures.

b. because of a chronic disease involving the digestive tract that has interfered markedly with the oral intake of food or when the latter is contraindicated for pathological or therapeutic reasons.

From the point of view of hormonal balance this *type three* situation, whether due to the first circumstance without complications or to the second, again closely resembles a protracted starvation situation.

A decrease in insulinemia without a concomitant decrease in the glucoganemia can be expected to accentuate the cell consituent losses associated with gluconeogenesis. Severe deficiencies will develop, including enzyme, vitamin, trace element and electrolyte deficiencies.

Here again, the *I/G* ratio appears to be a representative indicator of the anabolic versus catabolic activity.

4. TYPE FOUR SITUATION – Before circumstances lead some patients into one of the previous three situations, they may initially suffer from some form of acquired or genetic disease of more or less marked severity.

These diseases carry their own specific metabolic disturbances which will be superimposed on, and generally further complicate, those inherant in the clinical situation into which they have subsequently fallen. Special therapeutic problems may thus result with respect to parenteral nutrition which deserve a specific approach which will not be discussed here. Diabetes, renal and liver failure, specific enzyme deficiencies, hyperlipemias, Crohn's disease, etc. are but a few examples.

REMARK

Special therapeutic problems may also result from initial metabolic differences of a physiological nature. This refers to the differences between infants, children, adolescents, adults, the aged, males and females. They deserve to be studied with the same approach as suggested here.

Stage three

In general, parenteral nutrition should be able to perform the following functions: a) help control the release of endogenous energetic substrates as well as the mechanisms which induce this process; b) improve the utilization of their excess when present, either by stimulating their catabolic utilization or inducing their storage or both (if this is not achieved, intolerance phenomena may develop); c) provide the type of substrate best adapted to nutritional requirements and most likely to cause the re-orientation of metabolism away from predominantly catabolic toward predominantly anabolic activity, or to maintain an even balance between anabolic and catabolic activities.

Parenteral nutrition supplies the nutritional substrates which under physiological situations can maintain the desired balance between anabolism and catabolism when administered in normal amounts. Under certain clinical situations as defined in *stage two*, however, difficulties which vary qualitatively and quantitatively with the type of situation concerned may be encountered. The aim of this *third stage* is to determine the origin of these difficulties in order to be able to improve the approach to nutritional therapy. It should include the study of: 1) the repercussions of the disturbances described in *stage two* on the metabolism and effects of the various substrates used in parenteral nutrition as studied in *stage one*; 2) the ability of the same substrates to correct these disturbances, including their ability to induce a switch from their predominantly catabolic toward their predominantly anabolic orientation for both the energy and the nitrogen balance.

The approach will be based initially on the analysis of the models proposed which revealed in both cases a common component, the *I/G* ratio; the metabolic significance of this ratio has already been mentioned. In these models, in which *GH* is absent, *I* and *G* are for all practical purposes the only substrate-responsive components which normally react quantitatively to glucose and amino acid administration. It now appears that the difficulties mentioned above are due to interference with the reactions by other factors which will be reviewed.

In a type one situation, it is well-known that depending upon the severity of the situation, more calories and nitrogen than would be normally expected are required to achieve the desired anabolic response. A delay in response or the "inertia" phenomenon can also be observed.

An explanation of these observations can be the contribution of *CA* + *GC* to the model denominator, i.e. their catabolic and anti-insulin properties, and to feed-back regulation disturbances.

These factors will lead to a diabetic-like *glucose* intolerance and I resistance not only because of interference with glucose phosphorylation mechanisms but also because of the increase in *FFA* that they induce. The positive glucose effect on *I* and the negative one on *G* secretion are depressed. More glucose will be needed to produce them, so that the need for exogenous *I* is then better understood.

Amino acids when administered alone will find a set of hormonal and enzymatic activities oriented mainly toward catabolism and gluconeogenesis. Absence of glycogen reserves will lead to further *G* secretion, without compensating *I* release, a situation favorable for further amino acid catabolism. Any nitrogen sparing will most likely be due mainly to the direct non-hormonally mediated amino acid effect. *GH* stimulation can also be anticipated, contributing more to lipolysis, as well as increased *FFA* and glucose intolerance both due to the "glucose fatty acid cycle" phenomenon (9) and hexokinase depletion (21).

Amino acid and *glucose* administration is thus necessary to stimulate directly and reciprocally the respective anabolic utilizations, although a depression of the substrate effect will still cause a need for a larger supply than normal, and a continued need for exogenous insulin.

Lipids should never be administered alone but always in the proper proportion with amino acids and carbohydrates because of the possible adverse affects of their excess on anabolic acitivity. Due to the absence of substrate effect on *I* and *G*, they can contribute to the improvement of anabolic activity without a further increase in the *I/G* ratio. Their use in a situation of high lipolytic activity should be considered with caution.

In conclusion, both the increased substrate needs and the "inertia" phenomenon are essentially induced by hormonal disturbances associated with stress and starvation. It must be noted that if substrates and exogenous *I* can contribute toward an increase in the model value and anabolic activity, pharmacological depression of the *CA* + *GC* factor can further improve the anabolic substrate effect and shorten the "inertia" phase (22).

In a type two situation, provided *type one* has not been too intense and/or prolonged, the metabolic situation moves toward that of a plain starvation situation with a decrease in the influence of *CA* + *GC*. As a result *I* and *G* return to normal substrate responsiveness. In fact metabolic response to substrate administration comes close to or equals that expected physiologically. Nevertheless, as in starvation, a diabetic-like situation with initial glucose intolerance and *I* resistance can be observed together with some degree of "inertia" of the anabolic response.

Interaction of the metabolic features of type two situation with substrate administration and vice versa will not be discussed since they are approximately the same as those observed in starvation and those discussed in stage one. A few remarks are nevertheless in order.

In a type one situation, it can be considered that the diabetic-like situation and "inertia" phenomenon are initially due essentially to hormone regulation disturbances. In type two, however, although increased *FFA* utilization is a contributing factor, starvation-induced depletion of certain glucose metabolizing enzymes – including hexokinase and some of the pentose pathways ones – and amino acid anabolizing enzymes appear to be the major factors in the diabetic and "inertia" phenomena, with time needed for resynthesis.

Finally it must be noted that this type two situation has been knowingly or fortuitously selected by many investigators for parenteral nutrition studies. Their conclusions must be analyzed in this light, and cannot be extrapolated to type one, three of four situations.

The type three situation concerns a situation in which advanced chronic starvation has been allowed to develop, as yet still encountered too frequently in severely sick hospitalized patients.

The metabolic characteristic of primary importance is an overall cell constituent deficiency. In a *type two* situation, as substrate administration proceeds the body contains enough elements to adapt its enzymatic and hormonal machinery to increased metabolization of the administered substrates to overcome the "inertia" phenomenon described.

This time, the "inertia" phenomenon is due not only to the slowing down of metabolic processes, but essentially to the fundamental deficiency of the elements required to rebuild the enzymatic and hormonal machinery. Hypophosphatemia is only one of the many aspects of this depletion.

The major problem that must be solved, the practical aspects of which are outside the scope of this study, is to adopt the best program of progressive administration of complete balanced parenteral nutrition supplying not only carbohydrates, amino acids and fats but also trace elements, electrolytes and vitamins; otherwise a hyperalimentation syndrome will develop.

DISCUSSION

On the basis of the approach suggested, a few selected practical observations will be discussed.

Concerning glucose metabolism, it is clear that what is a harmonious control under physiological conditions can become a source of problems under certain pathological situations. In a *Type One* situation especially, numerous factors contribute to throw off glucose homeostasis mechanisms with negative metabolic consequences. These mechanisms operate mainly at the level of hexokinase activity and glucose phosphorylation.

A glucose substitute that by-passes this initial step could be utilized without the need for increased insulin activity or secretion with overall beneficial consequences similar to those of glucose plus insulin administration. Among various available glucose substitutes, orbitol proves to be such a substrate.

Sorbitol administration should lead to an increase in the lowerd *I/G* ratio to within the physiological range. It has been shown that sorbitol achieves an overall metabolic response similar to that of glucose, to achieve the same result glucose must cause an increase above this range, which anti-insulin factors can hinder.

Concerning *amino acid metabolism* in the presence or absence of various calorigenic substrates five studies can be mentioned (15, 16, 23, 24, 26). Three (15, 16, 26) can be taken as examples of a definite attempt to link the substrate effects on several hormonal parameters with overall nitrogen retention.

In the study by Jeejeebhoy et al. (16) the patients seem to belong to the *Type Two* situation. Two different groups of patients were studied from the standpoint of overall nitrogen balance, *I* and *G* levels, and the levels of other blood constituents.

The patients were divided into two groups. All received 1 g/kg/day of amino acids plus 40 kcal/kg/day. One group received these calories in the form of 50% glucose and the other group in the form of lipid emulsion and glucose, representing 83 and 17% of these 40 kcal, respectively. The random crossover technique was used. Both regimes gave an equivalent overall positive nitrogen balance. In the first regimen, high *I* and insignificantly changed *G* levels were maintained. With the second regimen, much lower *I* levels and practically unchanged *G* levels (with a slight tendency toward a rise) were maintained. These hormone profiles are in agreement with the information presented in *stage one*. Thus an equivalent calorie supply in the form of either glucose or mainly lipids, together with amino acids, can yield similar overall nitrogen balances with different *I* and *G* profiles.

The study by Greenberg et al. (15) compares the nitrogen sparing effects of glucose alone, and of amino acids either alone or in combination with either lipids or glucose in four different groups of patients. It appears that the patients generally represented the *Type One* situation. Each group received the same amount of calories, i.e. 450 in the form of glucose or lipids, except for the amino acid alone group who received 1 g/kg/day of amino acids. Thus, this latter regimen constituted a partial starvation diet from the caloric standpoint.

The nitrogen balance was markedly negative in all groups and did not differ significantly for the three groups receiving amino acids, irrespective of the concurrent infusion of glucose or lipids. In contrast, the nitrogen balance was significantly more negative for the patients receiving only glucose.

The *I* levels in the protein and protein plus lipid groups were the lowest and did not differ significantly with respect to each other. In both glucose groups this value was significantly higher than in the non-glucose group. The highest level measured was in the protein plus glucose group.

G levels tended to be higher in groups not receiving glucose. Protein plus lipid administration gave levels significantly higher than those measured for glucose alone, protein alone and protein plus glucose. The high level for protein alone was significant only when compared with that for protein plus glucose.

The authors conclude that the protein sparing effect of amino acids appears to be a function of the infused amino acids alone.

The *I* and *G* profiles are again in agreement with the information discussed in *stage one*.

In the past couple of years it has been claimed (23, 24) that with a supply of 1 g of amino acid/kg/day without added calories patients could be maintained at a near zero nitrogen balance. These studies, however, lacked precision on many points including the type of patients. From what could be deduced from the very limited information, they appear to belong in the *Type Two* situation. Other authors have tried to duplicate these results without success (15).

On the basis of the information presented in *stage one*, it is apparent that a supply of amino acids alone would lead to no change in or a slight lowering of *I* levels and a rise in *G* and *GH* together with hyperlipemia and hyperkenonemia. The study of Kaminski et al. (26) supports this deduction.

The above-mentioned studies call for further comments.

The first and most interesting one is that regardless of the *I* and *G* profile, the administration of amino acids either alone or with a minimum caloric requirement or with adequate calories, regardless of their nature and possible reciprocal proportion, exerts a significant nitrogen sparing effect. This would appear so far to apply to both *Type One and Type Two* situations.

It is thus tempting to deduce that the non-hormonally mediated positive effect of amino acids on protein metabolism is far from being negligible. It constitutes an essential part of the positive effects of parenteral nutrition.

A clear distinction must be made however between nitrogen sparing effects that can be exerted through a limited number of mechanisms, and the return to a zero or positive nitrogen balance which in addition must involve a complete set of balanced physiological mechanisms requiring qualitatively and quantitatively balanced nutritional measures especially in a *Type One situation.*

In addition, it is possible that the relative participation in overall nitrogen retention by each type of mechanism might vary depending upon the *Type of situation* the patient is in.

The second observation is that the administration of amino acids alone is likely to induce a *diabetic-like hormone* profile which cannot be considered metabolically desirable, even if some overall protein spring effect can be observed. This is particularly true in *Type One* situations. Resumption of a glucose-containing regimen after administration of only amino acids is most likely to result in marked glucose intolerance and *I* resistance.

The third observation concerns the different sensitivities of the various organs and tissues to hormones as pointed out in *stage one.*

It has been seen that similar degrees of overall nitrogen retention or balance can be achieved in the presence of different *I* and *G* profiles, both being hormones which are known to have an influence on protein, carbohydrate and fat metabolisms. It has also been seen that a not unimportant portion of the positive effects of amino acids on nitrogen metabolism can be due to mechanisms which apparently are not significantly hormone-sensitive. As already mentioned, this obviously leaves a portion of this effect under hormonal control, the importance of which can be expected to increase as the nitrogen balance is improved, especially with increased calorie supply. It is known finally that different organs and tissues react differently not only to variations in absolute hormone level but also to the relative variations.

This all leads to the conclusion that, whereas the overall nitrogen balance can be similar with different regimes, not only amino acid utilization but also carbohydrate and lipid metabolism must differ among organs and tissues depending upon the composition of the regimes. The clinical importance of this situation should be determined.

It remains, however, a fact that since many metabolic disturbances of diabetes are known, such as impaired healing, any regime inducing a diabetic-like hormone pattern is to be considered with great caution especially in surgical patients. This applies in particular to the amino acid alone regime.

SUMMARY

As a means to further improve the efficacy and tolerance of parenteral nutritional therapy, the author suggests and summarizes a three-stage study approach.

The first stage outlines the hormonal regulation of the metabolism of the three major substrates used in parenteral nutrition. This includes: hormonally mediated substrate effects of glucose, fats and amino acids at the level of insulin (*I*), glucagon (*G*), catecholamines (*CA*), glucocorticoids (*GC*) and growth hormone (*GH*); various substrate-hormones and hormone-hormone feed-back regulation mechanisms; positive substrate effects which apparently are not hormone-mediated; the relative metabolic significance of the *I/G* ratio and the absolute requirement of amino acid supply for zero or positive nitrogen balance and the basis for concomitant glucose administration.

The second stage outlines first the need for, and then suggests, a patient classification using four types of clinical situations, based on a distinction between the different hormonal disturbances induced by the various major pathological situations for which parenteral nutrition is indicated. Metabolic consequences are reviewed, including their effects on endogenous substrate mobilization, induced feed-back regulation disturbances among the substrates and hormones mentioned above, the development of a diabetic-like situation and cell constituent losses. For the first three situations models are suggested based on the hormone profile reflecting the anabolic/catabolic activities.

The third stage outlines briefly the possible interactions of the metabolic effects of substrates and the metabolic disturbances of the first three types of situation on the basis of the data presented in the first two stages of the study, in order to determine favorable and possibly unfavorable metabolic interactions. The various mechanisms that can induce an "inertia phenomenon" in the positive metabolic response to substrate administration are suggested with respect to the first three types of clinical situation.

The discussion focusses on recent studies which indicate that, on the one hand, the nitrogen sparing effect of amino acids can be independent of calorie supply regardless of its nature and that on the other hand, a similar positive nitrogen balance can be obtained with the same amount of amino acids whether administered with glucose or mainly lipids as the calorie source. Since *I* and *G* profiles are then different and these hormones are known to affect protein metabolism differently depending on the organs considered, it is tentatively concluded that, although overall nitrogen retention can be similar, metabolic effects may differ at the levels of the different organs and tissues not only from the standpoint of hormonally mediated mechanisms but perhaps also non-hormonally mediated ones. Attention is directed to the need to consider possible clinical repercussions, in particular the possible adverse effects of the administration of substrates or substrate combinations capable of inducing a diabetic-like hormonal profile, such as amino acids either alone or with lipids.

REFERENCES

1. Carlo, P. E., Hormonal control of substrate utilization in parenteral nutrition. A model proposal. In: Proceedings of the "International Symposium, Australian Society for Parenteral Nutrition", 29, Melbourne, Australia, March 1974.
2. Parilla, R., Goodman, M. N. and Toews, C. J., Effect of Glucagon: Insulin Ratios on Hepatic Metabolism, *Diabetes 23*: 725 (1974).
3. Cahill, G. F., Glucagon, *New Engl. J. Med. 288*: No 3, 157, (1973).
4. Marks, V. and Samols, E., Glucagon Mediated Insulin Release in Man. *Acta Diab. Latina 5*: suppl. 1, 285 (1968).
5. Oliver, J. R. and Wright, P. H., Interactions between Glucose and Glucagon Secretagogues in perfused Rat Islets of Langerhans. *Diab. 24*: 2, (1975).
6. Cain, J. P., Williams, G. H. and Dlucky, R. G., Glucagon stimulation of human growth hormone. *J. Clin. Endoc. 31*: 222 (1969).
7. Geser, C. A., Felber, J. P., Brand, E. and Shultis, K., Untersuchungen zur Glucagon-induzierten Sekretion von Wachstumshormon und Insulin und deren Einfluss auf Parameter des Kohlenhydrat- und Fettstoffwechsels nach einem Operationsstress. *Klin. Wochenschr. 49*: 21, 1175 (1971).
8. Wise, J. J., Hendler, R. and Felig, Ph., Influence of Glucocorticoids on Glucagon

Secretion and Plasma Amino Acid Concentrations in Man. *J. Clin. Invest. 52*: 2774 (1973).
9. Randle, P. J., Garland, P. B., Hales, C. N. and Newsholme, E. A., The Glucose Fatty Acid Cycle. Its Role in Insulin Sensitivity and the Metabolic disturbances of Diabetes Mellitus. *Lancet 1*: 7285, 785 (1963).
10. Fulks, R. M., Li, J. B. and Goldberg, A. L., Effects of Insulin, Glucose, and Amino Acids on Protein Turnover in Rat Diaphragm. *J. Biological Chemistry 250*: No 1, 290 (1975).
11. Jefferson, L. S. and Korner, A., Influence of Amino Acid Supply on Ribosomes and Protein Synthesis of Perfused Rat Liver. *Biochem. J. 3*: 703 (1969).
12. Woodside, K. H. and Mortimore, G. E., Suppression of Protein Turnover by Amino Acids in the Perfused Rat Liver. *J. Biol. Chem. 247*: No 20, 6474 (1972).
13. Neely, A. N., Nelson, P. B. and Mortimore, G. E., Osmotic Alterations of the Lysosomal System during Rat Liver Perfusion: Reversible suppression by Insulin and Amino Acis. *Bioch. Biophys. Acta 338*: 458 (1974).
14. Unger, R. H., Progress in Endocrinology and Metabolism. Alpha- and Beta-cell Interrelationships in Health and Disease. *Metabolism 23*: No 6, 581 (1974).
15. Greenberg, G. R., Marliss, E. B., Anderson, G. H., Langer, B., Spence, W., Tovee, E. B. and Jeejeebhoy, K. N., Protein-Sparing Therapy in Postoperative Patients. Effects of Added Hypocaloric Glucose or Lipid. *New Engl. J. of Med. 294*: No 26, 1411 (1976).
16. Jeejeebhoy, K. N., Anderson, G. H., Nakhooda, A. F., Greenberg, G. R., Sanderson, I. and Marliss, E. B., Metabolic Studies in Total Parenteral Nutrition with Lipid in Man. *J. of Clin. Invest. 57*: No 1, 125 (1976).
17. Kissebah, A. H., "Stress" Hormones and Lipid Metabolism. *Proc. roy. Soc. Med. 67*: 665 (1974).
18. Ketterer, H., Powell, D. and Unger, R. H., Growth hormone response to surgical stress. *Clin. Res. 14*: 65 (1966).
19. Oyama, T. and Takazawa, T., Effects of methoxyflurane anesthesia and surgery on human growth hormone and insulin levels in plasma. *Canad. Anaesthe. Soc. J. 17*: 347 (1970).
20. Carlo, P. E., Nutrition parentérale et équilibre hormonal. Int. Cong. Parenteral Nut., Montpellier 12-14 Sept. 1974, 169, Deehan Ed., Montpellier, 1976.
21. Cahill, G. F., Physiology of Insulin in Man. *Diabetes 20*: No 12, 785 (1971).
22. Setbon, L., Le métabolisme azoté sous neuroleptanalgésie postopératoire. *Cahiers d'Anesthésiologie 18*: 8, 981 (1970).
23. Kaminski, M., Dunn, N., Wannemacher, R., Dinterman, R., DeShazo, R., Wilson, W., Earll, J. and Carlson, D., Mechanism for protein sparing during postoperative dextrose free amino acid infusions. *Am. J. Clin. Nut. 29*: No 4, 463 (1976).
24. Blackburn, G. L., Flatt, J. P., Clowes, G. H. A. and O'Donnel, T. E., Peripheral Intravenous Feeding with Isotonic Amino Acid Solutions. *A. J. Surg. 125*: 447 (1973).
25. Blackburn, G. L., Flatt, J. P., Clowes, G. H. A., O'Donnel, T. F. and Hensle, T. E., Protein Sparing Therapy during Periods of Starvation with Sepsis or Trauma. *Ann. Surg. 177*: 588 (1973).
26. Howard, L., Dobbs, A., Chodos, R., Chu, R. and Loludice, T., A comparison of administering protein alone and protein plus glucose on nitrogen balance. *Am. J. Clin. Nutr. 29*: No 4, 463 (1976).

Requirements for protein and amino acids: applications to parenteral nutrition

Hamish N. Munro

INTRODUCTION

In several clinical conditions, such as cancer, injury, burning, and malabsorption, there is often significant loss of body protein, and in some other diseases, notably hepatic cirrhosis and uremia, there are abnormalities of protein metabolism. In the treatment of all these conditions, the maintenance or restoration of body protein content and the correction of metabolic abnormalities become major therapeutic objectives. In order to reverse these pathological changes in protein metabolism, an important strategy is the adjustment of the diet, and a potent way of ensuring this is by parenteral nutrition. It is therefore important to design nutritional treatment for these various clinical conditions along lines that will take advantage of our current knowledge of protein metabolism and protein requirements. This contribution to the symposium will describe three areas of significance for these objectives:

(i) current concepts of the regulation of protein metabolism in the body;

(ii) requirements by normal subjects for protein and amino acids, alterations in requirements caused by disease and modifications in nutrient intake that may be required for delivery by the parenteral route;

(iii) parameters for measuring protein depletion and repletion.

CURRENT CONCEPTS OF THE REGULATION OF PROTEIN METABOLISM

Digestion, absorption and the role of the liver

Figure 1 provides an overall view of the role of digestion and absorption in protein metabolism as currently understood (1). The first step involves proteolytic enzymes which attack and degrade dietary protein. In the case of trypsin, there is evidence (2) for a regulatory mechanism in which the protein to be digested combines with the digestive enzyme. That is to say, if most of the trypsin is bound to the protein undergoing digestion, little free trypsin will be present and the pancreas will continue to secrete more, but will stop when free trypsin accumulates. Another point of significance relates to the mechanism of amino acid absorption by the gut. Free amino acids used to be regarded as the only end-products of protein digestion which were absorbed by the mucosal cells of the small intestine. It is now known that a significant and perhaps even a major part of absorption occurs not as free amino acids but as peptides (3) which are then hydrolyzed to free amino acids within the mucosal cell for absorption as such into the portal vein.

It must be recognized that the gut wall actively carries out a number of important metabolic reactions. Thus, transamination of glutamic and aspartic acids occurs, giving rise to the corresponding keto acids. This may exert a protective effect. Another important feature shown in Fig. 1 is the secretion of endogenous protein. This occurs mainly from shed mucosal cells, the contribution of the intestinal juices being relatively small. A figure of 70 grams per day has been estimated for the amount of endogenous gut protein found in a normal adult man ingesting 100 grams of dietary protein daily (4). Since fecal protein represent about 10 grams daily, the total amount of protein absorbed by the gut thus becomes about 160 grams daily.

This load of amino acids passes up the portal vein to the liver which is the

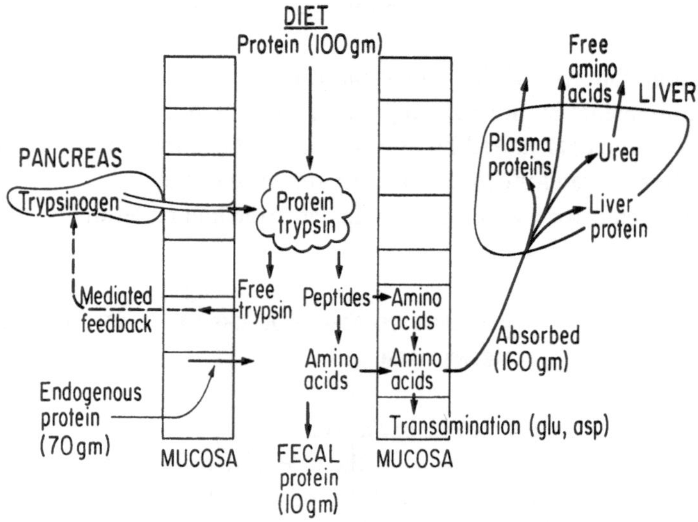

Fig. 1. Diagram showing the fate of dietary protein, the secretion of endogenous protein, feedback control of pancreatic enzyme secretion and passage to the liver [From Crim and Munro (1)].

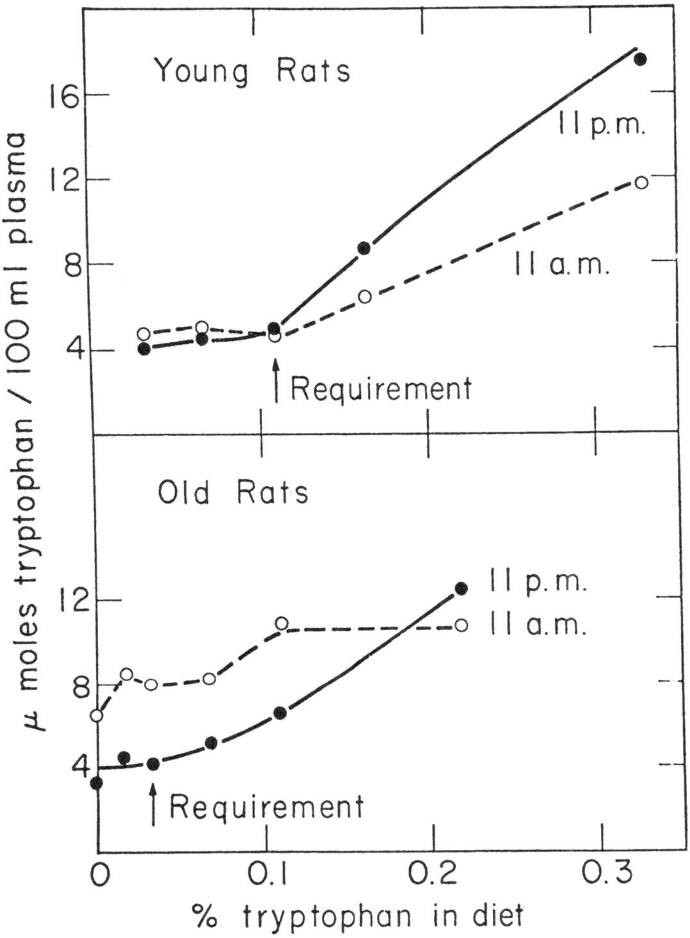

Fig. 2. Plasma tryptophan levels of young and mature rats fed diets containing various levels of tryptophan [Young and Munro(6)].

main or exclusive site of oxidation of seven of the essential amino acids whereas the branched-chained amino acids are oxidized in kidney and particularly in muscle, while the nonessential amino acids readily enter many metabolic pathways and their oxidation occurs at many different tissue sites. When the dietary intake of essential amino acids is increased, an induction of liver enzyme activity occurs. In at least some such cases this induction shows a break point occurring at levels of intake beyond the needs of the body (5). This implies that the liver is sensitive to general requirements and does not destroy essential amino acids extensively below that level of intake. When the dietary intake increases beyond that point, induction of the appropriate enzymes occurs. This general pattern for the essential amino acids is not shared by the enzymes responsible for metabolism of the nonessential amino acids, which are degraded in proportion to intake (5). Thus, there is a sensitive mechanism modulating amino acid metabolism in the liver in relation to body needs.

Impact of diet on plasma amino acid levels

Although the liver thus monitors the amounts of free amino acids passing into the general circulation, it does not completely eliminate a rise in plasma levels of amino acids when excess of an essential amino acid is consumed. Below requirements for that amino acid, intake often has little effect on systemic levels, whereas above requirements, the level in the plasma starts to rise. The point of inflection when the plasma level starts to rise has been used as an index of requirements. For example, we (6) gave young and mature rats various levels of dietary tryptophan, varying from insufficient to excess, and measured the response of plasma tryptophan at 11 a.m. and 11 p.m. (Fig. 2). Up to the level of requirement for tryptophan, there was little change in plasma tryptophan level, but above this, the concentration rose, especially at 11 p.m. (feeding time). The point of inflection varied with age, occurring at lower dietary concentrations for older rats that need less tryptophan. This procedure has also been used to determine amino acid needs of humans but some doubts have been expressed about its precision. However, shifts in the inflection point could be valuable for study changes in requirements with disease.

The plasma levels of amino acids are also affected by dietary carbohydrate through an insulin-dependent mechanism (Fig. 3). Within an hour of consuming carbohydrate, most plasma amino acids decrease, due to deposition in muscle through insulin-mediated transport (7). This response to carbohydrate is maximal for branched-chain amino acids. A similar metabolic interaction occurs between dietary protein or amino acids and carbohydrate consumed in the same meal (8), presumably due to the same insulin-dependent mechanism. A similar interaction is known to occur between infused amino acids and glucose in parenteral nutrition (9).

The alterations in plasma free amino acid patterns caused by the amino acid and carbohydrate components of a meal or a parenteral infusion can have significance for the availability of amino acids to the peripheral tissues. In particular, it has been shown that entry of tryptophan into the cells of the brain is determined by the plasma levels of other competing neutral amino acids, notably the branched-chain amino acids (10). The extensive reduction in plasma levels of branched-chain amino acids caused by carbohydrate results in greater passage of tryptophan into the brain and more serotonin is synthesized (11). This mechanism is not only significant in regulating serotonin metabolism but is also critical to brain function under pathological conditions. As shown in Fig. 4, hepatic cirrhosis results in a series of meta-

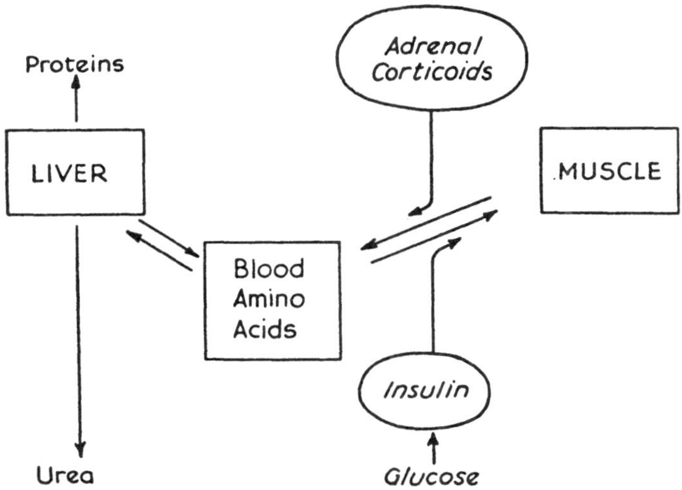

Fig. 3. The mechanism of action of dietary carbohydrate on plasma free amino acids [from Munro (8)].

bolic alterations relating to protein metabolism (12). Ammonia and amines formed in the intestines are no longer removed by the liver, but pass into the systemic circulation and enter the brain. Next, amino acids normally degraded exclusively in the liver, such as tryptophan and phenylalanine, are no longer subject to hepatic control and their levels tend to rise. Finally, the liver no longer inactivates part of the insulin as it passes through, and the higher system levels of insulin drive the branched-chain amino acids into muscle, thus accounting for the low plasma levels of branched-chain amino acids observed in cases of cirrhosis. Because the levels of the branched-chain amino acids in the plasma are subnormal, a larger proportion of the plasma tryptophan passes into the brain and the resulting excessivè production of serotonin contributes to hepatic coma. This theory of the role of excess serotonin formation as a factor in hepatic coma receives some confirmation from

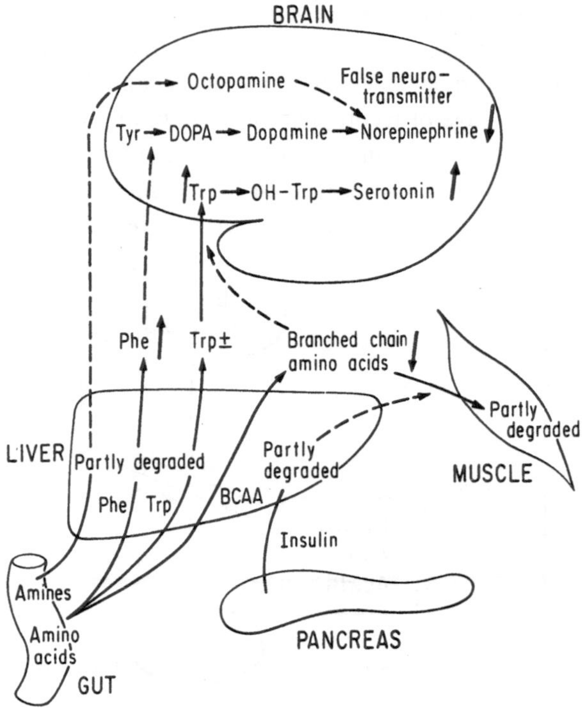

Fig. 4. Role of branched-chain amino acids in hepatic coma. Owing to unrestricted passage of insulin into the general circulation in hepatic coma, branched-chain amino acids are removed excessively by muscle. In consequence of this lowering of plasma branched-chain amino acids, there is less competition with tryptophan for entry into the brain and thus more serotonin is synthesized (from Crim and Munro (1)].

the demonstration that administration of branched-chain amino acids to animals with hepatic coma can reverse the comatose state (13).

Role of skeletal muscle in protein metabolism

Muscle is the major depot for retention of free amino acids in the body (14) and is also the major component of whole body protein, so that metabolism of amino acids in this tissue are of considerable significance for the body as a whole. The daily turnover of muscle protein, estimated by studying the rate of release of alanine, glutamine and other amino acids into plasma, has been put at 75 gm per day for a subject fasting up to 24 hrs (15). This estimate is probably too low because it does not allow for intracellular reutilization of amino acids liberated by muscle protein breakdown. Accordingly, it would be useful to measure the true rate of muscle protein breakdown by having an amino acid released from the protein which was not reutilized. Urinary output of 3-methylhistidine appears to provide such an index. In order to monitor muscle protein breakdown rate without reutilization, we have used 3-methylhistidine output in the urine (Fig. 5). Methylation of histidine in actin and myosin occurs only after the muscle protein backbone has been synthesized. However, this methylhistidine is not reused when muscle protein breaks down but is quantitatively excreted in the urine (17). Thus 3-methylhistidine appears to fulfill all the requirements of an index of myofibrillar breakdown.

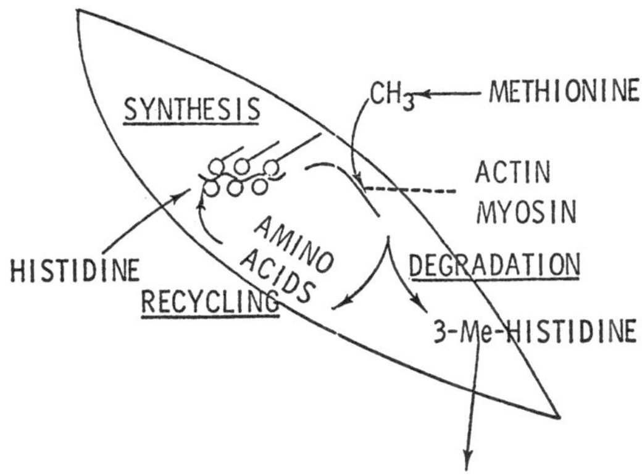

Fig. 5. Synthesis and release of 3-methylhistidine in muscle (from Munro [16)].

The content of methylhistidine of various tissues and organs of the rat shows that skeletal muscle is the overwhelming reservoir of methylhistidine in the body (18). In addition, changes in methylhistidine excretion have been examined in young growing rats receiving either a normal diet or diets deficient in either protein alone or protein and calories (19). This study showed that breakdown of muscle protein in the growing animal is sensitive to protein depletion (reduced breakdown) or caloric insufficiency (increased breakdown). Thus 3-methylhistidine appears to provide an index of muscle protein turnover that is sensitive to nutritional factors. In this connection, it may be noted that malnourished children in India show a low output of methylhistidine, which rises when recovery occurs (20). We have also observed that grossly obese subjects undergoing prolonged fasting show a progressive reduction in 3-methylhistidine output (21).

The current status of our knowledge can be summarized as follows. Most of the methylhistidine in the body occurs in myofibrillar protein. It has a low renal clearance and thus is rapidly excreted. Nearly all of a test dose given

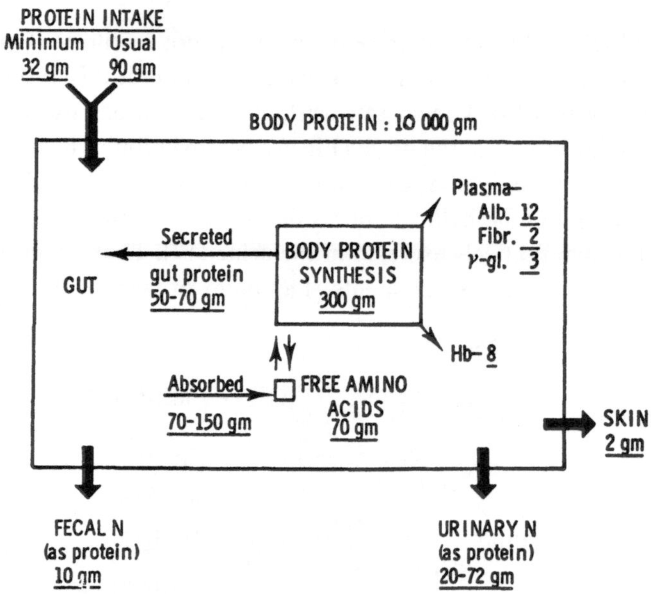

Fig. 6. Over-all protein metabolism in a 70 kg man [from Munro (16)].

to the rat or to the human subject has been recovered in the urine. The responsiveness of urinary output to protein-calorie deficiency varies according to whether protein alone is deficient or whether protein and calories are both deficient.

Overall body protein metabolism

From the preceding information, a composite picture of the daily flux of amino acids in the body of an adult man can be obtained (Fig. 6). The customary protein intake in Western countries is about 100 gm daily, to which is added at least 70 gm of protein secreted into the gastro-intestinal tract, and thus the total protein for absorption is at least 160 gm. Pools of free amino acids in the tissues are at least 70 gm. Experiments with ^{15}N suggest that some 300 gm of protein are synthesized daily by the adult (22). The difference between the intake of 100 gm protein and the daily turnover of 300 gm indicates the amount of amino acid reutilization involved in protein metabolism. More accurate estimates of amino acid fluxes are needed, not only in adult healthy subjects but also in patients with injuries or debilitating diseases.

PROTEIN AND AMINO ACID REQUIREMENTS IN HEALTH AND DISEASE

Protein and amino acid needs in health

The dietary allowances for protein at different ages are shown in Table 1. For optimal growth, the newborn infant needs about 2 gm protein per kg per day and this requirement diminishes as one approaches the adult level. After correction for variations in the quality of dietary protein, the adult requirement turns out to be about 0.8 gm per kg body weight per day (23).

Table 1. Safe levels of protein and essential amino acids at different ages [adapted from FAO/WHO Report (23)]

Age group	Protein* g/kg	Essential amino acids (% total protein)
Infant (6-11 months)	1.75	37%
Male adolescents (10-12 year)	1.01	33%
Male adults	0.81	15%

Requirements for the eight essential amino acids add up to about 39% of the total protein needs of the healthy infant, but they account for only 15% of the proteins needs of the healthy adult (23). This, does not mean that the depleted adult (e.g., after injury) still requires this relatively small proportion of essential amino acids. Probably the adult in a state of repletion has essential amino acid needs that once more resemble those of the growing subject. This is supported by studies carried out many years ago (Table 2), in which adult rats were depleted of protein and then repleted (24). Repletion after depletion raised the requirement for each of the essential amino acids threefold. We can thus conclude that the demands for tissue growth in repletion are likely to be similar to those of childhood.

The importance of energy intake is emphasized in Fig. 7. The figure shows the effects of different levels of energy intake upon nitrogen balance (8). On a diet of adequate protein content (upper line), there is a linear effect of energy on N balance, even at excess caloric intakes. The lower line in the figure shows the effects of limiting the amount of protein in the diet; at a certain point, the restriction of protein intake prevents further improvement in N balance in response to increased caloric intake. Thus N balance cannot

* Quality score of 80 for mixed dietary protein.

be defined only in terms of protein intake but is the resultant of both protein and energy intake.

Protein requirements in disease

Changes in protein and amino acid requirements in disease are difficult to estimate, especially because diseases are not constant in intensity. Table 3 provides some rough estimate of changes in the need for protein in several major diseases (25). In several important disease states (e.g. fever, fracture, burning, post-operatively), body protein is lost during the disease process and replaced during convalescence. In some of these states, the requirement of dietary protein to compensate for such losses can be double the needs of the healthy subject. For example, a loss of 0.3 kg body protein by an adult can occur from simple disuse atrophy during bed rest, and to this can be added 0.4 kg body protein after gastrectomy, 0.7 kg after fracture of a femur and 1.2 kg following a 35% burn. These losses have to be replaced during convalescence. On the other hand, some diseases (renal failure, liver failure) require restriction of protein intake.

In view of our increasing knowledge about optimal intakes of amino acids, it has been possible (26) to recommend a rational formula for the amino acid content of parenteral solutions for general use in the parenteral feeding of infants. Such a solution provides a pattern of essential amino acids similar

Table 2. Repletion requirements of amino acids by repleting mature rats [calculated from Steffee et al. (24)]

Amino acid	Repleting	Normal (mg/kg/day)	Ratio
Histidine	120	35	3.4
Isoleucine	345	180	1.9
Leucine	415	110	3.8
Lysine	330	60	5.5
Methionine	220	90	2.4
Phenylalanine	255	50	5.1
Threonine	245	85	2.9
Tryptophan	80	30	2.7
Valine	290	120	2.4

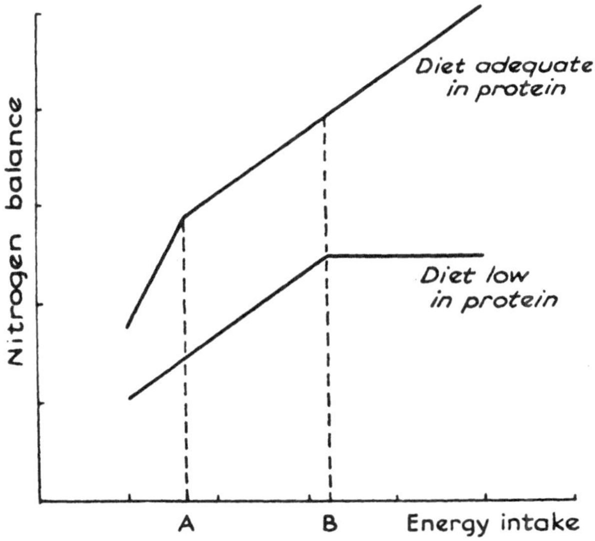

Fig. 7. Relationship of N balance to energy intake on diets of differing protein content [from Munro (8)].

Table 3. Protein requirements in specific disease [from Munro (25)]

I. Normal adult –
   (a) for N equilibrium; 0.6 gm/kg raised to 0.8 gm/kg by protein quality correction (80%)
   (b) customary intake: 1-2 gm/kg
II. Metabolic response to severe injury and burning –
   (a) Acute phase – 2-4 gm/kg + cals
   (b) Convalescence – 2+ gm/kg
III. Malabsorption and g.i. diseases –
   (a) Malabsorption syndrome: 1 gm/kg
   (b) Ulcerative colitis: 1-1.4 gm/kg**
   (c) Ileocecostomy: 1-1.4 gm/kg**
IV. Liver disease –
   (a) Acute hepatic encephalopathy: very low*
   (b) Recovered encephalopathy – 1-1.5 gm/kg
   (c) Chronic encephalopathy – 0.5 gm/kg*
V. Renal disease –
   (a) Uremia: 0.5 gm/kg*
   (b) Nephrosis: 1-1.4 gm/kg**
VI. Malignant disease –
   Increased protein and energy

* Intake restricted on clinical grounds.
** In each condition, losses of protein can double minimal requirements.

to that established as the dietary needs of the infant and constituting 40% of the total amino acids present, and also contains a representative mixture of non-essential amino acids. It should thus be suitable for use in rehabilitation of depleted patients whose needs for essential amino acids are greater than those of healthy adults. Indeed, a mixture of synthetic amino acids resembling the above has been used parenterally by Anderson *et al.* (27) to rehabilitate adults with gastrointestinal diseases. With this mixture, they obtained nitrogen retentions comparable to those observed when animal protein was fed in comparable amounts. A casein hydrolysate was much less effective than the synthetic mixture. Further exploration of optimal mixtures for parenteral administration should include a wide range of indicators of repletion, as discussed below. Such formulations can be modified for use with cases of hepatic and renal failure.

ASSESSMENT OF PROTEIN DEPLETION AND REPLETION

There remains the important question of the best criteria of protein depletion and repletion. A variety of indices has been suggested (1). The plasma essential-to-nonessential amino acid ratio declines, but this changes too readily in response to transient alterations in intake, so that it does not represent the state of depletion. Plasma albumin level is insensitive to depletion, and in consequence does not fall until there is significant depletion. Plasma enzymes mainly indicate liver damage and are not much used nowadays. Changes in antibody-forming cells are of growing importance. Leukocyte metabolism shows changes in malnutrition but is technically difficult to do.

Table 4. Protein-energy malnutrition and endocrine functions [see Crim and Munro (28) for evidence]

Hormone	Kwashiorkor (protein deficiency)	Marasmus (protein-calorie deficiency)
Growth hormone	Elevated	Sometimes raised
Somatomedin	Reduced	–
Insulin	Reduced	Normal
Cortisol	No change	Often elevated
TSH	No change	Much reduced
Thyroxine	Reduced (protein carrier less)	Normal or raised

Finally, changes in methylhistidine excretion may be helpful, as our rat studies (19) suggest.

An additional area of interest concerns changes in hormone levels. Crim and Munro (28) have recently reviewed the effects of protein-energy malnutrition on endocrine function, as reflected in changes in plasma hormone levels (Table 4). Some hormone levels undergo striking changes in malnutrition with increments in growth hormone in kwashiorkor but not in marasmus. A reduction in somatomedin level has been noted in kwashiorkor and might be a useful index of changes in the liver in response to diet. A reduction in plasma insulin level might also be helpful. Cortisol is elevated in the marasmic patient but not usually in the kwashiorkor case, whereas TSH is a very sensitive index of calorie deficiency. These alterations are obtained under extreme conditions of dietary deficiency, but suggest that endocrine changes deserve more attention in less severe malnutrition.

CONCLUSIONS

Some of the challenges faced by nutritional science in relation to parenteral nutrition can be summarized as follows:

(1) Protein and amino acid requirements following trauma have to be more firmly established. (2) The role of energy intake in amino acid utilization needs greater clarification. (3) Better and more sensitive methods for measuring depletion and repletion of body protein are required. (4) Using more sensitive measurements of protein depletion, reassessment of the protein needs in chronic diseases should be investigated.

REFERENCES

1. Crim, M. C. and Munro, H. N., Protein and amino acid requirements in relation to defined formula diets. In: *Defined Formula Diets for Medical Purposes* (editor M. Shils). Amer. Med. Assoc., Chicago (1977).
2. Green, G. M., et al., Protein as a regulator of pancreatic enzyme secretion in the rat. *Proc. Soc. Exp. Biol. Med. 142*: 1162-1167 (1973).
3. Adibi, S. A. and Soleimanpour, M., Functional characterization of dipeptide transport system in human jejunum. *J. Clin. Invest. 53*: 1368-1374 (1974).
4. Munro, H. N., A general survey of techniques used in studying protein metabolism in whole animals and intact cells. In: *Mammalian Protein Metabolism*, Vol. 3, pp. 237-262 (H. N. Munro ed.). Academic Press, New York (1969).
5. Harper, A. E., Diet and Plasma Amino Acids. *Am. J. Clin. Nutr. 21*: 358-366 (1968).
6. Young, V. R. and Munro, H. N., Plasma and Tissue Tryptophan Levels in Relation to Tryptophan Requirements of Weanling and Adult Rats. *J. Nutr. 103*: 1736-1763 (1973).
7. Munro, H. N., Black, J. G. and Thomson, W. S. T., The mode of action of dietary carbohydrate on protein metabolism. *Brit. J. Nutr. 13*: 475 (1959).
8. Munro, H. N., General aspects of the regulation of protein metabolism by diet and

by hormones. In: *Mammalian Protein Metabolism*, Vol 1, pp. 267-319 (H. N. Munro and J. B. Allison eds.). Academic Press, New York (1964).
9. McNair, R. D., O'Donnell, D. and Quigley, W., *Arch. Surg. 68*: 76 (1954).
10. Fernstrom, J. D. and Wurtman, R. J., Brain serotonin content physiological regulation by plasma neutral amino acids. *Science 178*: 414-416 (1972).
11. Fernstrom, J. D., Madras, B. K., Munro, H. N. and Wurtman, R. J., Nutritional control of the synthesis of 5-hydroxytryptamine in the brain. In: *Ciba Foundation Symposium on Aromatic Acids in the Brain.* (G. E. W. Wolstenholme, ed.) p. 153 (1974).
12. Munro, H. N , Fernstrom, J D. and Wurtman, R. J., Insulin, plasma amino acid imbalance, and hepatic coma. *Lancet 1*, p. 722 (1975).
13. Fischer, J. E., Funovics, J. M. and Aguirre, A., The role of plasma amino acids in hepatic encephalopathy. *Surgery 78*: 276 (1975).
14. Munro, H. N., A general survey of mechanisms regulating protein-metabolism in mammals. In: *Mammalian Protein Metabolism*, Vol 4, p. 3 (H. N. Munro, ed.). Academic Press, New York (1970).
15. Pozefsky, T., Felig, P., Tobin,‘· J., SoeJdner J. S. and Calhill, G. F., Amino acids balance across tissues of the forearm in post absorptive man. Effects of insulin at two dose levels. *J. Clin. Invest. 48*: 2273-2282 (1969).
16. Munro, H. N., Control of plasma amino acid concentrations. In: *Aromatic Amino Acids in the Brain*, p. 5-24, (Ciba Foundation Symposium 22) Elsevier, New York (1974).
17. Young, V. R., Alexis, S. D., Baliga, B. S. and Munro. H. N., Metabolism of administered 3-methylhistidine. *J. Biol. Chem. 247*: 3592-3600 (1972).
18. Haverberg, L. N., Omstedt, P. T., Munro, H. N. and Young, V. R., N^t-methylhistidine content of mixed proteins in various rat tissues. *Biochem. Biophys. Acta 405*: 67-71 (1975).
19. Haverberg, L. N., Deckelbaum, L., Bilmazes, C., Munro, H. N. and Young, V. R., Myofibrillar protein turnover and urinary N^t-methylhistidine output: Response to dietary supply of protein and energy. *Biochem. J. 152*: 503-510 (1975).
20. Narasinga Rao, B. S., Nagabhushan, V. S., Urinary excretion of 3-methylhistidine in children suffering from proteincalorie malnutrition. *Life Sciences 12* (II), 205-210 (1973).
21. Young, V. R., Haverberg, L. N., Bilmazes, C. and Munro, H. N., Potential use of 3-methylhistidine excretion as an index of progressive reduction in muscle protein catabolism during starvation. *Metabolism 22*: 1429-1435 (1973).
22. Munro, H. N., Regulation of protein metabolism. *Acta anaesth. Scand.* Suppl. 55, 66-73 (1974).
23. FAO/WHO Expert Committee Report: Energy and Protein Requirements. *WHO Technical Report Series* No. 522, WHO Geneva (1973).
24. Steffee, C. H., Wissler, R. W., Humphreys, E. M., Benditt, E. P., Woolridge, R. W. and Cannon, P. R., Studies in amino acid utilization. V. The determination of minimum daily essential amino acid requirements in protein-depleted adult male albino rats. *J. Nutr. 40*: 483-496 (1950).
25. Munro, H. N., Protein Metabolism in response to injury and other pathological conditions. *Acta Anaesth. Scand.*, Suppl. 55, 81-86 (1974).
26. Winters, R. W. and Hasselmeyer, E. G. (editors). *Intravenous Nutrition in the High Risk Infant*. Wiley, New York (1975).
27. Anderson, G. H., Patel, G. N., Jeejeebhoy, H. N., Design and evaluation by nitrogen balance and blood aminograms of an amino acid mixture for total parenteral nutrition of adults and gastrointestinal disease. *J. Clin. Invest. 53*: 904-912 (1974).
28. Crim, M. C. and Munro, H. N. (1976), Protein-energy malnutrition and endocrine function. In: *Metabolic Basis of Endocrinology* (editors L. J. De Groot et al.) (in press).

Parenteral nutrition of clinical patients with special regard to the biological value of amino-acid patterns

Friedrichkarl Jekat

INTRODUCTION

Clinical patients frequently show high protein losses. The catabolic state associated with major operations, multiple fractures, burns as well as insufficient intake of nutrients can bring the patient into a critical condition. This can cause functional and structural changes in tissues and organs, increased rates of infection, delayed wound healing and convalescence.

In many preoperative and postoperative situations, parenteral nutrition has proven to be the only possibility to supply patients with calories and nutrients, to diminish catabolism.

The substitution of aminoacids or proteins is extremely important. Starvation and stress not only cause wasting of muscle mass but also affect the essential enzymes.

With parenteral nutrition, protein substitution is possible by means of cristalline aminoacids. Differences in the capability of protein derived from oral food or an aminoacid mixture to compensate for losses in the organism are determined by the nitrogen balance and are expressed as the biological value (B.V.). The whole egg protein (given orally) with a biological value of 100 is taken as the reference substance. This means that 100 gm of degraded body protein can be replaced by the intake of 100 gm of egg protein.

CLINICAL COLLABORATIVE TRIAL

Since 1969 more than 5,000 daily nitrogen balances involving 250 male and female patients, ranging between one and seventy years of age, have been recorded for this investigation (3, 4, 6, 7, 8, 9, 10, 11, 12, 18, 21, 22, 23, 24, 25). Plasma amino acids, blood urea, nitrogen, liver functions and electrolytes were determined in addition to analyses of nitrogen intake and output. To date 24 hospitals have participated in this investigation, including 9 university hospitals specialized in surgery, neurosurgery, intensive care, internal medicine, nephrology and pediatrics.

The extent of the study made it possible to form homogeneous groups of patients. The objectives of the study were:

1. an examination of the specific conditions of patients as compared to healthy persons or laboratory animals.
2. the determination of the optimal nutrient supply under these specific conditions to avoid stress due to surplus or deficiency.

BIOLOGICAL VALUE (B.V.) OF PROTEINS

The results of nutritional physiological studies on the B.V. of protein mixtures (5, 12, 13) (i.e. the defined requirement for certain combinations of aminoacids) were taken into consideration during the development of new infusion preparations. The highest B.V. so far is 137.6 for a mixture of 65% potato protein plus 35% egg protein (14) when given orally.

For parenteral use, a modification of this aminoacid pattern is necessary for physiological as well as technical reasons. These variations concern the nonessential part of the aminoacid pattern, especially the very high levels of ammonia and glutamic and aspartic acid. Olney et al. (20) maintain that the latter are related to brain damage in growing organisms.

RESULTS

The collaborative trial has confirmed the medical demands for a parenteral infusion solution are best met by a very valuable pattern.

The requirements for a good aminoacid solution are:

- physiological tolerance and a high Biological Value
- total compensation of nitrogen losses
- fast compensation of nitrogen losses
- safety in use
- reproducibility of results
- minimal stress for patients
- meeting of all requirements also for uremic patients
- acceptable requirements for patient care
- economical in use

a. Physiological tolerance as well as a high Biological Value.

The B.V. of a modified potato-egg aminoacid-pattern is 131.4 when given parenterally and 134.4 when given orally, as was shown in three studies by Semler (26).

A lower B.V. for humans is that of the Rose-pattern (B.V. = 71) or solutions based on the plasma pattern (B.V. = 84 and 86) (19).

Recently, these results have been criticized (17). However, we can substantiate our experiments with the following arguments:

1. The nitrogen balances with egg-protein are within the normal range, known from the literature (e.g. the oldest test person of the group (26) (female, 42 yrs) had the highest N requirement, but it was lower than the value determined by Kofrányi in a self-experiment) (16).

2. The nitrogen balances in the experimental results are insignificantly different from zero; in addition to this, they were mathematically balanced exactly for the analysis of these experiments. Thus the method satisfies the requirements for metabolic studies and exceeds the conditions that are recommended for parenteral nutrition I, 7 (2).

3. The results are reproducible with a very low egg protein input, associated with a slightly negative nitrogen balance. This is especially important, because in this balance range there is a linear correlation between N balance and either N intake or N absorption (1).

The results show that the qualitative as well as quantitative composition of the aminoacid-pattern is very important. The route of entry (oral, parenteral) is of no importance for the biological value. It is necessary however that the aminoacids required are available in a practical way, in sufficient amounts, in the correct proportion, at the right time, at the right place (cell or organ).

b. Total compensation of N losses by reaching equilibrium or – even better – a positive N balance.
Usually one liter of a potato-egg solution containing 9.2 gm N is administered per person per day (= 50 gm aminoacids). The infusion dose can be regulated according to the protein deficit: 0.6 l are sufficient to reach equilibrium or an acceptable negative balance. 2 l per person per day are easily tolerated and compensate large protein losses (3, 18, 21, 22). The potato-egg-principle is practical and effective in a low, medium and high intake range.

c. Fast replacement of N losses by utilizing the rapid and unconstrained kinetics of the steady-state between N input and output.
With a K.E. solution, a positive N balance was obtained within 2 to 5 days (10) (half life < 1 day). With oral administration it takes 10-14 days to reach a steady-state (15).

d. Safety in use, good reproducibility of results, far-reaching knowledge of cause (input) and effect (metabolic reaction), avoiding in particular uncontrolled or critical conditions.
   The clinical study with more than 5,000 observations in different groups and under different conditions confirms the practicability and validity of the K.E. (= potato-egg) solution (3, 18, 21, 22, 25). The reproducibility of the results with a K.E. solution is more accurate than with a Rose solution, as a comparison of the dispersion of the observation points shows (10, 11, 12).
e. Minimal stress for the patients by using the optimal concentrations and volume of this solution.
   The K.E. solution is free of ammonia or ammonia-producing nitrogen carriers; it contains neither aspartic nor glutamic acid. Because of the high B.V. of the aminoacid combination (B.V. parenteral 131.4) it is suitable for all input ranges and it ensures the N supply quantitatively as well as qualitatively. Incompatibility was not observed. Positive results have been obtained in pediatrics (24).
f. Especially in uremic patients: complete satisfaction of specific N requirements, even with minimal N supply.
   Exact and fast kinetics of a N balance in the small range between slightly positive and slightly negative values as well as a reproducible balance at a low intake can be achieved. In uremic patients it becomes extraordinarily clear that a high intake of aminoacids is not always necessary; it can even be disadvantageous if it causes stress in the organism and if it works uneconomically. Noneconomical aminoacid mixtures result in an increased production or urea which has to be handled by the diseased kidney (4, 5).
g. Acceptable requirements for patient care, and
h. economy

These two last points have become increasingly important for progress in parenteral nutrition: uneconomical, insufficient or physiologically inadequate preparations (e.g. protein-hydrolysates or D, L aminoacid mixtures of the older types) are now rapidly being replaced by newly developed products. These are scientifically determined and their effects can be measured objectively. In addition to infusion preparations, crude fiber-free synthetic diets have been studied successfully. Now more than ever, the physician can fight successfully and avoid N catabolic conditions in patients as well as restore normal metabolic conditions.

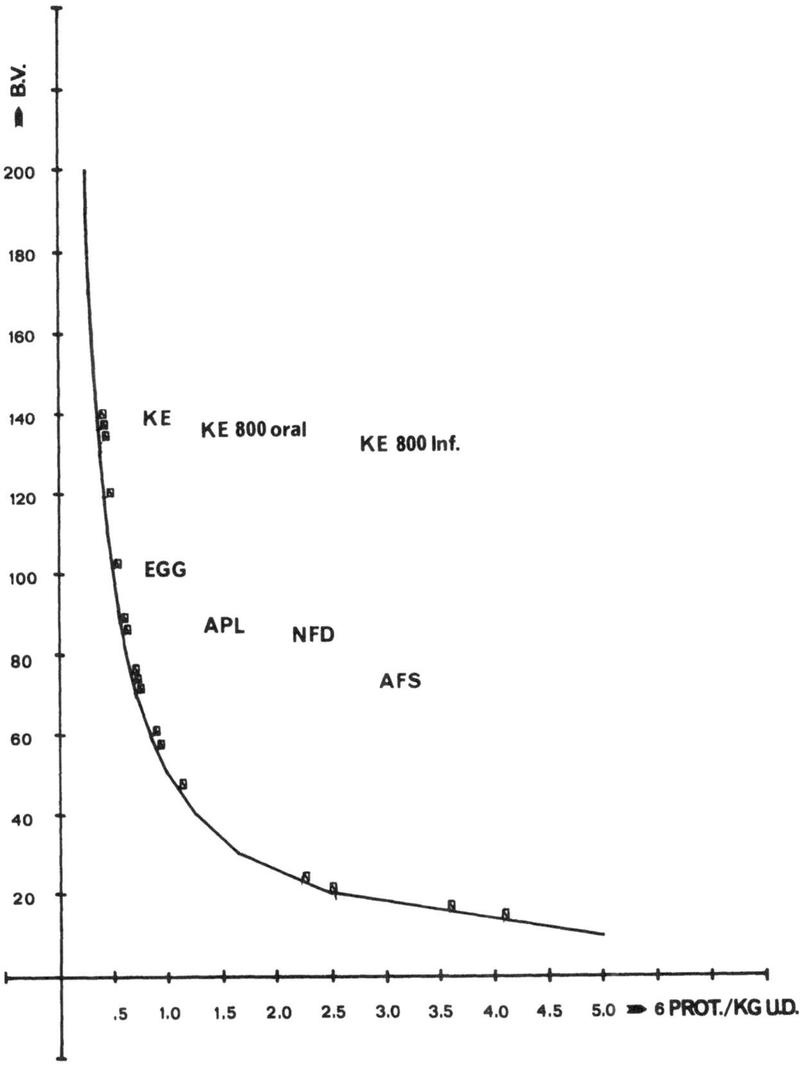

Figure 1. Biological value and protein requirement. Along the x-axis are the human requirements for proteins; along the y-axis are the biological values.

Requirements and biological value of proteins for humans

K.E.	=	potato-egg protein mixture (65% potato-N + 35% egg-N) with oral input (14)
Egg	=	whole egg protein (reference) with oral input (14, 19, 26)
K.E. 800 oral	=	K.E. (= potato-egg) aminoacids with oral input (26)
K.E. 800 Inf.	=	K.E. (= potato-egg) aminoacids with parenteral input (26)
APL, NFD	=	aminoacids derived from plasma pattern with parenteral input (19)
AFS	=	aminoacids according to W. C. Rose's results with parenteral input (19).

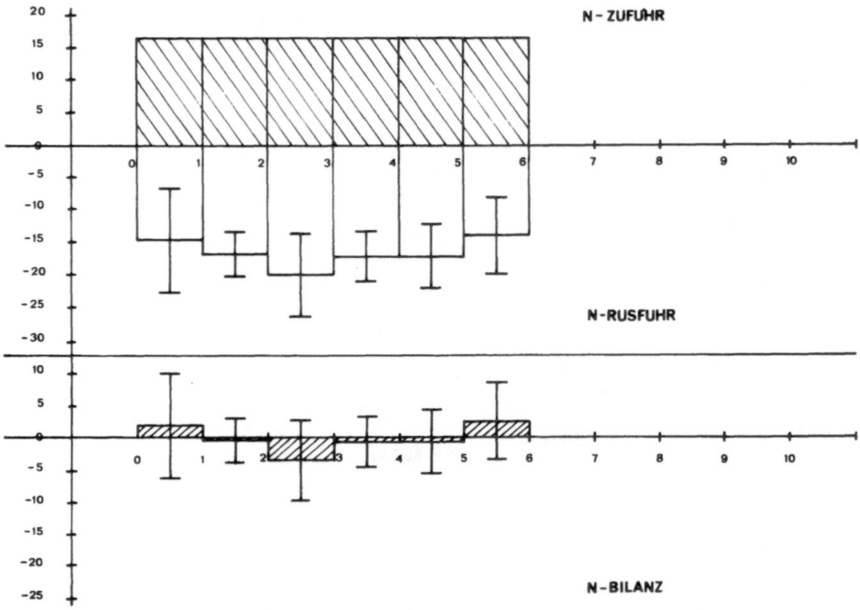

Figure 2. 6 days of postoperative nitrogen balances. Intake 16.4 gm nitrogen per person per day with an aminoacid pattern according to K.E. = potato-egg protein. Output and balances (average and standard deviation ± s) for seven surgical patients.

REFERENCES

1. Allison, J. B., Biological Evaluation of Proteins. Adv. in *Protein Chemistry*, Vol. V, p. 195.
2. Bäßler, K. H., Berg, C., Beisbarth, H., Burri, C., Demling, L., Dolif, D., Erdmann, G., Fekl, W., Förster, H., Halmágyi, M., Heidenreich, O., Heller, L., Jürgens, P., Lang, K., Opderbecke, H. W., Schnell, J., Schultis, K. und Wolf, H., Empfehlungen zur parenteralen Ernährung. Recommendations for Parenteral Nutrition. *Med. u. Ern. 11*: 201 (1970); Gg. Thieme-Verl. Stuttgart.

zur parenteralen Ernährung. Recommendations for Parenteral Nutrition. *Med. u. Ern. 11*: 201 (1970); Gg. Thieme-Verl. Stuttgart.

3. Carstensen, E., Jekat, F. und Krafft, W., Die Therapie der Hypoproteinämie chirurgischer Patienten. *Actuelle Chirurgie 7*: 135 (1972).
4. Hansen, H. und Bünger, P., Parenterale Ernährung bei Nierinsuffizienz. *Med. u. Ern. 13*: 106 (1972).
5. Frank, P., Neuere Erkenntnisse über Aminosäuren-Infusionslösungen. *Pharmazeut. Ztg. 118*: Nr. 3 v. 18. Jan. 1973.
6. Jekat, F., Stickstoffversorgung des Menschen durch parenterale Ernährung unter besonderer Berücksichtigung der Bilanzverhältnisse. In: *Parenterale Ernährung und Infusionstherapie in der klinischen Medizin.* Hrsg. Meyer, J., Gg. Thieme-Verl. Stuttgart 1973.
7. Jekat, F., Parenterale Ernährung des klinischen Patienten. *Infusionstherapie 1*: 106 (1973).
8. Jekat, F., Der spezifische Stickstoffbedarf des Menschen und seine Deckung durch

parenterale Zufuhr – Bilanzergebnisse und ernährungsphysiologische Gesichtspunkte. In: *Grundlagen und Praxis der parenteralen Ernährung*. Hrsg. Heller, K. L., Schultis, K. und Weinheimer, B., Gg. Thieme-Verl. Stuttgart 1974.
9. Jekat, F., Stickstoffbilanzen im Rahmen einer klinischen Gemeinschafts-Untersuchung über parenteral verabreichte Aminosäuren-Lösungen. *Intensivmedizin 11*: 284 (1974).
10. Jekat, F. und Hahn, F., Die Einstellungskinetik der Stickstoffbilanz bei parenteraler Nährstoffzufuhr. *Ernährungs-Umschau 17*: 451 (1970).
11. Jekat, F. und Hahn, F., Über die theoretischen und experimentellen Grundlagen der parenteralen Aminosäurenversorgung des Menschen. *Ernährungs-Umschau 18*: 420 (1971).
12. Jekat, F. (Hrsg.) unter Mitarbeit von Büsing, G., Droste, H., Hahn, F. und Hawickenbrauck, R., Parenterale Nährstoffversorgung des Menschen unter besonderer Berücksichtigung der Zufuhr von Aminosäuren. *Wissenschaftl. Informationen Fresenius*, Bad Homburg v. d. H. 1. Aufl. April 1971.
13. Karlson, P., Kurzes Lehrbuch der Biochemie für Mediziner und Naturwissenschaftler. Gg. Thieme-Verl. Stuttgart 1972, p. 353.
14. Kofrányi, E. und Jekat, F., Zur Bestimmung der biologischen Wertigkeit von Nahrungsproteinen, VIII Die Wertigkeit gemischter Proteine. Hoppe-Seyler's *Z. f. physiol. Chem. 335*: 174 (1964).
15. Kofrányi, E. und Jekat, F., Die biologische Wertigkeit von Kartoffelproteinen. *Forschungsberichte des Landes Nordrhein-Westfalen*, Nr. 1582, Westd. Verl. Köln u. Opladen 1965.
16. Kofrányi, E. und Müller-Wecker, H., Zur Bestimmung der biologischen Wertigkeit von Nahrungsproteinen, IV. Der Vergleich der Wertigkeiten von Milch-, Roggen- und Weizeneiweiß mit Vollei und ihre Berechenbarkeit aus der Bausteinanalyse. Hoppe-Seyler's *Z. f. physiol. Chem. 320*: 233 (1960).
17. Malchow, H., Optimale Eiweißsubstitution bei intravenöser Ernährung. *Dtsch. med. Wschr. 101*: 1203 (1976).
18. Metzel, E., Friedrich, H. und Elgert, K., Die parenterale Ernährung mit D, L- und L-Aminosäuren in der postoperativen Phase neurochirurgischer Patienten und ihr Einfluß auf die postoperative Katabolie. *Wissenschaftliche Informationen Fresenius*, Beih. 5, 49 (1972).
19. Müller-Wecker, H. und Kofrányi, E., Zur Bestimmung der biologischen Wertigkeit von Nahrungsproteinen, XVII. Die biologische Wertigkeit verschiedener Aminosäurelösungen nach oraler und parenteraler Verabreichung. Hoppe-Seyler's *Z. f. physiol. Chem. 354*: 527 (1973).
20. Olney, J. W., Ho, O. L. und Rhee, V., Brain-damaging potential of protein hydrolysates. *New. Engl. J. Med. 289*: 391 (1973).
21. Quirin, H., Droste, H., Jekat, F. und Kluthe, R., Vergleichende Stickstoffbilanzuntersuchungen als Grundlage für eine optimale parenterale Aminosäurenversorgung. *Verh. Dtsch. Ges. f. Inn. Med. 77*: 187 (1971).
22. Rittmeyer, P., Zur Frage der Utilization einer nach dem Kartoffel-Ei-Muster zusammengesetzten Aminosäurenlösung im Rahmen der operativen Behandlung der Colitis ulcerosa und anderer Darmerkrankungen. *Wiss. Inform. Fresenius*, Beih. 6, 74 (1972).
23. Sattler, R. W., Hantschmann, N. und Jekat, F., Bilanzierte synthetische Diät in der präoperativen Phase der Colon-Carcinom-Chirurgie. *Actuelle Chirurgie 9*: 1 (1974).
24. Schmidt, G.-W., Komplette Stickstoff-Bilanzen und Aminosäuren-Analysen bei Säuglingen - unter Oralkost sowie parenteraler Ernährung mit Aminosäuren-Infusionslösungen auf der Basis der Kartoffel-Eier-Eiweiße. *Fortschr. Med. 89*: 351 (1971).
25. Schröter, J. und Jekat, F., Parenterale Ernährung mit Aminosäuren-Lösungen. *Med. Welt 25*: 1147 (1974).
26. Semler, P. und Jekat, F., Optimale Eiweißsubstitution bei intravenöser Ernährung. *Dtsch. med. Wschr. 101*: 579 (1976).

The organization of a hyperalimentation unit

Josef E. Fischer, M.D.

There are basically two ways to approach parenteral nutrition. The first is to have the team as the primary physician. The second is to insure hospital-wide quality-control of parenteral nutrition with the team serving as the quality control center, but having each patient under the care of their own primary physician. With the first approach the team assumes primary control over the patient with the possibility of other disease states being cared for by consultants, such as the patient's original primary physician. In some situations this demands geographic segregation of all patients undergoing parenteral nutrition, although this is not an integral aspect of the scheme. By the second approach, the team may or may not assume primary control over the patient, depending on a given situation. There is no geographical segregation and the patient is cared for in any of the patient care areas throughout the hospital.

In the first approach (Table 1) there seem to be slightly more disadvantages than advantages. There is little question that more absolute control of the patient will allow a more careful control of parenteral nutrition, perhaps with a lower sepsis rate. On the other hand, it is wasteful of space, provides less exposure of other hospital personnel, and the overall care might not be as good, although this is questionable. This perhaps is summarized best in the

Table 1. The team as primary physician

Advantages
1. More absolute control
2. ? Lower sepsis rate

Disadvantages
1. Less exposure of hospital personnel
2. Wasteful of space
   a. If patients are segregated
3. Overall care may not be as good
4. No cross-fertilization of ideas
5. Physician jealousy = denial of TPN to patients

first figure (Figure 1). With the second approach, it is our feeling that this may provide the patient with better overall care. There is more general nursing staff involvement throughout the hospital, there is less physician jealousy, patients are considered candidates for parenteral nutrition more easily, as physicians do not lose control of their patients. It is less expensive as far as space is concerned and there is cross-fertilization of ideas. Collaboration is more easily carried out. There is little question that this is much more difficult to do and that sepsis rate is perhaps higher and quality control is more difficult to achieve because of the large number of individuals involved in a patient's care. This approach is best typified by Figure 2, which is (Figure 3) the approach we have chosen to take at the Massachusetts General Hospital. I would emphasize that the most important factor in any team approach is the team itself and that one should adapt whatever policy is suitable for that institution, as institutions are different in character. The basic approach remains the same, to make it safe for the patient (Table 2, Figure 2).

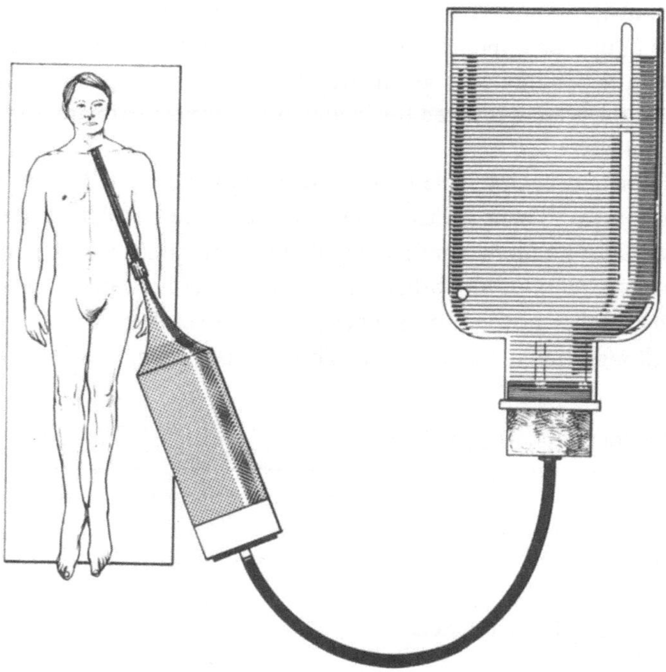

Figure 1. The approach in which the team is the primary physician. Note that the needs of parenteral nutrition take precedence over the overall care of the patient. We do not believe that a system such as this provides the best care for the patient.

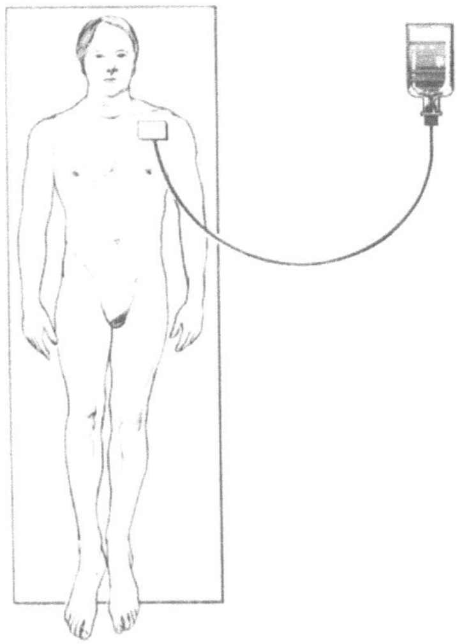

Figure 2. A graphic description of the approach utilized at the Massachusetts General Hospital in which parenteral nutrition is simply another means of therapy which takes its place among the other means of therapy in the care of a patient.

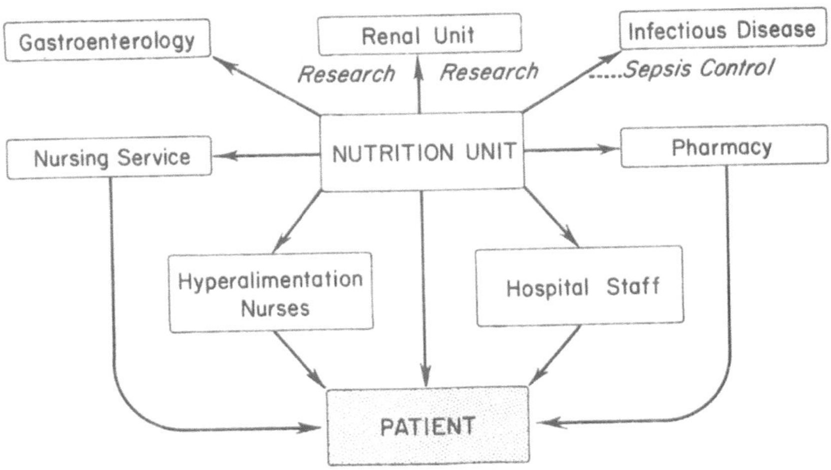

Figure 3. Organizational chart of the Hyperalimentation Unit at the Massachusetts General Hospital. Note that a large number of groups interact with the nutrition unit in order to provide excellent patient care.

Table 2. The team as consultant

Advantages

1. Better overall care?
2. More general nursing staff involvement
3. Less physician jealousy
4. Greater collaboration, more cross-fertilization
5. ? Less expensive
   a. No segregation

Disadvantages

1. Safety more difficulty to achieve
2. Greater opportunity for error

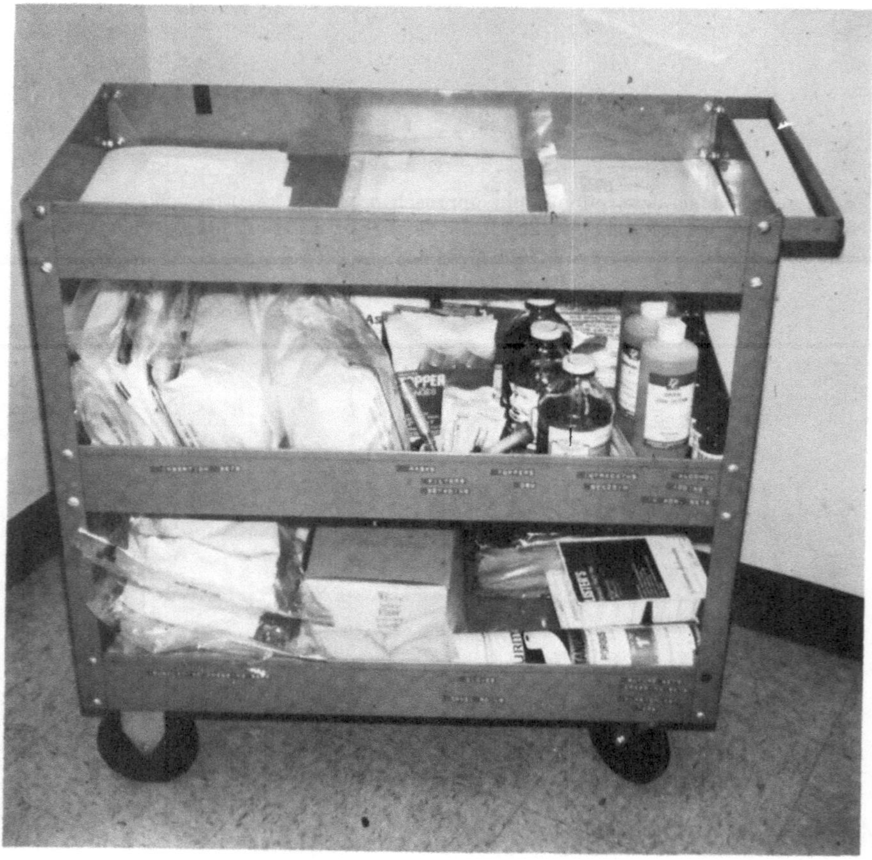

Figure 4. Hyperalimentation Cart stationed at intervals throughout the hospital contains all the materials one needs to start a parenteral nutrition infusion.

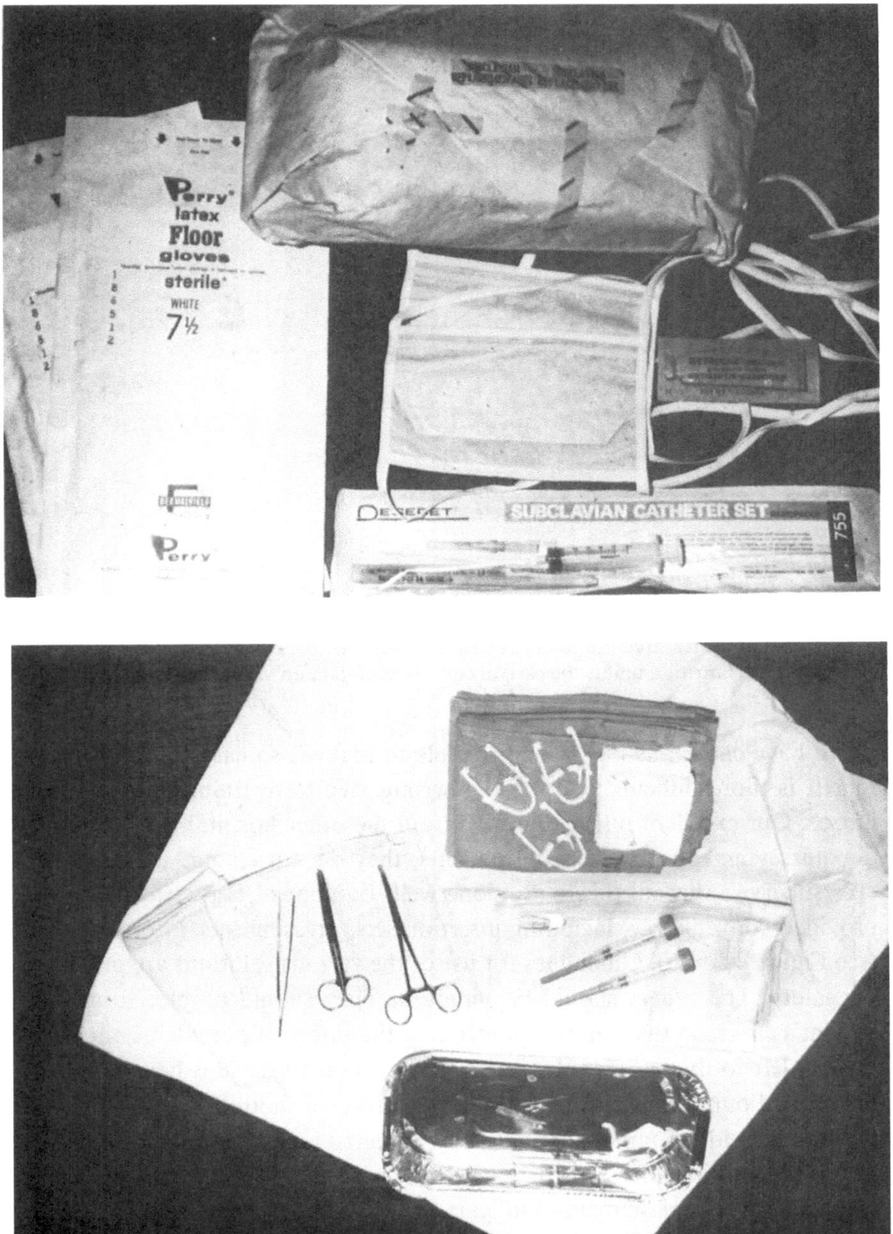

Figure 5. The open contents of a subclavian or internal jugular placement set in which all materials needed for the safe and sterile insertion of a hyperalimentation line are contained.

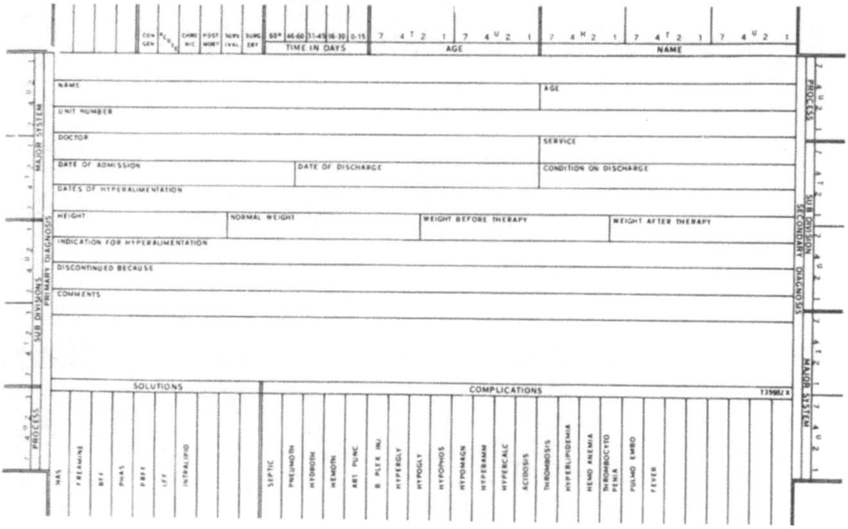

Figure 6. A punch card used in the collation of data from the Hyperalimentation Unit, Massachusetts General Hospital. Every patient is collated and punch carded for retrieval of information for research purposes, as well as in general. We believe one of the functions of a parenteral nutrition unit is the careful collection of data on various disease states.

We have chosen as our basic principle to make it so easy to do properly that it is more difficult to do things wrong. We have trained the hospital nurses. Our excellent nurse clinicians train the other hospital nurses. While our nurses make rounds on the patients, they do not change the dressing, ever supervise that all things are done well. Equipment is prepackaged and provided conveniently, including insertion sets, dressing sets, insertion carts (see Figure 4 and 5). Guidelines for use of the various solutions are provided for safety. The orders should be standard. They should be placed in each patient's chart, so that matters controlling the safety of parenteral nutrition are not left to the individual discretion of various physicians hospital wide, but carried out automatically. The nursing protocol should be used throughout and should be uniform. It basically concerns the inviolate nature of the hyperalimentation line, which is used for nothing else. And finally, some member of the hyperalimentation team should be empowered by the trustees or the director of the hospital to stop parenteral nutrition on any patient in the institution when he feels his or her life is endangered. This is a power which exists not to be used very freely, but only under dire circumstances. Most disagreements are deviations from protcol and can be solved amicably.

Under such a system, the physician's role is that of making the decision when the patient should be hyperalimented. The physician inserts the catheter and writes the orders daily. The nurses do approximately everything else from supervising the actual care of the lifelines to supervising the rates, to generally interacting with the patient and his family about the fears of parenteral nutrition.

Under such hospital wide protocol, the pharmacy can make available to the individual physicians, guidelines as far as mixing of various ionic additives on the basis of solubility so that any metabolic derangement may be managed by the use of the parenteral nutrition solution alone and not by IV's given peripherally.

In any rapidly growing field, such as parenteral nutrition, the importance of research is paramount. Although this should not be done in any way to endanger the care of patients, nonetheless it is worthwhile considering that in an area whose efficacy is less than a decade, it is important to continue testing by prospective studies. The unity of the hyperalimentation team is essential. Every patient who has been treated with hyperalimentation should be punch carded so that this information is available for retrospective and prospective studies (Figure 6). In such ways, the field of parenteral nutrition will be advanced the same time that patient safety is assured.

Nursing in parenteral nutrition

R. Colley

One thing basic to our Unit's function is respect for education and its relevance to physicians, patients and their families, pharmacists and nurses. I would like to spend this time discussing both technique and our philosophy of patient care. As Dr. Fischer said, we have a special teaching program and a certification process for nurses. This means that each nurse in our hospital attends an orientation program and may also attend the special "Hyperalimentation Workshop". The Workshop is an 8 hour course conducted every 2 months. In this course both theory and nursing care are presented and discussed. The course is available to selected applicants (nurses) within the hospital as well as to outside visitors.[1]

The anticipated learning outcome of the Workshop may formally be described as follows:

I. An increased depth of knowledge in the following areas:
   a. History and development of total parenteral nutrition.
   b. Rationale for use.
   c. Anticipated physiologic response of the body to hyperalimentation therapy in health and disease.
   d. Pharmacologic aspects of hyperalimentation solutions.
   e. Exploration of possible complications of hyperalimentation with emphasis on prevention.
   f. Projected trends in total parenteral nutrition including studies in progress.
   g. Nursing intervention in the management of the hyperalimented patient.
      1. Subclavian catheterization.
      2. Dressing change.
      3. Intravenous tubing and filter change.
      4. Metabolic nursing management.
      5. Catheter sepsis.

[1] Colley, Rita, "Education of the Hospital Staff", in TOTAL PARENTERAL NUTRITION, editor - Josef E. Fischer, M.D., Little, Brown and Company, Boston, 1976.

6. Procedures and policies at Massachusetts General Hospital.
7. Resources.
8. Case examples.
9. Group processing.
10. Testing.
11. Project.

II. Development of skill in planning, administering and evaluating the nursing care of the hyperalimented patient.

III. Increased recognition of the importance of continued learning relative to hyperalimentation therapy and a concomitant willingness to assume the responsibility for continued study.

IV. Development of the understanding of the psychologic needs of the patient undergoing hyperalimentation therapy.[2]

Although we encourage all nurses to attend this conference, we particularly desire that leadership people attend. This is because participation in the

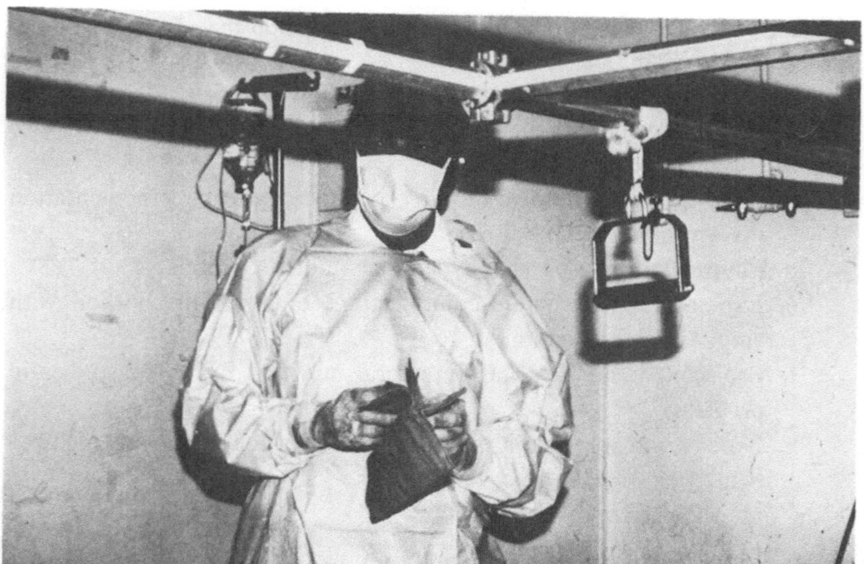

Figure 1

[2] Hyperalimentation Work Conference: Description, Purpose and Objectives. Boston: Massachusetts General Hospital, Department of Nursing, Staff Education, July, 1973.

workshop imparts better understanding of the subject matter and increased capability to perform skills and practice the care these patients require.

It is very important to prepare a patient prior to catheter placement. The patient should be told what to expect – that the doctor will be wearing a mask, gown and gloves (fig. 1), that a towel roll will be placed along the cervical-thoracic vertebrae, that the patient will be placed head down in Trendelenberg position, that surgical drapes will be placed around the area of catheter insertion, that the surgical prep includes a scrub with strange smelling solutions (particularly the acetone, which smells like ether) and that the local anesthetic injection feels similar to a bee sting.

Patients are very afraid if they haven't been told how a subclavian and or jugular catheter differs from normal i.v.'s. Teaching ahead of time can also prevent physical complications because if the patient is relaxed during catheter placement, he is more able to remain still and cooperative. If one knows a patient well and can determine that he is very anxious, or if the patient usually receives tranquilizers, it is a good idea to suggest premedication. We stress the importance of support; an act as simple as holding the patient's hand can be enormously comforting.

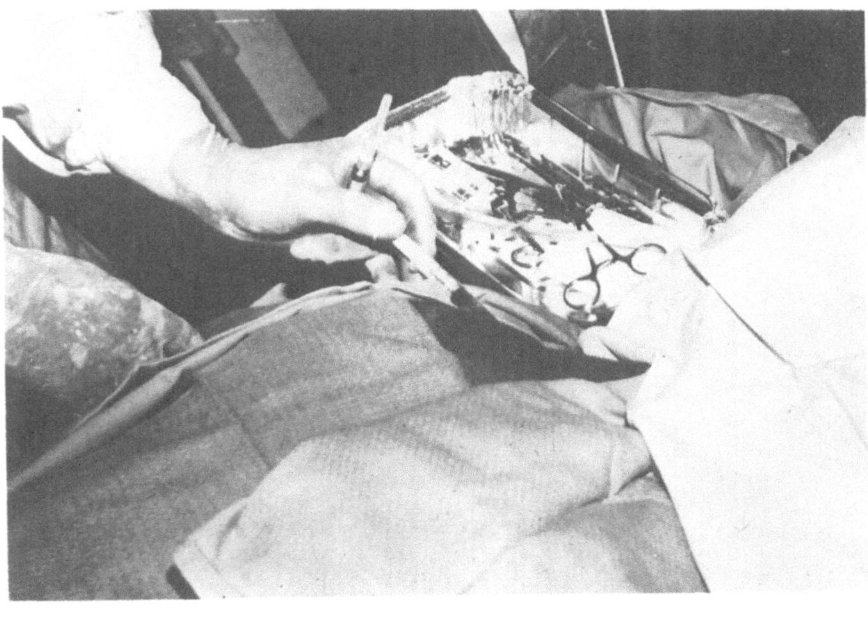

Figure 2

The importance of air embolus precautions cannot be over-emphasized. When there is direct communication between the venous system and the atmosphere the danger of air embolus always exists. In order to avoid this complication the following precautions should be taken: either instruct the patient to perform the Valsalva maneuver (forced exhalation with a closed glottis) or compress the patient's abdomen and achieve the same result. Remember that direct communication between the venous system and the atmosphere exists both when the syringe is disconnected (fig. 2) from the needle during catheter placement and when the intravenous tubing is separated from the catheter hub during tubing changes.

After the catheter has been placed, an x-ray is taken immediately. This is done to confirm catheter tip location in a central vein – ideally the superior vena cava. Until this confirmation, isotonic solution is infused at a slow rate. Although complications of catheterization are infrequent, the patient should be observed carefully for the most common symptoms, which are: respiratory distress, pain or a slowly growing hematoma. Reported complications of subclavian or jugular catheterization include pneumothorax, hemothorax, hydrothorax, arterial puncture, brachial plexus injury, thoracic duct injury and a sheared catheter embolus.

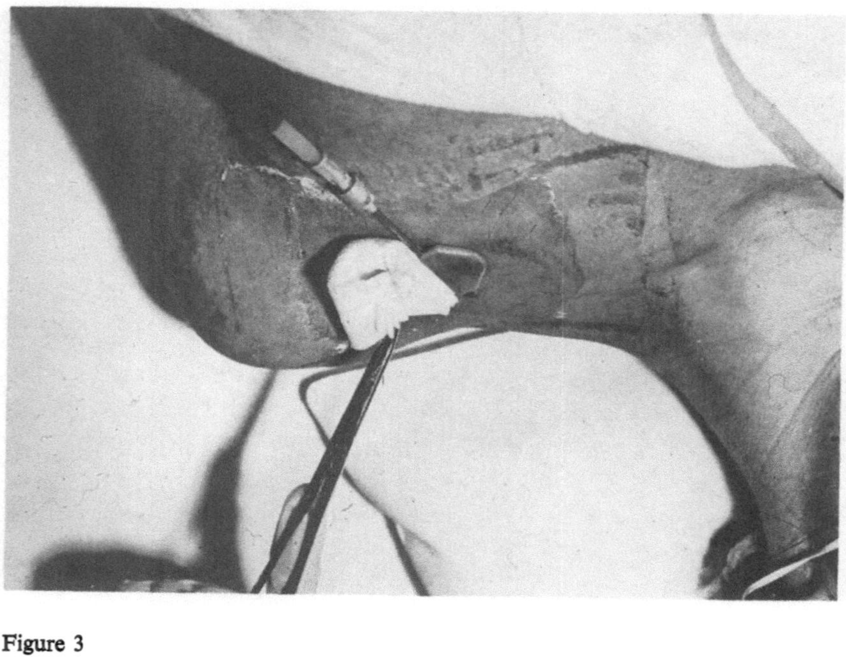

Figure 3

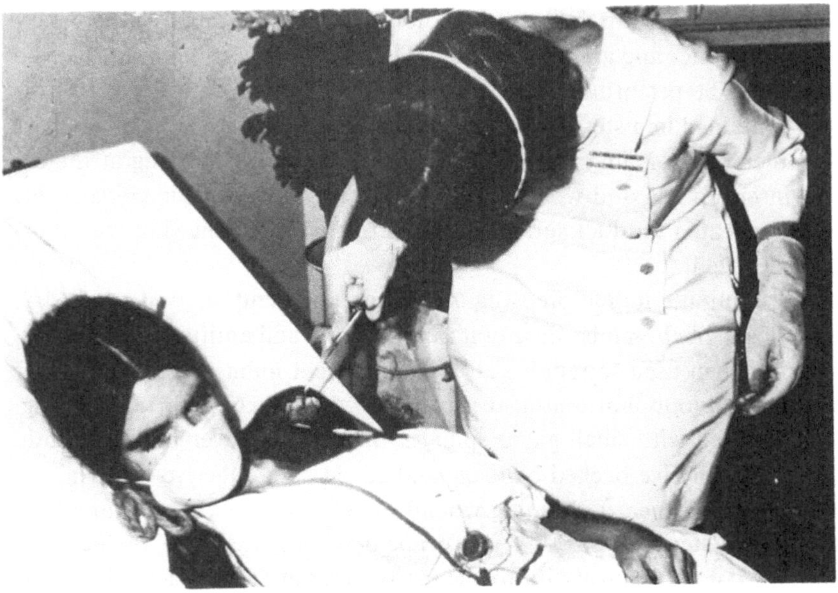

Figure 4

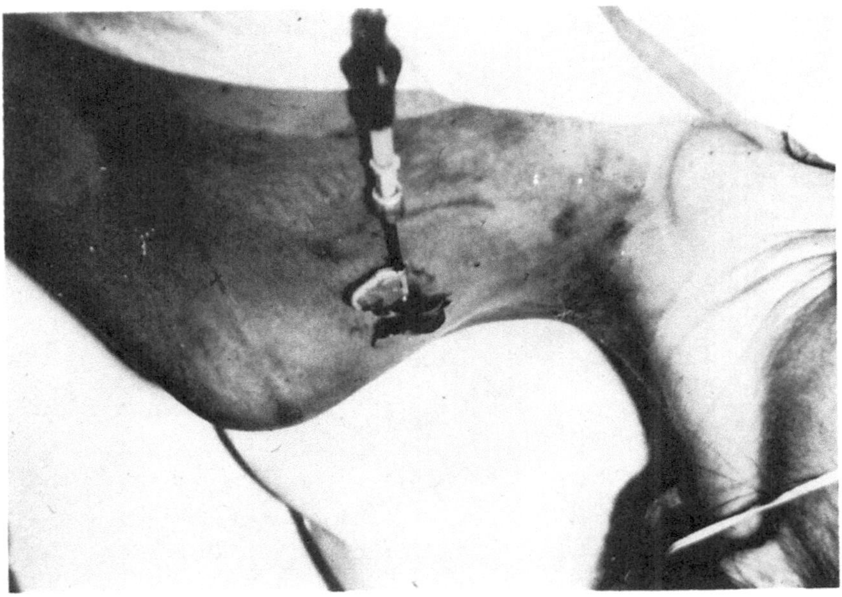

Figure 5

Dressing changes are done every 48 hours or more frequently if necessary to maintain water and air occlusiveness. This is a sterile technique and aseptic procedure. The performer wears a mask and sterile gloves and uses instruments contained in a sterile prepackaged kit. The patient also wears a mask. The catheter area is first washed with acetone (fig. 3), beginning at the catheter insertion site and working outward in larger concentric circles. This scrub is repeated until all surface debris is removed and the skin area thoroughly defatted.

A full 2 minute iodine prep (fig. 4) is then done and allowed to air dry. Iodine has been chosen because of its antibacterial and antifungal properties. Alcohol is then used to remove all iodine, prevent iodine burn and further antisepsis. An iodophor ointment is placed at the catheter insertion site (fig. 5) and covered with small gauze sponges. The area is covered with a cloth, elasticized, adhesive-backed bandage and edged with adhesive tape (fig. 6). If the bandage is near a draining wound or subjected to a moist humid environment, a sterile plastic adhesive drape may be placed over the bandage to waterproof it. If sensitivity to the elasticized bandage occurs, the sterile plastic drape may be used as a substitute. All i.v. tubing junctions are se-

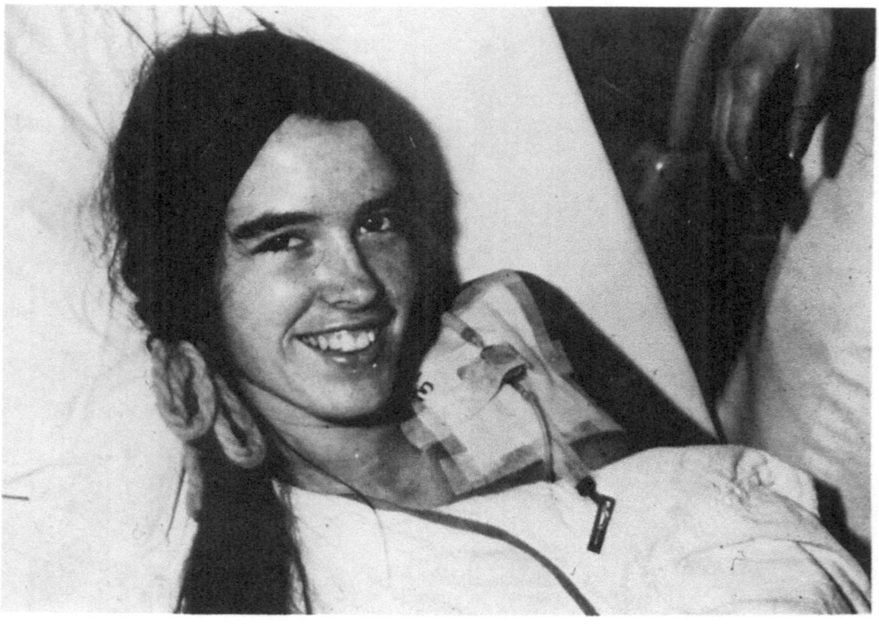

Figure 6

cured with either adhesive or plastic tape. This prevents accidental tubing separation; it can be a lifesaving maneuver when one considers the catheter hub – i.v. tubing junction.

Special slides illustrate our pediatric dressing change procedure, specifically, the infant's dressing. This is different because an infant catheter has a tunnel exit to the scalp, after placement via a jugular cutdown (fig. 7). Infant catheter placement is done in the operating room. Over the catheter site, we place a very small gauze. Instead of covering this with an elasticized bandage, we place a small, adhesive, sterile plastic drape to form a dry, occlusive seal.

We do exactly the same prep as described for the adult: acetone, iodine

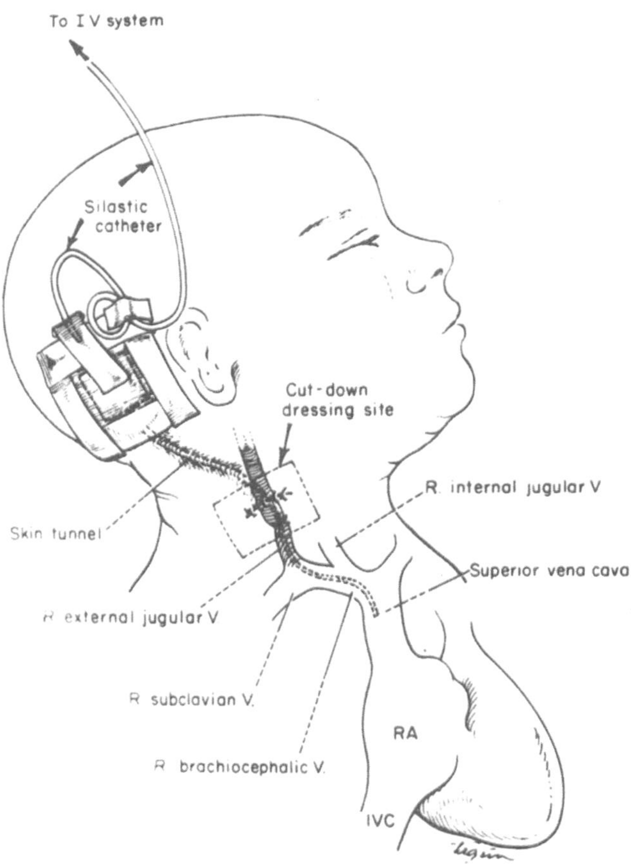

Figure 7

and alcohol, followed by iodophor ointment. We place a slit piece of tape up under the catheter hub in order to make a good seal, so that when the i.v. tubing is changed, dressing occlusiveness is not disturbed. Plastic tape is placed over the exposed catheter to secure it, so that if there is tension on the i.v. line, the catheter will not be dislodged. We anchor the i.v. tubing (both in adults and in children) to the basic dressing. This also prevents external tension from dislodging the catheter (fig. 8, 9). The nurses date and sign the dressing and then write a note in the patient's record. This note states the condition of the skin and catheter site, as well as any deviation from normal.

Another aspect of infection control is the policy regulating use of i.v. tubing and filters. We use regular i.v. tubing and .22 micron inline filters. These are changed every twenty-four hours. Special care must be taken not to contaminate the new i.v. tubing before it joins the catheter hub. The .22 micron filters available (fig. 10) are capable of infusing hypertonic solutions by gravity drip.

Physicians are responsible for deciding whether or not a hyperalimentation catheter is infected. However, relevant nursing responsibilities are important: if the patient shows even a slight temperature elevation, the nurse should notify the doctor at once. Also, if the hyperalimentation system has been violated in any way, nurses should do everything in their power to have a new nutritional catheter inserted.

Our protocol for catheter care has been very successful. We did a prospective study of 200 consecutive patients to measure its effectiveness.[3] This took almost a year and involved 355 catheters. If the catheter care was according to protocol it was called "good". On the other hand, if there was even one protocol violation, the care was termed "poor". We found that 275 catheters received good care and had an infection rate of only 3%. The 80 catheters which were not cared for according to protocol had a very high infection rate – 20%!

The protocol is very rigid. A catheter must be placed for hyperalimentation and not used for anything else. Only the jugular or subclavian veins are acceptable as vessels for placement, (the brachial approach involves a longer catheter and often results in thrombophlebitis). Blood must not be withdrawn from these catheters, central venous pressure manometers are not connected to the system, piggy-back infusions are not given through the i.v.

[3] Ryan, J. A., Jr., Abel, R. M., Abbott, W. M., Hopkins, C. C., Chesney, T. McC., Colley, R. Phillips, K., and Fischer, J. E., "Catheter complications in total parenteral nutrition: A prospective study of 200 consecutive patients", NEW ENGLAND JOURNAL OF MEDICINE, 290: 757, 1974.

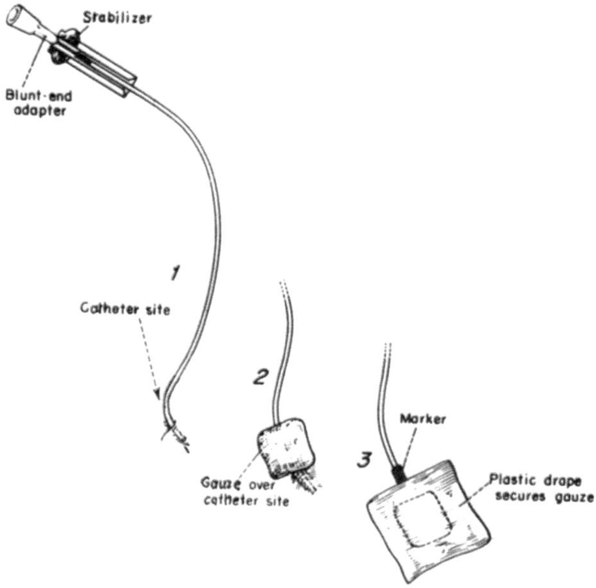

Figure 8

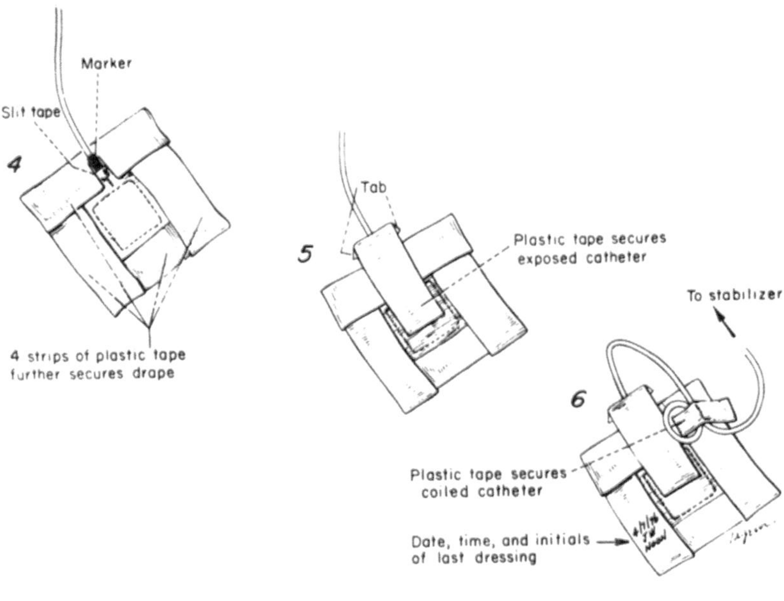

Figure 9

tubing – the system must be considered totally inviolate in order to protect the patient from infection.

Metabolic management of hyperalimented patients is greatly enhanced by nurses who understand the need for careful observation and care. Enlightened nurses will respect the need for maintaining constant solution flow rates. "Double clamping" the i.v. tubing (using a second screw type clamp), times taping the bottles, and frequently checking the solution rate, may prevent the danger of a "runaway" i.v. which is always possible with gravity delivered infusions. Urinary glucose testing should be done at least every 6 hours and noted, especially during the first days of therapy. This assists in determining the patient's glucose tolerance. A urinary glucose measurement of 2++ or greater is reportable and should be considered as an indication of possible hyperglycemia.

Nurses should also be aware of the signs and symptoms of hypo- and hyperglycemia. Persistent hyperglycemia combined with a large fluid overload can lead to the devastating complication of hyperosmolar nonketotic coma.

Accurate charting of the patient's daily weight and intake and output will provide valuable information for the physician as he determines daily nutritional requirements.

We have learned some interesting things from our patients. Their psychological needs have been fascinating to share and wonder about. So many patients have reported both dreams and obsessive conscious thoughts about

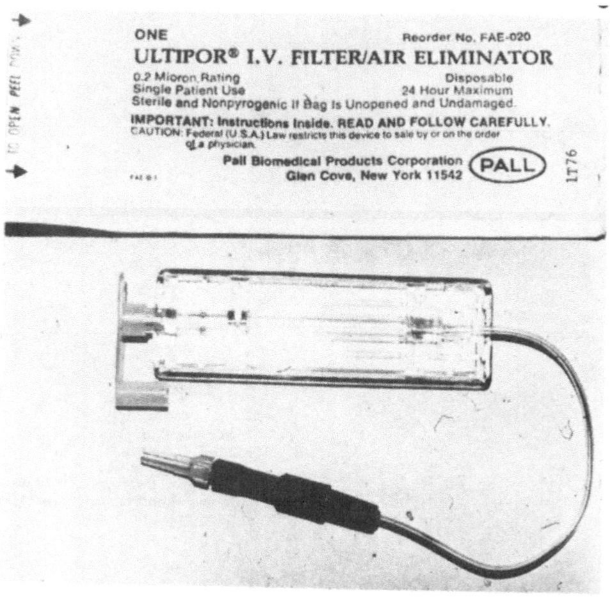

Figure 10

food that we now automatically expect it. They have also reported hallucinations of taste and smell – often related to a particular food craving. Other patients have a strong desire to steal food from a roommate's tray. I think these phenomena could be considered analytic aspects of oral deprivation but this has not yet been proven.

Nursing considerations here relate to the issues. It is good to tell the patient that these things sometimes happen. Then, if they do, it isn't cause for great alarm. Also, it's probably a considerate gesture to locate the patient's room away from the kitchen.

Small comfort measures are very important to these patients. A study[4] we did in our hospital revealed that the incidence of psychiatric consultation in this population was sixteen times greater than that of the general house patients. I do not necessarily imply a cause-effect relationship between total parenteral nutrition and psychiatric upset. On the other hand, this certainly demonstrates that these patients are very stressed and can benefit from a calm understanding approach.

Perhaps it's relevant here to also focus on a few specific fears and fantasies related to the hyperalimentation catheter. Many people have an unrealistic concept of what is inside their body after catheter placement. One woman believed that a needle was "sitting directly in my heart and if I move suddenly it will penetrate my heart!" Another person thought that his heart was in danger of being punctured during catheter insertion. Many patients express this common fear indirectly with the anxious question, "Will you put the catheter on the right side, Doctor?" The actual procedure (catheter placement) has been misunderstood as "emergency surgery being done on me right here in my bed". This is a logical misconception if one considers that (to those who have not been pretaught) the drapes, surgical gloves, gown and mask, prepackaged kits and instruments, surgical prep (especially the acetone wash, which smells like ether!), and the routine, careful behavior of the doctor and nurse does mimic a surgical procedure. Patients also wonder about the catheter removal and are relieved to learn that it's quick, simple and painless.

In conclusion, I would like to thank you all for your kind attention. There hasn't been time to cover every aspect of total parenteral nutrition nursing but I hope these points have provided useful information. Basically, we believe that with a complete protocol for care and an educational effort that teaches people *why* as well as *how*, you get very good results.

[4] Colley, Rita, unpublished data.

2

Specific aspects of management

Parenteral nutrition and gastro-intestinal fistulas

Peter B. Soeters

In their classic paper in 1960 Edmunds, Williams and Welch reviewed 157 patients with external gastro-intestinal fistulas treated at Massachusetts General Hospital (M.G.H.) in Boston between 1947 and 1960 (1). They reported a high overall mortality (43%) despite antibiotics and intravenous replacement.

From the 1947-1960 series, it was concluded that high output fistulas (especially gastroduodenal and small bowel fistulas) were associated with many complications and a higher mortality (Table 1). Since many of the fistulas resulted from surgical complications, prevention was considered to be essential. They recommended that high-output fistulas should be treated surgically with minimal delay by radical resection rather than a bypass or lesser procedure. It was suggested that the advent of antibiotics had not produced a decrease in mortality.

In 1964, Chapman, Foran and Dunpy (2) were the first to attribute low mortality in a series of gastro-intestinal fistula patients to adequate nutrition; later many others followed (3, 4, 5, 6) (Table 2). Evidently, none of these series were randomized in any way, which makes it difficult to assess the relative merits of intravenous nutrition and other aspects of the sixties, like general advances in fluid and electrolyte therapy, respiratory physiology and acid-base balance as well as therapeutic lessons from the past. We recently reviewed all patients with gastro-intestinal fistulas (7) which were treated at M.G.H. from 1960 to 1970, a total of 119 patients. None of these patients re-

Table 1. Mortality of fistula patients 1947-1960

Gastroduodenal fistulas	(55)	Mortality	62%
Small bowel fistulas	(46)	Mortality	54%
Large bowel fistulas	(56)	Mortality	16%
Overall Mortality	(157)		43.3%

Mortality of all fistula patients treated at Massachusetts General Hospital, Boston, U.S.A. from 1947 to 1960.

ceived hyperalimentation and somewhat to our surprise, mortality turned out to be 15%.

Many suggestions put forward in the papers of Edmunds group (1) proved to be of value:

1. Sepsis largely determines mortality.
2. Patients with abdominal sepsis and patients with high-output fistulas should be treated surgically and without delay.
3. Radical surgery should be attempted.
4. Prevention of hard-to-treat gastro-duodenal fistulas contributed to a decrease in mortality. A catheter duodenostomy was considered to be beneficial.
5. Good intensive patient care contributed to a decrease in mortality.
6. The role of the rather liberal use of antibiotics could not be assessed.
7. Electrolyte imbalances had no influence on mortality.

Finally, we reviewed all patients with gastro-intestinal fistulas treated at M.G.H. from 1970 to 1975, a total of 128 patients (Table 3).

Seventy-three patients received hyperalimentation, fifty-five did not. Of the patients on hyperalimentation, the fistulas closed spontaneously in 17 cases and were closed surgically in 24 cases; thus in 50 patients the fistulas were closed (one patient died after closure of the fistula).

Table 2. Mortality of fistula patients on hyperalimentation

Chapman (1964)	16%
Sheldon (1971)	12%
Aguirre (1974)	21%
MacPhayden (1973)	6.45%

Mortality of patients with gastro-intestinal fistulas on hyperalimentation, recorded in the literature.

Table 3. Results fistula patients 1970-1975

	Hyperalimentation	No hyperalimentation
128 patients	73 (100%)	55 (100%)
Spontaneous closure	17 (23.3%)	3 (5.4%)
Surgical closure	34 (46.6%)	35 (63.6%)
Overall closure rate + alive	50 (68.4%)	36 (65.4%)

Results for all patients with gastro-intestinal fistulas treated at Massachusetts General Hospital, Boston, U.S.A. from 1970-1975.

Of the patients who were not on hyperalimentation, only three fistulas closed spontaneously; 35 were closed surgically. For this group therefore 36 patients survived with a closed fistula (2 patients died after closure of the fistula). Fifteen of these patients were not operated on; only 3 of the fistulas closed spontaneously.

Table 4 represents the factors for the group without hyperalimentation,

Table 4. Factors influencing fistula closure in 55 fistula patients (1970-1975) without hyperalimentation

	Esoph. gastroduod.	Biliary pancreat.	Small bowel	Large bowel	Total
Cancer	1	2	1	4	8
+ radiation	1			4	5
+ chemotherapy				1	1
+ both	1				1
Regional enteritis			4	1	5
+ steroids			3	3	6
Leukemia					
+ radiation				1	1
+ chemotherapy				1	1
+ steroids				1	1
Lupus erythematodes disseminatus					
+ steroids				1	1
Total					30

Factors that may have influenced closure rate in 55 fistula patients without hyperalimentation treated at Massachusetts General Hospital, Boston, U.S.A. from 1970-1975.

Table 5. 128 fistula patients (1970-1975).

	Hyperalimentation	No hyperalimentation
Patients	73 (100%)	55 (100%)
Mortality	18 (24.7%)	9 (16.3%)
Surgical	59 (80.8%)	22 (40%)
High output	59 (80.8%)	21 (38.2%)
Malnutrition	44 (60.3%)	21 (38.2%)
Uncontrolled sepsis	39 (53.4%)	11 (20%)

A comparison between patients with gastrointestinal fistulas (128 patients) on hyperalimentation (73 patients) and patients who were not on hyperalimentation (55 pts), with regard to mortality, etiology (surgical or non-surgical), output, malnutrition and uncontrolled sepsis.

which may have influenced closure rate. The mortality for the group on hyperalimentation amounted to 24.7% (Table 5). Fifty-nine of the 73 patients had surgical fistulas, and 59 had high-output fistulas. Forty-four showed malnutrition, and 39 had uncontrolled sepsis at some point in the course of their illness, all of which are high values.

For the group without hyperalimentation, mortality was lower. The group included fewer surgical and high-output fistulas. In addition, the patients in this group showed less malnutrition and less uncontrolled sepsis. These results suggest again that sepsis and malnutrition are primary determinants of mortality.

These results are somewhat different from other series, including our own series from 1960 to 1970. In contrast to other series however they reflect all patients with gastro-intestinal fistulas that were treated during that period.

In addition, this material does not reflect an average fistula population since an increasing number of patients is being referred from other hospitals with long-standing sepsis and severe malnutrition.

There may be a group of patients in whom the fistula might have closed spontaneously had a longer course of hyperalimentation been undertaken. No rigid protocol was followed because these patients were treated according to the personal views of several private surgeons and members of the house staff.

Through the decades, three factors seem to have determined mortality:

1. Electrolyte disturbances. Today this problem seems to have been solved.
2. Malnutrition may be caused by the primary disease, by a high output fistula or by associated sepsis. When sepsis does not occur, or in general when the patient is metabolically stable, many reports by now have demonstrated that hyperalimentation can restore the nutritional state, plasma albumin level and body cell mass.
3. Sepsis remains the most important cause of mortality and is associated with a high catabolic rate which as yet cannot be completely reversed with hyperalimentation. In other words, as long as sepsis exists, the nutritional state deteriorates despite hyperalimentation. Total body weight may be deceptive because of increases in total body water and total body fat.

It follows that it is of the utmost importance to treat uncontrolled continuing sepsis. If the source of the sepsis is located in the abdomen (abscesses, peritonitis due to a blow-out, anastomotic breakdown, etc.), the treatment of choice should be surgery, especially as the 1947-1960 series of Edmunds,

Williams and Welch suggested that the advent of antibiotics had no major impact on the results.

A good nutritional state is associated with good wound healing. In consequence, every fistula patient who is unable to take oral feeding or may not take oral feedings due to contra-indications may benefit from hyperalimentation. The underlying philosophy of the treatment of gastro-intestinal fistulas in general is that bowel rest is beneficial and that the decrease in the fistula output may be regarded as a sign of healing of the fistula. We often reverse that statement: decreasing the fistula output closes the fistula.

Wolfe et al. (8) showed in dogs with experimental enterocutaneous fistulas of the ileum that the volume lost in dogs fed by intravenous hyperalimenta-

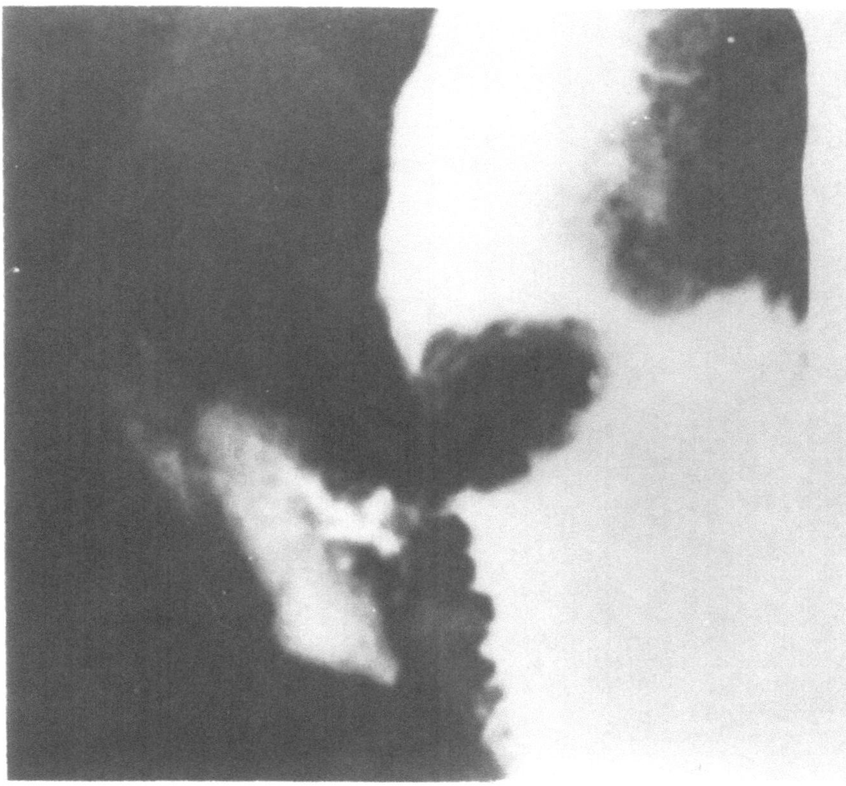

Figure 1. An example of a lateral fistula related to a gastro-jejunal anastomosis. The bowel appears normal and not inflamed. This type of fistula can be expected to close spontaneously with hyperalimentation.

tion was 93% lower than that in dogs fed regular canned dog food. This was demonstrated clinically by Hull and Barnes (9) as early as 1951 and subsequently by many others (5, 6).

MacFadyen, Dudrick and Rubey in particular have promoted this mode of treatment. They reported excellent results with conservative treatment: low mortality (under 5%) and a high spontaneous closure rate. Their results may not be comparable to those of other series however because their material appears to consist of different types of patients.

This does not reduce the merit of this remarkable series, but it is important that the more casual or less well-informed reader should beware of the false impression that as soon as the patient has received his caval catheter and

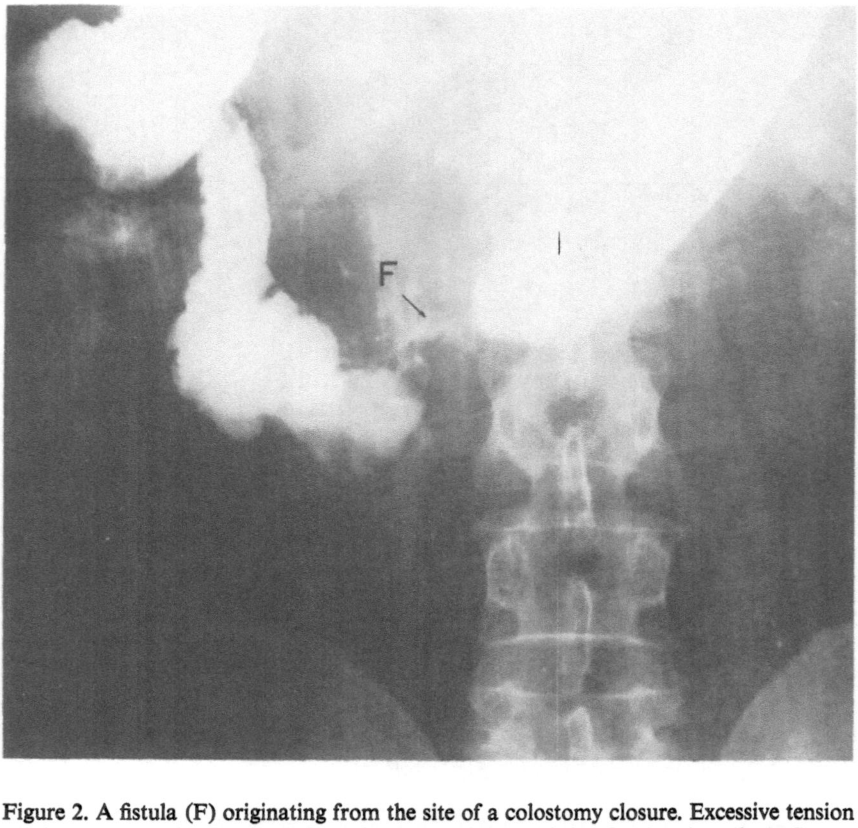

Figure 2. A fistula (F) originating from the site of a colostomy closure. Excessive tension on the anastomosis appears to have been the etiology of this fistula: the splenic flexure was not adequately mobilized. This type of fistula cannot be expected to close spontaneously with hyperalimentation.

the amino acids and calories are flowing in, the surgeon can turn his back on the patient.

It appears both from the literature and from our own material that strict criteria should be applied in selecting patients in which "conservative" treatment is warranted:

1. No continuing sepsis should exist. Uncontrolled abdominal sepsis should be treated surgically and without delay.

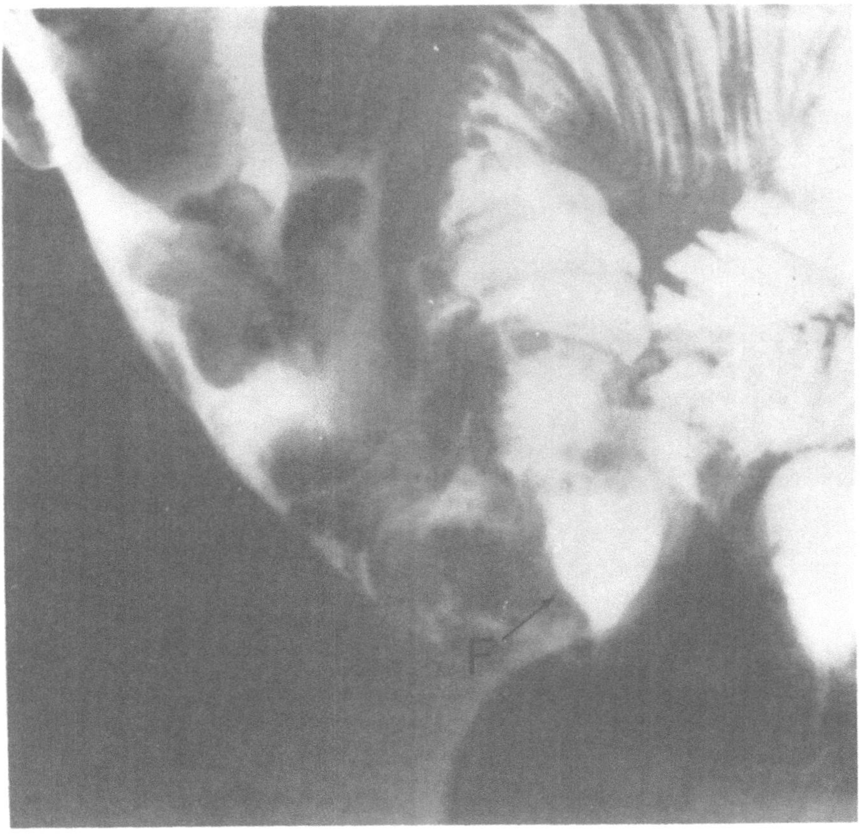

Figure 3. A fistula (F) due to rupture of an anastomosis. This is an example of an end fistula. The distal part of the bowel is not visualized. The bowel empties directly into an abscess cavity which communicates through a fistulous tract with the skin. Surgery was required to close this fistula.

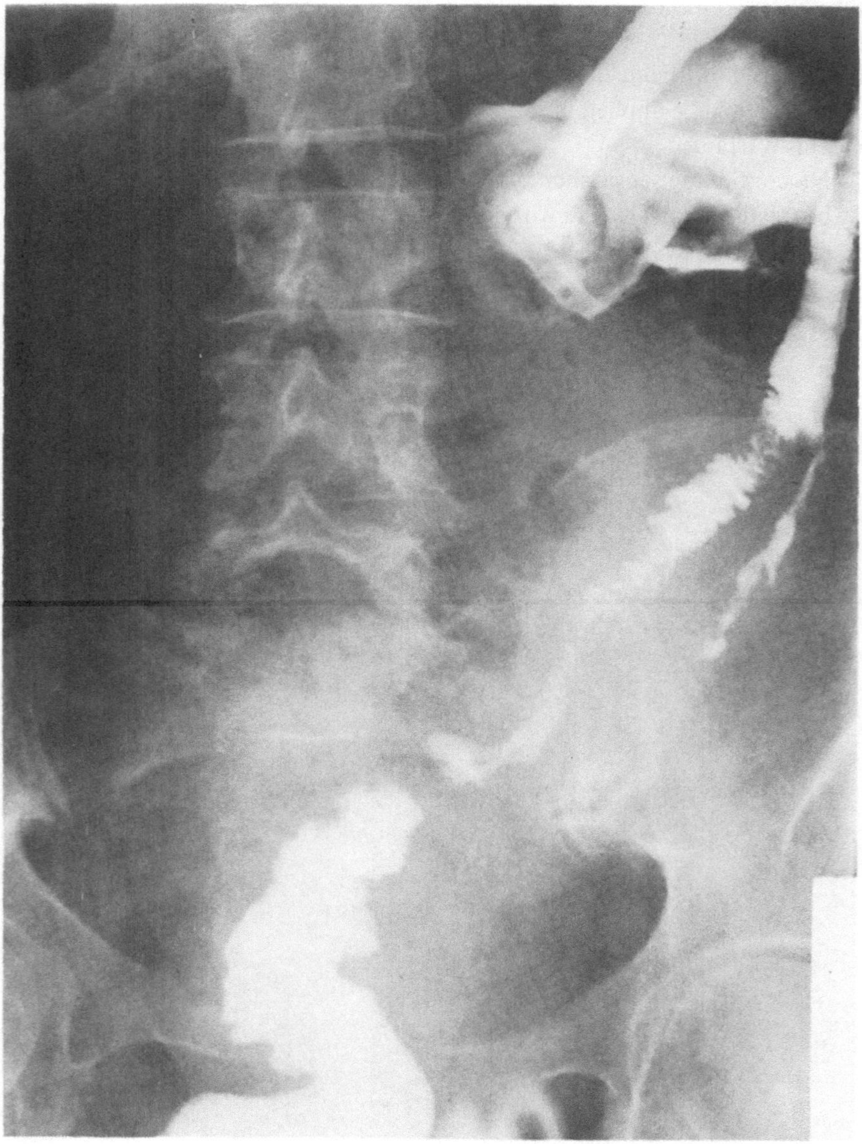

Figure 4. A lateral colocutaneous fistula in a patient with severe diverticulitis and peri-diverticulitis for which a colostomy and sigmoid-resection were performed. This fistula did not close with conservative means, probably because of the poor condition of the bowel and stricture at the site of the anastomosis.

2. The local situation of the fistula is another primary determinant in deciding what therapeutic course to take:
   - lateral fistulas (fig. 1) are more likely to heal with conservative treatment than end fistulas due to rupture of the bowel (fig. 3), anastomotic breakdown, etc. Lateral fistulas often arise from inflamed bowel which may explain the early spontaneous closure that is sometimes observed (3).
   - distal obstruction (fig. 4), poor condition of the bowel (fig. 2, 4) or abscesses (fig. 3) adjacent to the fistula constitute reasons for planning a surgical attack on the fistula.

Spontaneous fistulas are frequently lateral fistulas and are more amenable to hyperalimentation than surgical fistulas which are generally due to rupture of the bowel or wound dehiscence.

Ileal fistulas generally show a high failure rate (5) despite the recently reported beneficial effect of hyperalimentation (10, 11) in regional ileitis in contrast to granulomatous colitis or ulcerative colitis. Good results have always been reported for colon fistulas, regardless of the type of treatment. They are less liable to cause malnutrition and show a high percentage of spontaneous closure. When surgery is necessary however, equally satisfactory results are generally achieved.

Table 6. Complications of parenteral nutrition (1970-1975)

Positive catheter culture	10
Clinical catheter sepsis	8
Elevation of SGOT, LDH, ALK. PHOS.	2
Hypercalcemia (? of Vit. D. intox.)	1
Hyperglycemia	3
Overhydration	1
Hematoma neck	1
Phlebitis subclavian vein	1
Subcutaneous emphysema	1
Pneumothorax	4
Blood culture positive	2
Freamine intolerance with N.S. depression and NH_3 elevation	3

Complications of parenteral nutrition in 73 patients with gastro-intestinal fistulas on hyperalimentation treated at Massachusetts General Hospital, Boston, U.S.A. from 1970-1975.

COMPLICATIONS

Table 6 shows the complications of parenteral nutrition that were encountered in the fistula patients who received hyperalimentation in the period from 1970-1975.

Rita Colley went through the patients' histories and detected in most cases of catheter sepsis breaks in the protocol with regard to the aseptic technique. This once more emphasizes the importance of using strict aseptic and antiseptic techniques (12). However, it also demonstrates that in these seriously ill patients with septic wounds, tracheostomies and ventilatory support, a departure from the protocol is more likely to occur.

CONCLUSIONS

1. Hyperalimentation is a valuable supplement in the treatment of gastro-intestinal fistulas.
2. Sepsis is the principal cause of mortality. The advent of antibiotics does not seem to have led to a decrease in mortality. Hyperalimentation should not delay aggressive diagnosis and surgical therapy in case of continuing abdominal sepsis.
3. Parenteral nutrition provides us with the luxury of being able to improve nutritional state and body cell mass and to try to close fistulas conservatively, but only if the patient is metabolically stable. Some authors opt for a trial course of conservative treatment of 4-5 weeks. If no clinical improvement has occurred within this time, it can be assumed that the fistula will not close conservatively. Others opt for a shorter trial period, improving nutritional states and allowing the future site of surgery to rest, and attack the fistula surgically 2-3 weeks later. A specific group of fistulas seems to be susceptible to conservative treatment: lateral fistulas with good drainage and without adjacent abscesses or distal obstruction.
4. The low mortality observed in recent publications has been ascribed by some authors to the advent of good nutritional support. We agree with that statement, but the M.G.H. 1960-1970 series should teach us that improved intensive patient care and sound surgical principles have also contributed significantly to a decrease in mortality.

REFERENCES

1. Edmunds, L. H., Williams, G. M. and Welch, C. E., External fistulas arising from the gastrointestinal tract. *Ann. Surg. 152*: 455 (1960).
2. Chapman, R., Foran, R. and Dunphy, J. E., Management of intestinal fistulas. *Am. J. Surg. 108*: 157 (1964).
3. Aguirre, A., Fischer, J. E. and Welch, C. E., The role of surgery and hyperalimentation in therapy of gastrointestinal-cutaneous fistulae. *Ann. of Surgery 180*: 393 (1974).
4. Fischer, J. E., The management of high-output intestinal fistulas. *Adv. in Surg. 9*: 139 (1975).
5. MacFadyen, B. V., Jr., Dudrick, S. J., Management of gastrointestinal fistulas with parenteral hyperalimentation. *Surg. 74*: 100 (1973).

6. Sheldon, G. F., Gardiner, B. N., Way, L. W. and Dunphy, J. E., Management of gastrointestinal fistulas. *SGO 133*: 385 (1971).
7. Soeters, P. B., Fischer, J. E. and Franklin, Cynthia, 119 patients with gastrointestinal fistulas. *Archivum Chirurgicum*, vol. 29, nr. 1, pp. 19-31 (1977).
8. Wolfe, B. M., Keltuer, R. M. and Willman, V. L., *Am. J. Surg. 124*: 803 (1972).
9. Hull, H. C. and Barnes, T. G., *Ann. Surg. 133*: 644 (1951).
10. Fischer, J. E., Foster, G. S., Abel, R. M., Abbott, W. M. and Ryan, .J A., Hyperalimentation as primary therapy for inflammatory bowel disease. *Am. J. of Surg. 125*: 165 (1973).
11. Reilly, J., Ryan, J. A., Strole, W. and Fischer, J. E., *Am. J. Surg. 131*: 192 (1976).
12. Ryan, J. A., Abel, R. M., Abbott, W. M., Hopkins, C. C., Chesney, T. Mc.C., Colley, Rita, Phillips, K. and Fischer, J. E., *NEM 290*: 757 (1974).

Clinical and physiological consequences of total parenteral nutrition in the pediatric patient

Thomas L. Anderson, M.D., William C. Heird, M.D., and Robert W. Winters, M.D.

INTRODUCTION

Pediatricians share a long common historical tradition with their surgical colleagues in a concern for the provision of effective parenteral nutrition to patients in whom an adequate flow of enteral nutrients cannot be maintained. In the pediatric patient the problem is even more complicated than in adults, since in the former the nutritional requirements for normal growth and development are superimposed upon those for maintenance.

The technical breakthrough of Dudrick and coworkers (1) whereby central venous catheters could be inserted and maintained for long periods of time made it practical for the first time to provide a total nutritional regimen safely and effectively by the parenteral route. This route in effect solved the osmotic problem inherent in all parenteral nutritional infusates, namely, that in order to provide sufficient non-protein calories as glucose, a solution approximately six times the osmolality of the plasma is required (see Figure 1). Dudrick *et al.* showed that damage to the vein could be avoided if such a potentially damaging solution were given slowly and continuously through a vessel having a high blood flow (*e.g.*, the superior vena cava).

This seminal work aroused great interest among pediatricians, and over the past seven or so years, much effort has been expended in evaluating the efficacy as well as the safety of this method of feeding in the pediatric patient. Our group at the Babies Hospital of the Columbia-Presbyterian Medical Center has been actively involved in these research efforts, and this paper attempts to summarize some of our own experiences both with respect to the clinical usefulness of the technique as well as some of its metabolic complications.

* Supported by grants from the National Institutes of Health (HD-08434, HL-14218 and RR-00645).

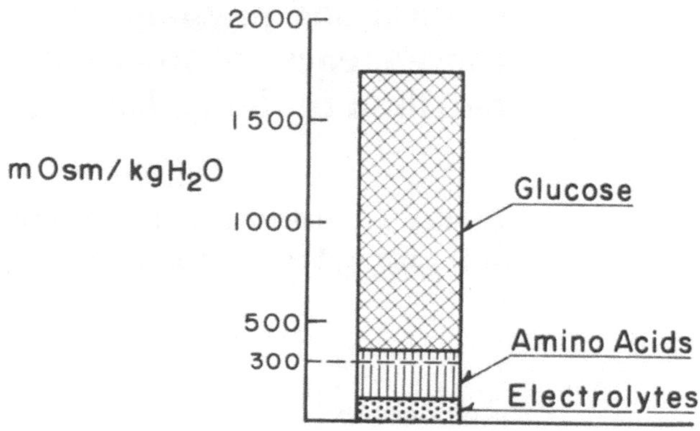

Figure 1. The osmolality of the conventional fat-free TPN infusate used in the US for infants. [Reproduced with permission from Heird and Winters (2)].

TECHNIQUE AND COMPOSITION OF INFUSATE FOR TOTAL PARENTERAL NUTRITION

The technique of inserting of central venous catheter in infants which we use is that described originally by Dudrick *et al.* (1) and is depicted in Figure 2. A silastic catheter is inserted through a small neck incision and threaded through the internal jugular vein into the superior vena cava. The location of the tip of the catheter must be verified radiographically. The other end of the catheter is tunnelled through a skin tunnel and exits behind the ear, a location which makes the tri-weekly dressing changes much easier and which removes the wound from the mouth area. All nutrient fluids are mixed by a registered pharmacist under a laminar flow hood; they are pumped continuously using a closed pump. A 0.22 μ millipore filter is added in the line as a further safeguard against the infusion of contaminated fluids.

Table 1 shows the usual composition of the conventional, fat-free nutritional infusate used for TPN in infants in the USA (2). It should be emphasized that the values shown here are average ones for the full strength solution; they often may require modification on a daily basis depending upon monitoring data in individual infants.

Glucose is the sole source of non-protein calories in the solution and in general at least 100 cal/kg/d are required. When initiating TPN, the glucose load must be slowly increased over a period of several days to the full strength in order to allow the infant to adapt to the high glucose loads of

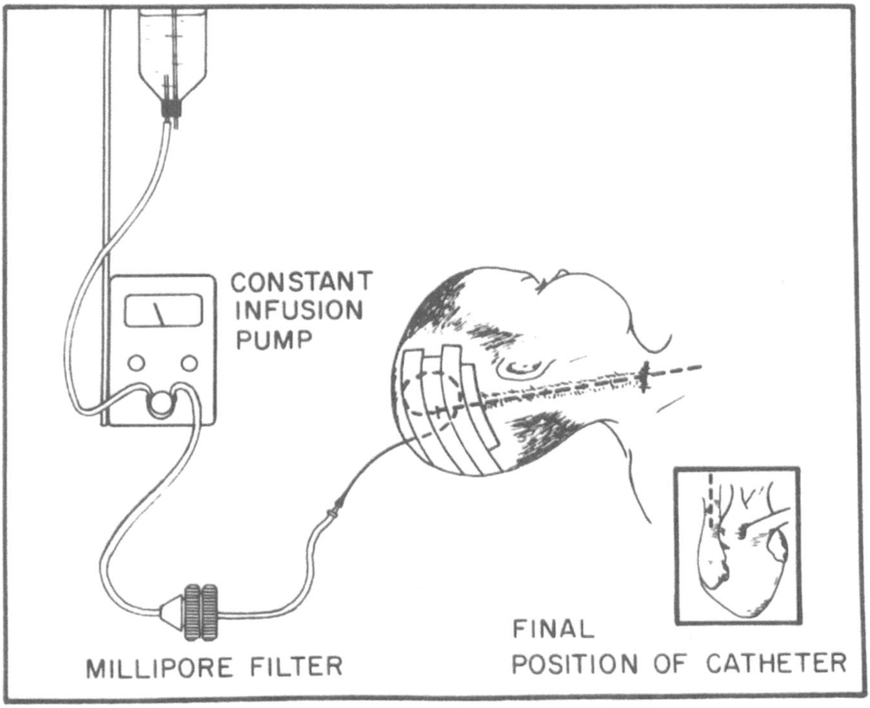

Figure 2. Technique of delivery of hyperosmolar TPN nutrient infusates in infants. The insert shows the tip of the catheter in the superior vena cava. [Reproduced with permission from Heird and Winters (2)].

Table 1. Usual composition of infusate

Constituent	Amount
Nitrogen source	2.5 gm/kg/day
Glucose	25-30 gm/kg/day
NaCl	3-4 mM/kg/day
KH_2PO_4	2-3 mM/kg/day*
Ca gluconate	0.25 mM/kg/day (0.5 mEq/kg/day)
$MgSO_4$	0.125 mM/kg/day (0.25 mEq/kg/day)
MVI	1 ml/day
Vitamin B_{12}	50 μg/day
Folic acid	50-75 μg/day
Vitamin K_1	250-500 μg/day
Total volume	130 ml/kg/day

* KH_2PO_4 should be limited to 2 mM/kg/day; additional potassium should be provided as KCl. [Reproduced with permission from Heird and Winters (2)].

the full strength solution. It is noteworthy that the solution contains no essential fatty acids (EFA) or trace minerals, potentially important omissions (see below).

SURGICAL NEONATES

One of the two general groups of patients in which TPN is definitely indicated is the group of infants which we have called surgical neonates. The group actually consists of several subgroups: (a) infants with major anomalies requiring multiple, staged operative procedures for complete repair (*e.g.*, gastroschisis), (b) infants with congenital or acquired anomalies of the gastrointestinal tract requiring removal of large segments of bowel (*e.g.*, long atresias), (c) patients with various surgical complications which preclude enteral feeding (prematurity, fistulas, etc.), (d) infants with non-mechanical obstruction of the small bowel, presumably due to a heretofore undescribed congenital disorder of motility, and (e) neonates with necrotizing enterocolitis.

We have had an extensive experience with this group of patients (2). Metabolically, they seem to require at least 100 cal/kg/d to show weight gain and positive nitrogen balance. But with that level of intake, a metabolic steady state is achieved and they show a good rate of weight gain (average 12.9 g/kg/d) and a brisk positive nitrogen balance (0.18 g/kg/d). Positive balances for other intracellular electrolytes (potassium, magnesium and inorganic phosphorus) are similar to the ratios seen for normal lean body mass (3). Indirect computation of the quality of weight gain of such patients shows that about two-thirds of the observed weight gain is normally hydrated, lean body mass (LBM). Of the remaining one-third, about half probably represents fat deposition and the other half represents "excess' extracellular fluid. These estimates are consistent with the clinical observation that if TPN is carried on long enough, physical evidence of fat deposition does indeed occur although detectable generalized edema does not.

Of our total experience with these patients, we have long term follow-up data on 21. At 2 to 4 years follow-up, 15 have shown normal growth patterns, normal bowel habits and are eating a normal diet; two are still being maintained on semi-synthetic formulas. Four died, all of causes unrelated to TPN. These overall results are very gratifying compared to the pre-TPN experience in which overall mortality of this group of patients was at least 75 percent.

CHRONIC INTRACTABLE DIARRHEA

A second category of infants who definitely seem to benefit from TPN are those with the syndrome(s) of intractable diarrhea. These are young infants, many of whom seem to have had diarrhea almost from birth. The diarrhea defies etiological identification and is resistant to virtually every change of formula. Malnutrition is often severe.

Keating (4) first explored the concept that such patients might benefit from a period of complete bowel rest by using a protracted period of TPN. He studied 16 such patients having an average age of 3 weeks who received TPN for a mean of 28 days. At long term follow-up, 15 of 16 had apparently regained normal gastro-intestinal function, with the exception of 6, all black, who were lactase-deficient. The remaining patient died of sepsis. These results are as spectacular as those obtained with the surgical neonates in that prior to TPN, mortality from this disorder(s) was about 75%. Keating's results have been fully confirmed by our group. In addition we have studied the metabolic responses of these infants and have determined that they are very similar to the surgical neonates in that 100 cal/kg/d seems to be the critical level for weight gain and positive nitrogen balance to occur. But once that level has been reached, the steady-state gains in weight and positive nitrogen balance are very similar to those seen in the surgical cases.

These interesting results with TPN raise a number of questions about the nature of this disease or diseases which masquerades under the general ap-

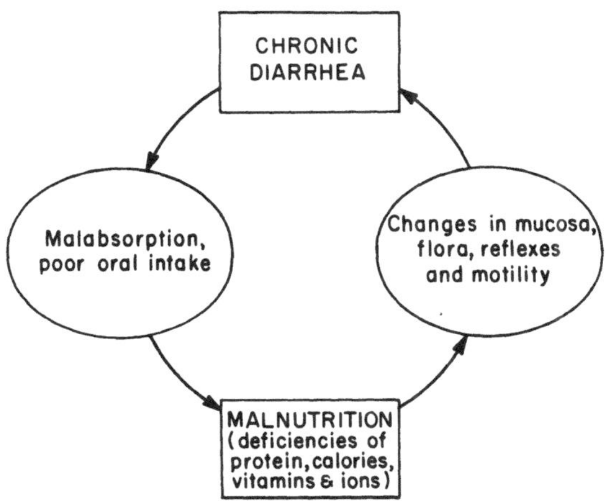

Figure 3. Postulated cycle between chronic intractable diarrhea and malnutrition. [Reproduced with permission from Heird and Winters (2)].

pellation of chronic intractable diarrhea. One suggestion is that chronic diarrhea through malabsorption and anorexia begets malnutrition, and malnutrition once well established then begets further diarrhea and the cycle is closed (see Figure 3). TPN appears to be one very effective way to break this cycle by resting the gut as well as nourishing the patient.

THE LOW BIRTH WEIGHT (LBW) INFANT

The feeding of the LBW infant remains a significant challenge to the neonatologist, particularly in the USA, where the rate of prematurity is relatively high compared to most western European countries. It is widely appreciated that the LBW infant is a significant nutritional risk, and there are several fundamental reasons for this. First, body composition studies show quite clearly that the degree of caloric reserve and probably the reserve of LBM as well is distinctly limited (5), so that relatively short periods of suboptimal nutrition could well be life-threatening. Second, the immaturity of the gastrointestinal tract of such infants is such as to entail a considerable risk in safely feeding enterally the relatively large amounts of nutrients needed for growth of such infants. In addition there is a high probability of poor digestibility and/or absorption of such enterally delivered nutrients. Finally there is the suspicion, based largely on animal work, that short-term nutritional deficiencies in early life may contribute to non-recoupable neurological deficits later in life.

In view of these considerations, much interest was aroused by the possibility that central venous TPN might be a significant adjunct to existing feeding practices of the LBW in overcoming the problems alluded to above. In order to explore this possibility, we conducted a feasibility study in which central venous TPN was administered for an average of 17 days to 14 infants, all having birth weights of less than 1,200 gm (6). This study was not controlled; rather it was directed at answering the question as to whether or not the very LBW infant could be safely and effectively fed by central venous TPN using the conventional techniques which had proven so successful in managing the older, larger infants with surgical disease or with diarrhea.

Early in this study we became aware of the very great degree of unpredictability of glucose intolerance in these infants. This was such as to make the most intensive monitoring of blood and urine glucose an absolute necessity in order to avoid serious hyperglycemia and osmotic diuresis. However, by careful titration of glucose intake against blood and urine glucose, we were able to achieve the desired intake of greater than 100 cal/kg/d in most such infants, although the time to achieve this goal varied from 2 to 15 days. Once this level of caloric intake had been achieved, however, gains in body weight and satisfactory positive nitrogen balance were obtained in all.

Of the original 14 infants involved in the study, 5 died of pulmonary insufficiency and 1 died of sepsis. In the survivors the neurological outcome was somewhat better than we would have expected from conventional management, but the results were not strikingly different. Based on a comparison with a group of non-concurrent controls who had been managed conventionally (7), we estimate that if the favorable differences in mortality and in neurologic outcome were to prevail in a concurrent controlled study, at least

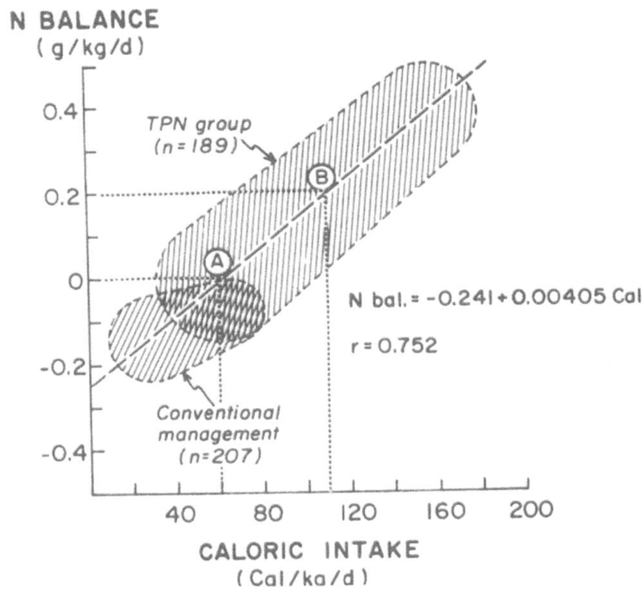

Figure 4. Regression line fitted to the authors' data on daily nitrogen balance as a function of daily caloric (glucose) intake in groups of LBW infants managed conventionally or by TPN. All infants were maintained at a thermoneutral environment. Point A represents the statistically average caloric intake (60 Cal/kg/d) at which nitrogen balance is zero. Point B represents the average value produced for a caloric intake in the range which we have used for infants with surgical disease or with chronic diarrhea (see text) as well as in our previous studies of LBW infants (6). It is evident that for this statistical treatment positive nitrogen balance need not demand intakes of 100 Cal/kg/d or more, but rather could be achieved at levels of about 60 Cal/kg/d. These observations form the basis for the approach of the authors in providing TPN by the peripheral rather than the central venous route (see text).

75 infants in the TPN and another 75 in the control group would be needed to show a statistically significant difference in favor of TPN. These large numbers would clearly require a collaborative study, and in view of our experience as well as that of others with fatal hyperglycemia in such infants (8) plus the inherently high risk of sepsis in the LBW infant fed by means of central venous TPN, we felt that mounting any such controlled collaborative study was simply not feasible.

Thus another safer approach was clearly needed if TPN were to go forward in this group of patients, and this was forthcoming as the result of two different lines of research which converged on this problem. First, in extensive balance studies of caloric intake versus nitrogen retention (see Figure 4), we (9) showed that the LBW infant kept at thermoneutral conditions could achieve positive nitrogen balance on a caloric intake of as little as 60 cal/kg/d rather than the higher level of at least 100 cal/kg/d which we originally established for the surgical and the diarrhea patients (see above). Second, a review of the entire literature [see, for example, Mestyan *et al.* (10)] on thermoregulation showed that the total caloric expenditure of LBW infants maintained at thermoneutrality rarely exceeded 60 cal/kg/d during the first one or two weeks

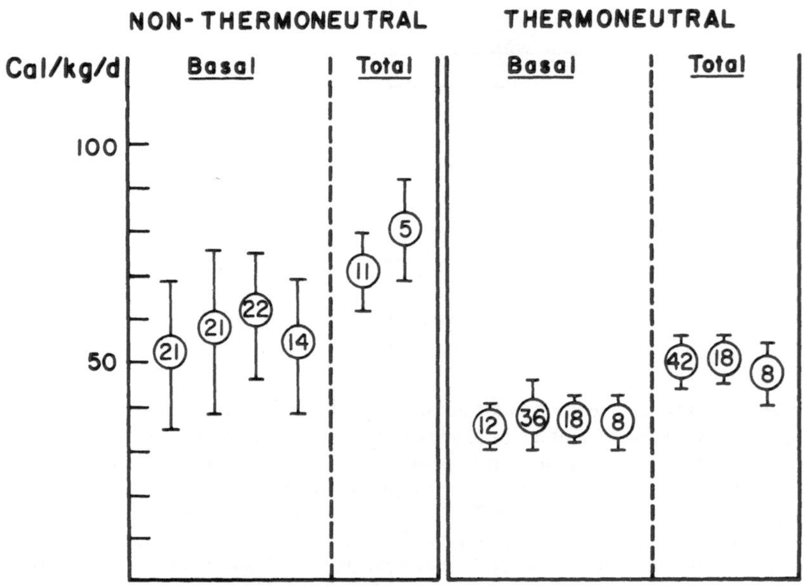

Figure 5. Summary of literature on basal and total metabolic rate in LBW infants (1.1 to 2.4 kg) during the first several weeks of life under non-thermoneutral and thermoneutral conditions. [Literature quoted by Mestyan et al. (10)].

of life whereas much higher values were seen when thermoneutral conditions were not maintained (see Figure 5).

In other words, it seemed possible that 60 cal/kg/d would provide enough energy to meet the needs for maintenance, for SDA, for activity and for growth if the energy usually diverted for temperature regulation could be conserved. Put another way, on a limited energy intake energy would be preferentially directed towards thermoregulation at the expense of growth; but by insuring thermoneutrality, the energy intake could be dramatically reduced, and growth, at least growth of LBM if not of fat stores, could occur. This approach was especially attractive because the requisite 60 cal/kg could be provided by a reasonable volume of 10% glucose delivered by peripheral vein, thus eliminating the risks of central venous catheterization.

We (9) have now evaluated this approach in a controlled study in which randomly selected infants having body weights of about 1,650 $\pm$ 600 gm were given either 60 cal/kg/d from glucose or 60 cal/kg/d from glucose plus 2.5 g/kg/d of the crystalline amino acid mixture, Aminosyn (Abbott Laboratories). Electrolytes, minerals and vitamins were added to both groups. The nutrient infusions, having a final total osmolality of about 650 to 750 mOs/kg water, were given at rates of 150 ml/kg/d for 5 days by peripheral vein.

In both groups the nutrient regimes were started on the first or second day of life. In the "glucose alone" group, body weight fell and average nitrogen balance was – 130 mg/kg/d, while in the group receiving glucose plus amino acids, there were no significant changes in body weight and average nitrogen balance was 150 mg/kg/d. Although post-natal changes in hydration make body weight difficult to interpret in this study, the nitrogen balance data leave little doubt that there was definite anabolism of LBM in the group receiving glucose plus amino acids.

This conclusion was borne out by the data on the plasma aminograms. In the "glucose alone" group, the general pattern showed a lowered concentration of the total of all amino acids (TAA) and especially of the total essential amino acids (TEAA), so that the TEAA/TAA was low, a pattern faintly reminiscent of other states of protein malnutrition. In the "glucose plus amino acids" group, however, the absolute levels of both TEAA and TAA were generally higher so that the pattern resembled more closely the post-prandial pattern seen in otherwise normal, enterally-fed infants of comparable weight.

There were two noteworthy abnormalities, however, in the "glucose plus amino acids" group – namely the low levels of tyrosine and cystine. These are not unexpected in view of the fact that both of these amino acids are essential for the LBW infant, and because of their poor solubility, they cannot be included in the parenteral mixture in sufficient amounts to meet the estimated requirements. Yet despite these deficiencies, nitrogen balance was not impaired to the degree that positive balance was not obtainable. On the other hand, one may argue that had these amino acids been present in adequate amounts, an even larger positive balance would have been obtained.

Another interesting set of observations concerned the plasma EFA status in these two groups of infants. Infants receiving glucose alone showed a slight tendency for the plasma triene/tetraene ratio to rise. But in the infants receiving glucose plus amino acids, this rise was much more definite suggesting that EFA deficiency may occur in a period as short as 5 days if the infant is made anabolic in the absence of an exogenous EFA source.

These observations stress the interrelations between EFA status and anabolism which are diagramatically shown in Figure 3. When anabolism is promoted, EFA are taken up as components of new cell and mitochondrial membranes, and in the infants, there is a special need for EFA for deposition of brain lipids as well. Normally, the term infant has appreciable stores of depot EFA due to transplacental transfer of EFA which occurs late in pregnancy. The LBW infant, however, misses this late transplacental "boost" of EFA stores and lacking any exogenous intake of EFA is thus highly susceptible to depletion of his minimal reserves of endogenous EFA.

This chemical evidence of EFA deficiency is of more than academic interest. In a series of recent studies, we have shown that the newborn beagle puppy receiving 10 days of fat-free TPN beginning on the first day of life shows a significant increase in triene/tetraene ratio not only of the plasma and of the liver phospholipids but of the EPG (ethanolamine phosphoglyceride) fraction of the brain lipids as well (11). This lipid fraction is important in the myelinization of the developing nervous system and thus has considerable functional importance.

Our studies of peripheral TPN in the LBW reviewed above are being continued. One critical question is how intravenous fat emulsions should be used in such infants. There are two facets to this question: (a) use of such emulsions to provide the EFA requirements, likely to be in the range of about 4 cal/kg/d, and (b) use of these emulsions in calorically significant amounts (*e.g.*, 20 to 30 cal/kg/d). The first of these would seem to pose no significant practical risk and should be straightforward. But the second does pose interesting and unanswered problems. Whether a fat calorie is truly equivalent to a carbohydrate calorie in promoting nitrogen intake is a critical question in the definition of the role of intravenous fat emulsions in the pediatric patient receiving TPN. Despite the extensive clinical experience with Intralipid in pediatric patients in Scandinavia and in Canada, this question remains unanswered. There is the possibility, judging by the results of Long *et al.* (12) that isocaloric substitution of fat for carbohydrate results in a diminution of nitrogen retention in adults, that fat will not support anabolism as well as carbohydrate in the LBW infant. Work on this important question is currently underway in our laboratory and will be reported in due course.

METABOLIC COMPLICATIONS IN TPN IN INFANTS

In many ways the human infant is the most sensitive test organism available for the assessment of both the safety and the efficacy of TPN. This premise derives from the fundamental metabolic fact that per unit of body mass, the metabolic rate of the infants roughly three times that of the adult. It follows from this that in the infant compared to the adult there must be commen-

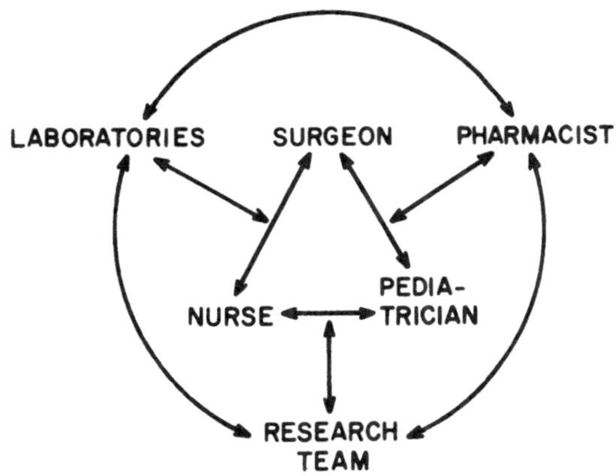

Figure 6. Composition of the TPN-team at the Babies Hospital, Columbia-Presbyterian Medical Center in New York. [Reproduced by permission from Heird and Winters (2)].

surate increases in the flow of substrates, in the rate of O_2 and CO_2 production and in the rate of excretion of end-products of metabolism by the kidney. Thus any complication which interferes with these normal processes will likely develop three times as fast and be three times as severe in the infant than in his adult counterpart.

Virtually every metabolic complication of TPN has been seen in the infant. Fundamentally these may be classified into two major groups depending upon the ability of the physician to rapidly correct them. The first group of such complications includes disorders of glucose, electrolyte, mineral and water metabolism. Basically, all of these come about because of a failure to match intake of these various constituents to their output or metabolic deposition. Intensive chemical and clinical monitoring of the patient will rapidly reveal the presence of these abnormalities, and treatment basically involves a readjustment of one or the other of the constituents of the nutrient infusate so that intake and output are again matched and plasma concentrations are normal.

To carry out such monitoring and readjustment of fluid composition requires a team approach (see Figure 6) in which the pediatrician and pediatric surgeon operating in concert conduct a daily review of each patient's status and based on close clinical and microchemical monitoring data, an individualized fluid prescription is generated each day for each patient. This "tailor-made" fluid is prepared in accordance with the usual aseptic techniques by a specially trained pharmacist. A specially designated TPN nurse changes all dressings, collates data and maintains close contact with all personnel who interact with the patient. We have used this team approach in our entire efforts in clinical TPN in infants. As a result in our series of nearly 100 patients we have been able to keep the incidence of serious metabolic complications involving glucose, electrolytes, mineral and water metabolism to less than 5% while our TPN-related sepsis rate has been kept to about 6%. We believe that this exemplary record achieved in a large group of very high risk patients can be obtained only by the team approach and we further believe that those pediatric institutions unwilling or unable to mount this type of team should not attempt to care for infants requiring central venous TPN.

The second group of metabolic complications are those which are inherent in the infusate itself and therefore are not readily manipulable by the therapist. Essential fatty acid deficiency is one such example and deficiency of trace metals is another. But it is the design of the amino acid composition of the infusate that poses the greatest challenges in this area. With this question we are concerned with nutritional efficacy as well as safety of such solutions; the latter is especially important in the infant where we may be dealing with possibility of a damaging effect of hyperaminoacidemia upon the immature nervous system.

The fundamental problem of defining both safety and efficacy of a given amino acid solution in the setting of TPN is to select appropriate benchmarks for the assessment of these properties. This is a well-nigh impossible task given the fact that in TPN the amino acids are being infused continuously, whereas in enteral nutrition intake is intermittent.

As a first step towards the rational definition of such benchmarks, we have proposed that the post-prandial rather than the fasting levels of amino acids seen in normal infants after normal feedings represent a reasonable approach (13). In developing this concept, we argued that the normal brain is exposed episodically to the normal post-prandial peaks and therefore they are harmless in this setting. We also believe that a convincing case can be made for the idea that the post-prandial levels are more efficacious for optimal tissue protein synthesis and thus these levels are reasonable ones to aim for with respect to nutritional efficacy. Thus our concept envisions that if a given plasma value obtained during TPN falls below the post-prandial limit it probably reflects a deficiency, whereas if it exceeds the upper limit, it is grounds for suspecting toxicity.

To date, we have applied this approach to an examination of 161 sets of steady-state plasma amino acid data obtained in growing infants on TPN receiving one of six different amino acid solutions and have been able to discern the distinctive patterns and the abnormalities induced by each (14). A few examples will suffice. As already mentioned, cystine and tyrosine are both essential amino acids for the LBW infant and probably for the term infant as well. Since their poor solubility prevents any significant parenteral intake, consistently low plasma levels of both are seen with all solutions studied to date. A second example is the low valine level seen with fibrin hydrolysate. This is hardly surprising since this particular mixture is known to provide less than the recommended requirement for this essential amino acid. Thirdly, we have accumulated sufficient data on the three solutions which have been implicated in hyperammonemia (*e.g.*, FreAmine, fibrin hydrolysate and casein hydrolysate) and in all three, borderline or frankly low levels of plasma arginine occurred.

On the high side, the most significant quantitative abnormality occurs with those amino acid solutions containing large amounts of glycine. Plasma glycine varies linearly with parenteral intake, and with large parenteral intakes the plasma level of glycine may range up to 10 times the mean post-prandial level.

We have constructed dose-response curves relating daily intake of each amino acid to its steady-state plasma level. In approximately half of the cases, good to excellent correlations were obtained, whereas with the others, little or no correlation was observed. These data will be potentially useful in the future in optimizing the existing mixtures to improve their nutritional efficacy while avoiding hyperaminoacidemia and possible adverse influence upon the normal development of the nervous system.

A good example of the sensitivity of the infant to metabolic complications in TPN is hyperammonemia. It is widely recognized that both casein and fibrin hydrolysates produce asymptomatic hyperammonemia; this has usually been attributed to their high preformed ammonia content. For this reason, some years ago we switched to the crystalline amino acid mixture, FreAmine, which contained no preformed ammonia. We were thus surprised to discover four infants, all of whom developed life-threatening degrees of hyperammonemia (blood levels up to 800 μg/100 ml) while receiving FreAmine (15). The hyperammonemia was very sensitive to either arginine or ornithine supplementation, suggesting that this particular amino acid mixture was relatively deficient in arginine. A similar though much less marked degree of hyperammonemia due to FreAmine was reported in adults receiving large amounts of FreAmine (16).

Recent further studies of this problem have uncovered presumptive evidence for a metabolic unity between hydrolysate-induced hyperammonemia on the one hand and FreAmine-induced hyperammonemia on the other. We have shown that as infants on FreAmine developed hyperammonemia, there was a fall in BUN and urea excretion, but total urinary nitrogen and the nitrogenous fractions attributed to ammonia, creatinine, uric acid and α-amino nitrogen remained fairly constant. This implied that some unidentified nitrogen-containing substance was appearing in markedly increased amounts in the urine as the hyperammonemia developed. Dr. Hans Böhles of our group has now identified this as largely orotic acid. This substance is an intermediate in the pyrimidine biosynthetic pathway, the first step of which is the reaction of ammonia, CO_2 and ATP to form carbamyl phosphate. This step, of course, is also the initial step in the urea cycle (see Figure 7). Thus it would appear that as anabolic demands deplete arginine from the urea cycle, ammonia is preferentially shunted down the pyrimidine pathway and orotic acid accumulates.

As this work was underway, Sunshine (17) discovered that infants with hydrolysate-induced hyperammonemia also show an augmented orotic acid excretion. Furthermore, the arginine intake delivered by either of the hydrolysates is similar to that delivered by FreAmine. Finally, both of the hydrolysates and FreAmine are associated with generally low arginine and ornithine levels in the plasma. All of this evidence points to a similarity of mechanism between the hyperammonemia due to the hydrolysates and that due to FreAmine. It is more severe in the infant, probably because his anabolic needs for arginine relative to arginine intake are greater than in the adult.

Yet another example of the thesis of a greater sensitivity of the infant to metabolic complications is to be found in our earlier work on metabolic acidosis in TPN. We discovered that this acid-base disorder occurred with regularity in infants given one of two crystalline amino acid mixtures (Neo-

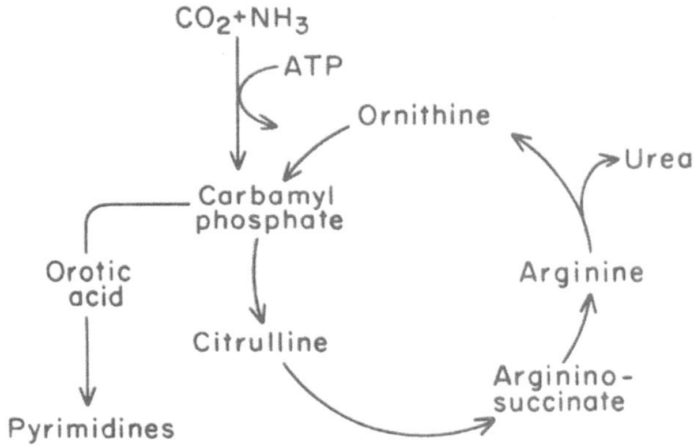

Figure 7. Metabolic pathways illustrating the relationship between ammonia metabolism via the urea cycle and via the pyrimidine biosynthetic pathway.

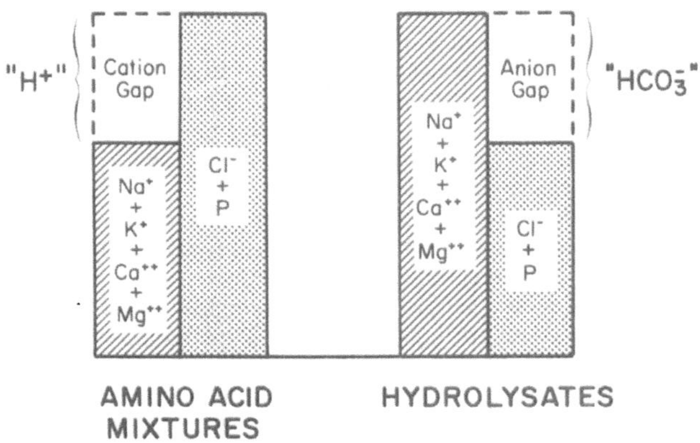

Figure 8. General cation-anion patterns of crystalline amino acids which produced hyperchloremic metabolic acidosis (left) and of protein hydrolysates which did not produce acidosis (right). The cation gap of the former is due to the positive charges contributed by arginine and lysine, which upon metabolism yield hydrogen ions. The anion gap of the hydrolysates is due to glutamate, aspartate and negatively charged peptides, all of which produce bicarbonate upon metabolism. [Reproduced by permission from Heird and Winters (2)].

Aminosol or FreAmine) whereas it did not occur with the hydrolysates (18). The acidosis was fairly severe in the infants. A much milder form occurred in adults, but like that of the infant, it was characterized by a hyperchloremia, a reduction in plasma bicarbonate and blood pH. Careful study of this problem demonstrated that the mechanism of the acidosis resided in the large potential acid load delivered by arginine and lysine, the principal cationic amino acids, which had been added as the hydrochloride salts to the crystalline mixtures (see Figure 8). Upon metabolism these amino acids yielded urea and hydrochloric acid. Substitution of chloride with acetate (a bicarbonate precursor) solved this problem, and all currently available solutions have since avoided this problem in this same general way. The infant's increased susceptibility to acidosis, of course, stemmed from the fact that the acid load delivered by the acidogenic amino acid solutions was proportionately greater than that delivered to the adult, and this, coupled with immaturity of the renal acidification mechanism, accounted for the more severe acidosis seen in the infant.

SUMMARY

Total parenteral nutrition has achieved an important, even life-saving role in the management of several groups of pediatric patients. Certainly this is the case with selected instances of anomalies of the gastrointestinal tract in the newborn and in older infants with the syndrome of chronic intractable diarrhea. The role of TPN in feeding the LBW infant remains to be accurately defined. Central venous TPN is probably too risky to be recommended as a practical alternative to conventional management. Recognition of the crucial interaction between thermoneutrality, energy intake and growth, however, has the potential of providing TPN by peripheral vein to the LBW infant. This new technique approaches a comprehensive clinical trial.

Metabolic complications are many and varied. In understanding these, much information can be gained by recognizing that the infant is relatively sensitive to the development of such complications. Rigid monitoring and the ability to rapidly readjust the nutritional infusate can effectively reduce serious metabolic complications due to glucose, electrolyte, minerals or water. The precise formulation of the amino acid mixture poses the greatest challenge for future study in TPN. The pediatric experience with both safety and efficacy of such solutions will undoubtedly be important in the future in pointing the way to better and safer mixtures. Elucidation of the mechanism of such complications as hyperammonemia and hyperchloremic metabolic acidosis are examples of the types of studies in infants which have general applicability to all patients receiving TPN. Similarly, the emerging metabolic picture of EFA deficiency observed in infants receiving fat-free TPN will likely provide important new generalizations for prevention and for treatment of this complication.

REFERENCES

1. Dudrick, S. J., Wilmore, D. W., Vars, H. M. and Rhoades, J. E., Long-term totel parenteral nutrition with growth, development, and positive nitrogen balance, *Surgery 64*: 134 (1968).
2. Heird, W. C. and Winters, R. W., Total parenteral nutrition, *J. Pediatr. 86*: 2 (1975).
3. Heird, W. C., Unpublished data.
4. Keating, J. P., Parenteral nutrition in infants with malabsorption, in: Winters, R. W. and Hasselmeyer, E. G., editors: *Intravenous nutrition in high risk infants*, New York, 1974, John Wiley and Sons, Inc.
5. Widdowson, E., Changes in body proportions and composition during growth, in: Davis, J. A. and Dobbing, J., editors: *Scientific foundations of paediatrics*, London, 1974, Wm. Heinemann Medical Books, Ltd., Chap. 12, p. 153.
6. Heird, W. C., Driscoll, J. M., Jr. and Winters, R. W., Total parenteral nutrition in very low birth weight infants. In: Dawes, G. (ed.): *Size at Birth*, Ciba Symposium 27. Elsevier-Excerpta Medica-North Holland, 1974.
7. Winters, R. W. and Hasselmeyer, E. G., editors: *Intravenous nutrition in high risk infants*, New York, 1974, John Wiley and Sons, Inc.
8. Chance, G. W., Results in very low birth weight infants (< 1300 gm birth weight), In: Winters, R. W. and Hasselmeyer, E. G., editors: *Intravenous nutrition in high risk infants*, New York, 1974, John Wiley and Sons, Inc.
9. Anderson, T. L., Nicholson, J. F. and Heird, W. C., Controlled trial of intravenous glucose vs glucose and amino acids in premature infants. *Pediatr. Res. 10*: 351 (1976) (Abst.).
10. Mestyan, J., Javai, F. and Fekete, T., The total energy expenditure and its components in premature infants maintained under different nursery and environmental conditions. *Pediatr. Res. 2*: 161 (1968).
11. Heird, W. C., Bieber, M. A., Bassi, J., Pulito, A. R. and Brasel, J. A., Effects of total parenteral nutrition on brain growth of beagle puppies. *Pediatr. Res. 10*: 323 (1976) (Abst.).
12. Long, J. M., Wilmore, D. W., Mason, Ad, Jr. and Pruitt, B. A., Jr., In press.
13. Winters, R. W., Heird, W. C., Stegink, L. D. and Nicholson, J. F., *Towards a rational interpretation of the nutritional significance of the plasma aminogram. A theoretical essay.* In press.
14. Nicholson, J. F., Heird, W. C. and Winters, R. W., Unpublished data.
15. Heird, W. C., Nicholson, J. F., Driscoll, J. M., Jr., Schullinger, J. N. and Winters, R. W., Hyperammonemia resulting from intravenous alimentation using a mixture of synthetic L-amino acids: A preliminary report. *J. Pediatr. 81*: 162 (1972).
16. Dudrick, S. J., MacFadyen, B. V., Jr., Van Buren, C. T., Ruberg R. L. and Maynard, A. T., Parenteral hyperalimentation: Metabolic problems and solutions. *Ann. Surg. 176*: 256 (1972).
17. Sunshine, P., Personal communication.
18. Heird, W. C., Dell, R. B., Driscoll, J. M., Jr., Grebia, B. and Winters, R. W., Metabolic Acidosis Resulting from Intravenous Alimentation Mixtures containing synthetic Amino Acids. *N. Engl. J. Med. 287*: 943 (1972).

Parenteral nutrition in trauma

M. Halmágyi

Parenteral nutrition in traumatized patients is not only a way of nourishment but also a therapeutical concept. The choice of substances and the dosage of nutrients have to be adapted to the specific metabolic state of the traumatized patient. For this reason, we should talk about intravenous therapy with nutrients instead of parenteral nutrition in trauma. The main problem in traumatized patients is to supply them with an adequate amount of calories with a minimum of complications and clinical risks.

Facing these problems we tried to find the most adequate source of energy-supply for severely traumatized patients treated in the ICU.

In our first study concerning severely traumatized patients, totalling a period of 330 days, all patients received 0.3 g of Nitrogen/kg body weight/day (Table 1). The nutrients were given via caval catheter. As amino-acid source, we administered Aminofusion 1 - forte. As a fat source Lipofundin S and Intralipid were used. Extra amounts of water and electrolytes were given according to each patient's requirements. Additional calories were supplied as glucose, fructose and xylitol.

Table 1. Frequency of daily positive nitrogen balance depending on caloric intake as a % of the B.M.R. during intravenous nutrition

Cal-Int. % of BMR	days of infusion	days of positive N-balance in %
without fat		
< 100	131	0
100-110	49	53.1
110-120	11	100.0
> 120	33	100.0
with fat		
< 100	–	–
100-110	21	0
110-120	18	0
> 120	67	0

In 100% of the cases, we found the daily nitrogen balance to be positive when only carbohydrate calories were supplied and when the total protein-free energy intake was about 120% of the basal metabolic rate of the patient. These results showed the protein-free caloric requirements of such patients to be about 1,600-2,000 calories per day. No positive nitrogen balance was observed when an isocaloric, isonitrogenous mixture was administered with 30% of the calories derived from fat (1).

However, we do not postulate that no positive nitrogen balance can be achieved at all in patients who receive fat emulsions. We observed positive nitrogen balances in patients who received fat emulsions. But this occurred only when the nitrogen and total caloric intake were increased and this depended on the amount of fat infused. The more fat administered, the more caloric supplements were necessary (Table 2).

In our opinion the results of our observations indicate that no fat emulsions should be used as caloric supply for severely traumatized patients; in the first place because more nitrogen and calories must be given and in the second place because the RES is blocked by fat, causing a reduced resistance to infection. On the other hand, essential fatty acids are needed during longer periods of artificial nutrition as documented by Collins et al. (2). For this reason fat emulsions should be administered not later than two weeks after the start of intravenous nutrition. Five hundred ml of 10% fat emulsion should be administered every second day.

In subsequent studies we tried to determine the best combination of carbohydrates for severely traumatized patients.

It is well-known that contrary to normal healthy persons, surgical patients have a disturbed glucose metabolism.

Table 2. Relationship between positive nitrogen balance and calorie, nitrogen and fat intake

N/kg BW	Cal % of BMR	Fat % cal/day	Balance
0.169	105.5	0	−
0.234	114.2	0	+
0.198	110.1	0- 8	−
0.256	120.9	0- 8	+
0.271	136.0	8-14.2	−
0.416	163.0	8-14.2	+
0.410	176.5	14.2-23.6	−
0.755	236.5	14.2-18.6	+

Zöllner et al. (3) found that in normal healthy persons the utilization rate of glucose was 99.1% 0.5 g glucose/kg body weight/h administered intravenously and 97.2% with 1.0 g glucose/kg body weight/h.

Weinstein and Roe (4) found a 82.3% utilization of glucose in patients in the immediate postoperative period. Bickel et al. (5) found different rates of glucose excretion in different patients when the same amount of glucose is given during the immediate postoperative period.

It is well-documented that hyperglycemia, glucosuria, insulin resistance and glucose intolerance accompany trauma.

We therefore investigated the utilization of glucose in 10 severely traumatized patients using the so-called steady-state method described by Müller (6, Fig. 1). Glucose was determined enzymatically. The patient data are summarized in Table 3. In two experimental studies we infused 10 patients with 0.5 g and 1.0 g glucose/kg body weight/h, respectively. In the first study we found an average metabolic rate for glucose of 78.7% of the infused amount, and in the second study we found only 60.3% (Table 4).

These metabolic rates of glucose allow the administration of 3,000 to 4,000 calories per day – sufficient to meet the requirements of the severely traumatized patient. But during the experiments we equally found a very high blood glucose level – in the first study more than 200 mg % and in the second more than 500 mg% during the steady-state in both cases without the administration of insulin (Fig. 2).

Although Lotspeich (7) has shown that the subcutaneous injection of in-

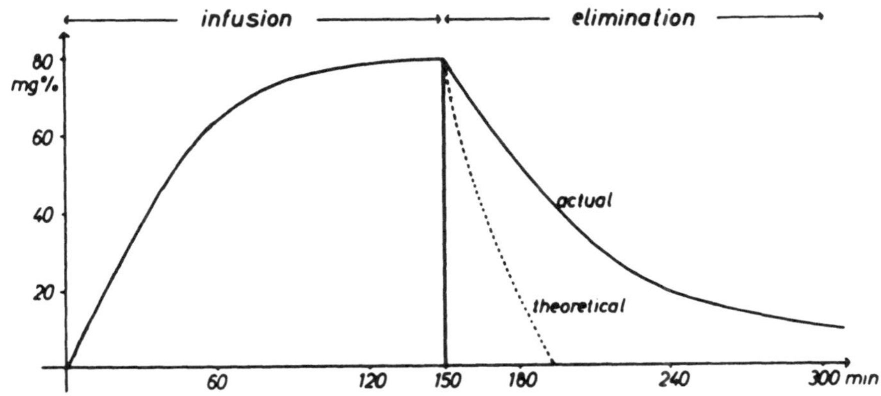

Figure 1. Kinetics of the elimination from the blood (steady-state technique according to Müller).

sulin lowers the blood glucose level in the post-traumatic phase, this does not improve nitrogen balance according to Schuberth (8).

From our own observations we concluded that the administration of high glucose loads should not be recommended in severely traumatized patients.

Obviously, as shown in the literature as well as in our own clinical studies, the results of parenteral nutrition in traumatized patients are better when glucose is combined with fructose to cover caloric needs.

Strauss and Hiller (9) reported that the rapid dissimilation of fructose provides increased amounts of ATP for the phosphorylation of glucose. This causes a rapid transfer of glucose into the cell and therefore decreases the glucose concentration in the blood.

Stuhlfauth and his coworkers (10) observed that post-operative nitrogen losses could be diminished by administration of fructose. They pointed out that fructose forms large amounts of pyruvic acid, and that therefore the hydrogen of the free sulfhydryl group, which is necessary for the activation of proteases, is used by the organism in increased amounts for the formation

Table 3. Patient data. Infusion of glucose, 0.5 g/kg/hour and 1.0 g/kg/hour

Nr.	Weight kg	Sex	Disease
1	79.3	♂	tetanus
2	72.5	♀	meningoencephal., bronchopneum.
3	62.0	♀	comm. cerebri, thoracic injury
4	72.5	♂	aspiration pneumonia
5	66.6	♂	thoracic injury
6	64.3	♂	respiratory insufficiency
7	57.4	♀	tetanus
8	102.0	♂	thoracic injury
9	56.0	♂	CO poison, cardiac arrest
10	80.3	♀	tetanus

Table 4. Metabolic rate of carbohydrates in traumatized and severely ill patients (infusion of single carbohydrates)

Dosage g/kg/h	Inf. phase mg/kg/h	Elim. phase mg/kg/h	Utilization % inf. amount
Glucose 1.0	493.7	215.7	60.3
Xylitol 1.0	483.7	327.1	82.3
Glucose 0.5	337.0	125.2	78.7
Fructose 0.5	410.0	182.2	91.0

of lactic acid from pyruvic acid. This may explain a decrease in the activity of the endocellular proteases as concluded by Carstensen (11).

For these reasons we first studied the utilization rate of fructose in severely traumatized patients. The data are summarized in Table 5. A metabolic rate was found of 410 mg/kg body weight/h during the infusion of 0.5 g/kg body

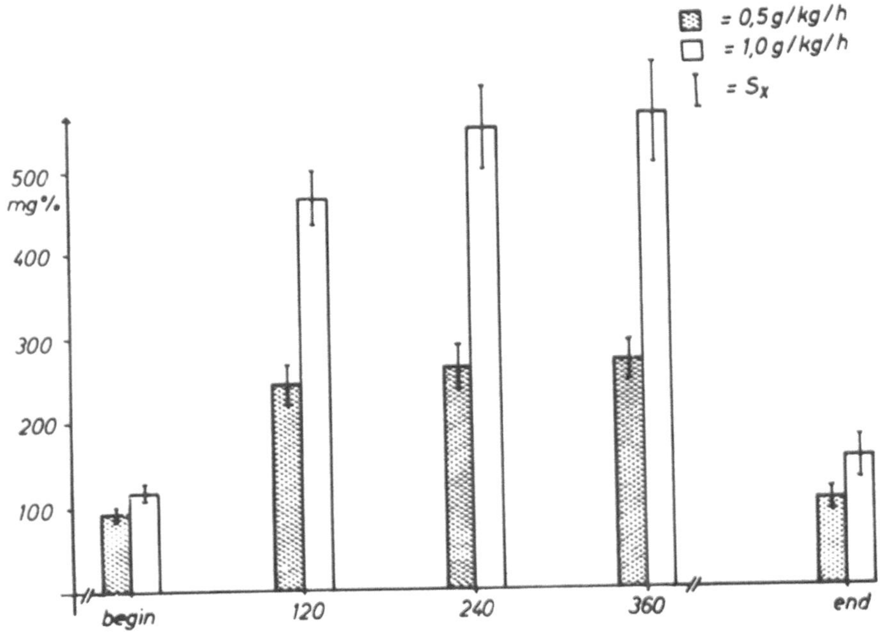

Figure 2. Blood glucose level in severely ill traumatized patients during the infusion of glucose, 0.5 g/kg/hour and 1.0 g/kg/hour.

Table 5. Patient data. Fructose 0.5 g/kg/hour

Nr.	Age years	Weight kg	Sex	Disease
1	72	56	♀	tetanus
2	74	82	♂	multiple rib fract.
3	37	90	♂	cerebral contusion
4	36	90	♂	multiple rib fract.
5	64	84	♀	tetanus
6	65	63	♂	tetanus
7	26	74	♂	cerebral contusion
8	25	72	♂	cerebral contusion
9	24	72	♂	cerebral contusion
10	60	88	♂	multiple rib fract.

weight/h fructose. The total amount utilized equaled 91.0% of the amount infused (Table 4). The blood glucose level remained about normal (Fig. 3). Lactate and pyruvate were only slightly elevated, phosphate was nearly unchanged (Fig. 4).

In spite of the small changes in lactate concentration in our experiments, we would like to point out that the use of fructose in high doses causes high lactate levels in the organism which can be especially dangerous in cases of hypoxia.

To be able to reduce these clinical risks during parenteral nutrition, we looked for additional carbohydrate sources which can be used as an intravenous caloric source.

Schultis and Geser (12) and also Yoshikawa (13) have shown that the administration of xylitol nearly normalizes the utilization of glucose in the posttraumatic period. It also reduces the production of ketone bodies and improves nitrogen balance. In spite of these facts, we infused xylitol in severely traumatized patients. The patient data are shown in Table 6.

When infusing 1.0 g xylitol/kg body weight/h, an average metabolic rate of 483.7 mg/kg body weight/h was found during the infusion and a total metabolic rate of 82.3% of the infused amount of xylitol (Table 4). The relatively high excretion of xylitol in these experiments as well as the meta-

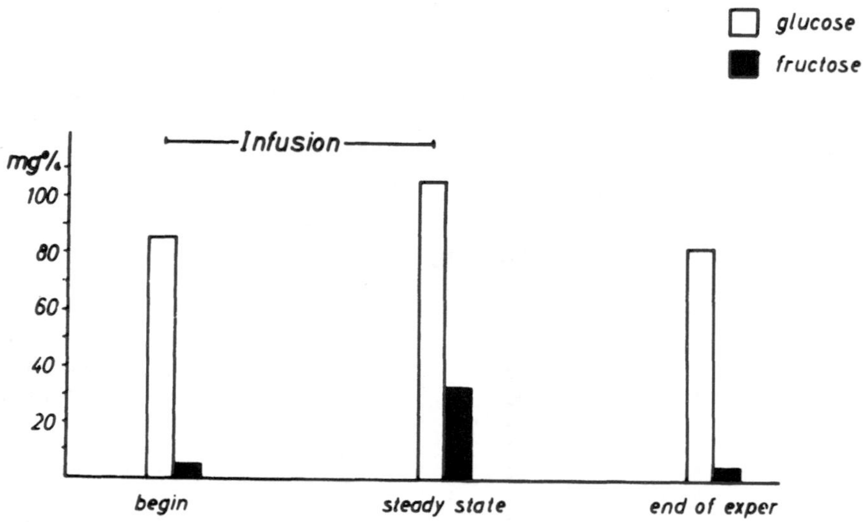

Figure 3. Concentrations of fructose and glucose in blood during and after the infusion of 0.5 g/kg/hour fructose in severely traumatized patients.

bolic rate during infusion indicates that it is not advisable to use xylitol alone as an energy source.

The results of all our clinical experimental studies as well as our clinical observations underscored the high risk of parenteral nutrition when high doses of a single carbohydrate are used to provide sufficient calories in severely traumatized patients. Consequently, it seemed preferable to us to administer combinations of carbohydrates in order to avoid metabolic complications.

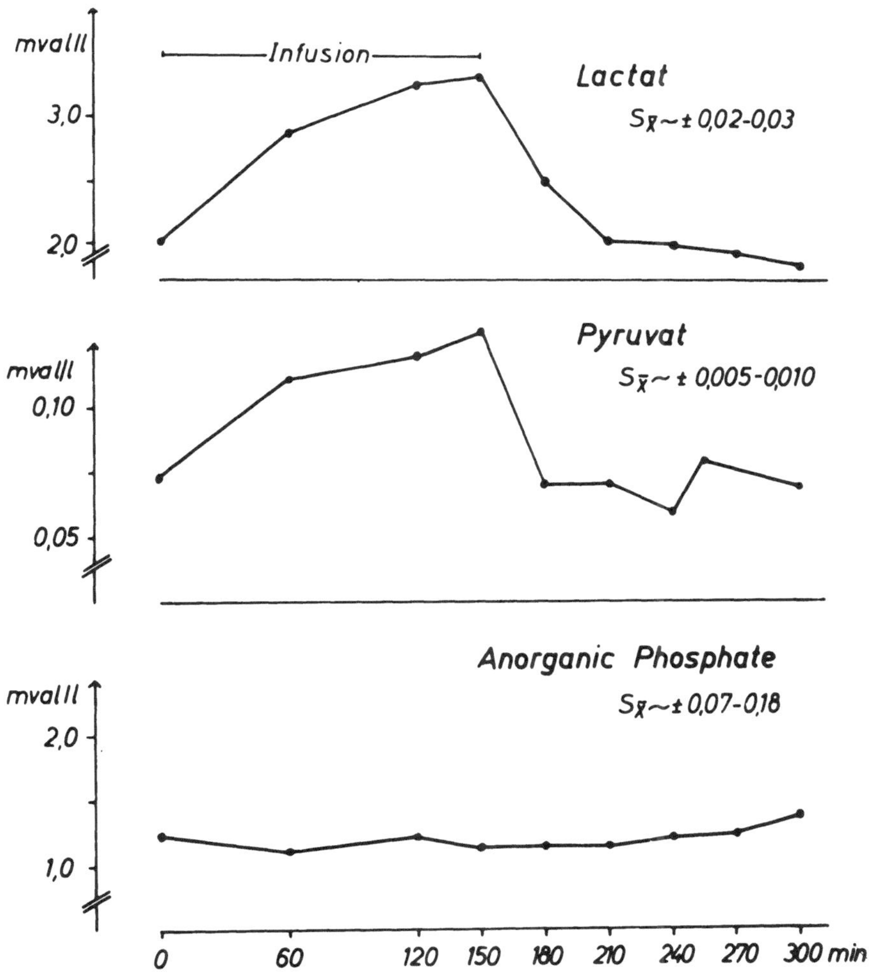

Figure 4. Concentration of lactate, pyruvate and anorganic phosphate in blood during and after the infusion of 0.5 g/kg/hour fructose in severely traumatized patients.

Table 6. Patient data. Xylitol 1.0 g/kg/hour

Pat.	Weight in kg	Habitus	Sex	Diagnosis
M.A.	82.0	obsese	♂	tetanus
D.M.	74.8	obese	♀	tetanus
K.M.	48.8	thin	♂	cerebral contusion
D.N.	63.6	normal	♂	tetanus
S.P.	68.9	normal	♂	tetanus
H.B.	80.7	obese	♂	tetanus
E.K.	74.1	normal	♂	gastric ulcer
S.N.	59.1	thin	♂	cerebral contusion
B.K.	63.9	thin	♂	cerebral contusion
M.L.	72.7	normal	♂	cerebral contusion

Table 7. Patient data. Infusion of a carbohydrate mixture lasting 150 minutes (fructose, glucose and xylitol - 2:1:1), 1.0 g/kg/hour

Nr.	Age years	Sex	Weight kg	Disease
1	24	♂	55	co intoxication
2	64	♀	78	tetanus
3	21	♀	45	cerebral contusion
4	61	♂	64	subdur. haem.
5	65	♂	63	Tetanus
6	23	♂	80	cerebral contusion
7	26	♂	78	cerebral contusion
8	25	♂	73	cerebral contusion
9	36	♀	60	cerebral contusion
10	36	♂	80	cerebral contusion

Table 8. Metabolic rate of carbohydrates in traumatized and severely ill patients during the infusion of a carbohydrate mixture lasting 150 minutes (fructose, glucose and xylitol - 2:1:1), 1.0 g/kg/hour

Dosage g/kg/h	Inf. Phase mg/kg/h	Elim. Phase mg/kg/h	Utilization % inf. amount
Glucose 0.25	178.4	64.4	97.0
Xylitol 0.25	178.8	48.8	91.1
Fructose 0.50	390.8	95.0	97.4

With that regard, we studied the metabolic rate of different carbohydrates given intravenously as a mixture. The patient data are given in Table 7.

We used a solution recommended by Bässler (14) containing 50% fructose, 25% glucose and 25% xylitol. This was infused at a dose of 1.0 g/body weight/h over a period of 150 minutes. During this period a steady-state was reached for each carbohydrate. The metabolic rate of these carbohydrates was calculated according to the suggestions of Müller (6). In these experiments we found a good metabolic rate for each carbohydrate. Fructose and glucose were metabolized at a rate of 97% of the infused amount, xylitol at a rate of 91% (Table 8). Blood glucose levels were slightly elevated (Fig. 5). Lactate and pyruvate concentrations rose slightly (1-2 meq/l). Anorganic phosphate remained at the basic level (Fig. 6).

The next problem to be solved was how this carbohydrate mixture was tolerated when given over a period of several days. In our attempt to answer this fundamental question, we studied the metabolic rate of the previously mentioned carbohydrates and their metabolic effects. The same carbohydrate mixture was infused continuously at a rate of 0.5 g/body weight/h for 5 days to severely traumatized patients. The patient data is summarized in Table 9.

In 8 out of the 10 patients examined, blood glucose levels were only slightly elevated. In two cases, however, there was a significant increase (Fig. 7). Fructose and xylitol concentrations in blood did not exceed the expected

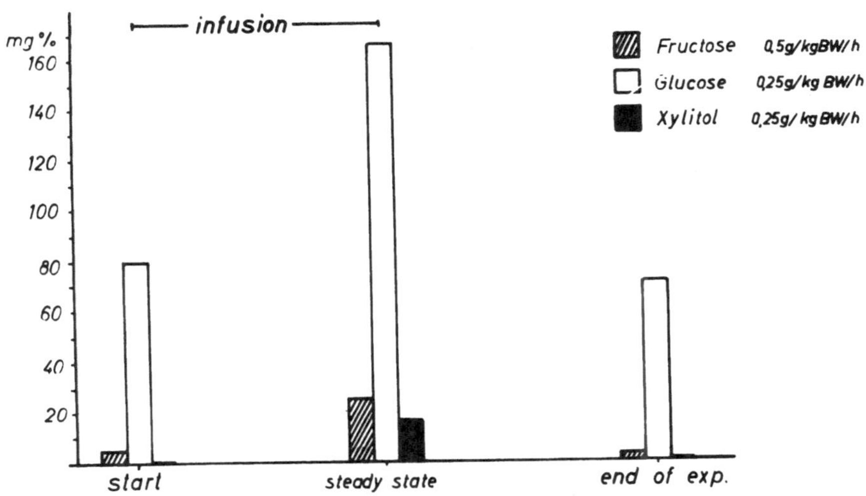

Figure 5. Concentration of carbohydrates in blood during and after the infusion of 1.0 g/kg/hour carbohydrate mixture in severely traumatized patients.

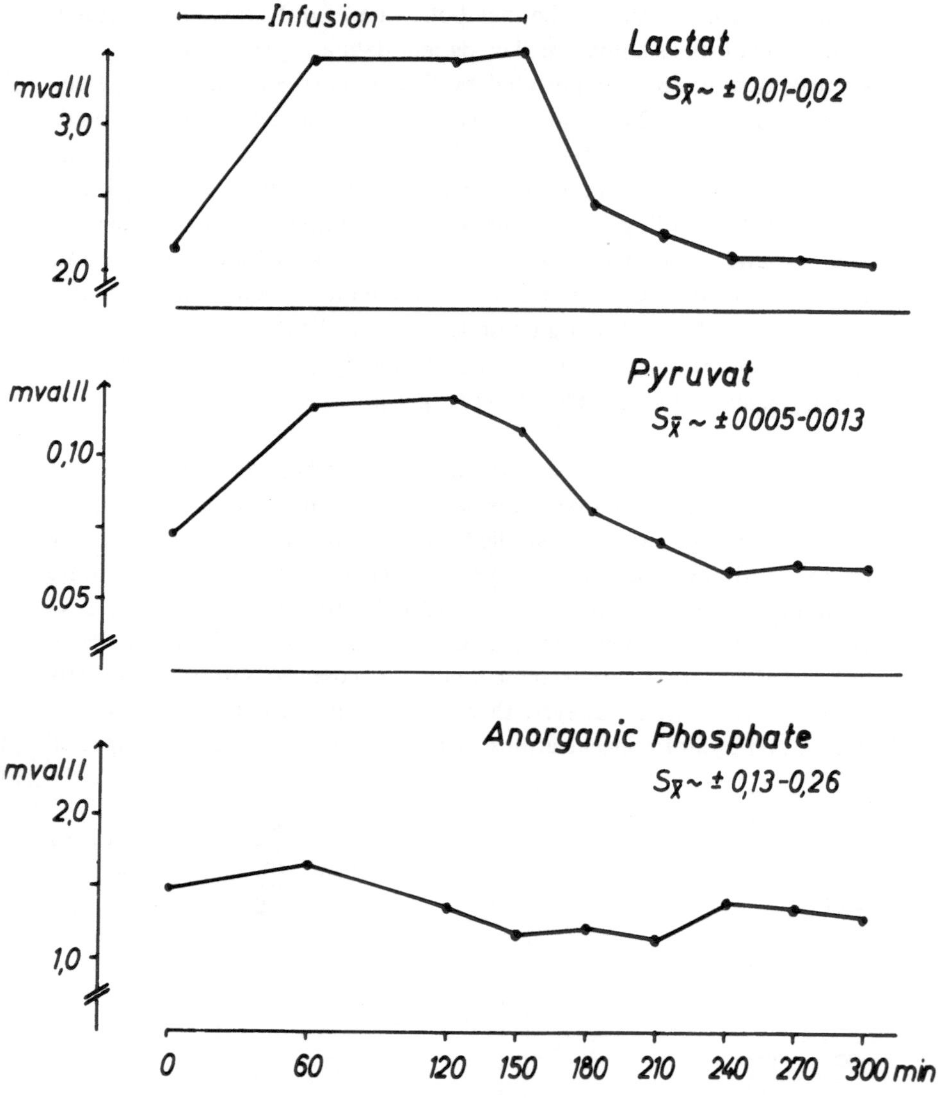

Figure 6. Concentrations of lactate, pyruvate and anorganic phosphate in blood during and after the infusion of 1.0 g/kg/hour carbohydrate mixture in severely traumatized patients (n = 10).

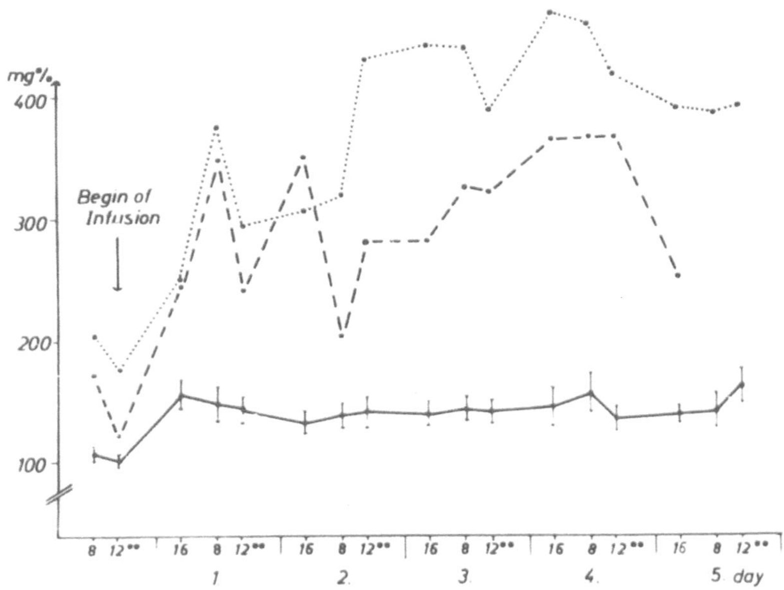

Figure 7. Glucose concentration in blood during the infusion of a carbohydrate mixture (0.5 g/kg/hour) for 5 days in severely traumatized patients.

Table 9. Patient data. Infusion of a carbohydrate mixture for 5 days (fructose, glucose and xylitol - 2:1:1), 0.5 g/kg/hour

No.	Weight kg	Sex	Disease
1	87	♂	multiple trauma
2	64	♂	multiple trauma
3	78	♂	multiple trauma
4	56	♀	multiple trauma
5	59	♂	intracran. bleeding
6	61	♀	tumor (postop.)
7	66	♂	multiple trauma
8	63	♂	tumor (postop.)
9	91	♂	intracran. bleeding
10	65	♂	multiple trauma

levels (Fig. 8 and 9). The total daily metabolic rate of each carbohydrate was about 97.98 (Table 10).

In these experiments lactate concentrations increased only by 1-2 meq/l (Fig. 10). The pH values and base excess values remained within the normal ranges (Fig. 11). Uric acid, anorganic phosphate and alkaline phosphate levels showed minor changes (Fig. 12). The insulin secretion was sufficiently stimulated (Fig. 13).

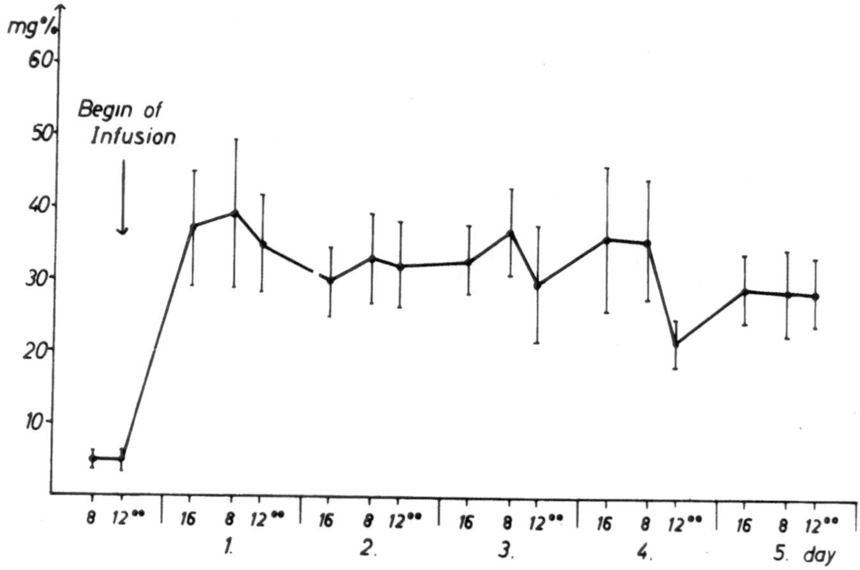

Figure 8. Fructose concentration in blood during the infusion of a carbohydrate mixture (0.5 g/kg/hour) for 5 days in severely traumatized patients.

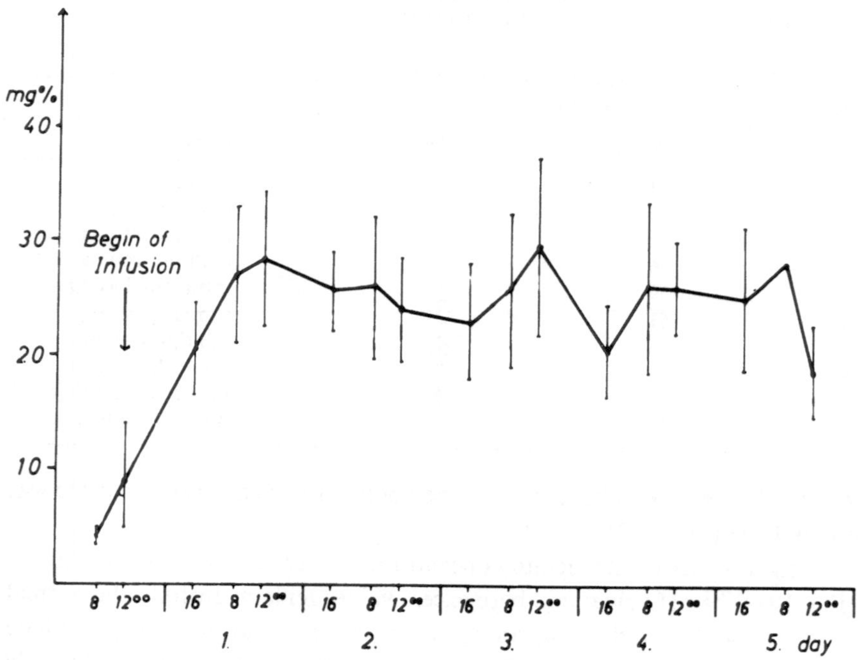

Figure 9. Xylitol concentration in blood during the infusion of a carbohydrate mixture (0.5 g/kg/hour) for 5 days in severely traumatized patients.

Table 10. Daily metabolic rate of carbohydrates during the infusion of a carbohydrate mixture for 5 days.

Dosage g/kg/h		1st day	2nd day	3rd day	4th day	5th day
Fructose 0.25	$\bar{x}$	98.28	97.51	97.72	97.77	98.01
	$S_{\bar{x}}$	0.35	0.49	0.73	0.58	0.52
Xylitol 0.125	$\bar{x}$	97.95	97.99	97.71	97.80	98.19
	$S_{\bar{x}}$	0.33	0.35	0.58	0.53	0.49
Glucose 0.125	$\bar{x}$	99.12	97.25	95.05	98.10	96.86
	$S_{\bar{x}}$	0.43	1.04	4.71	0.75	1.93

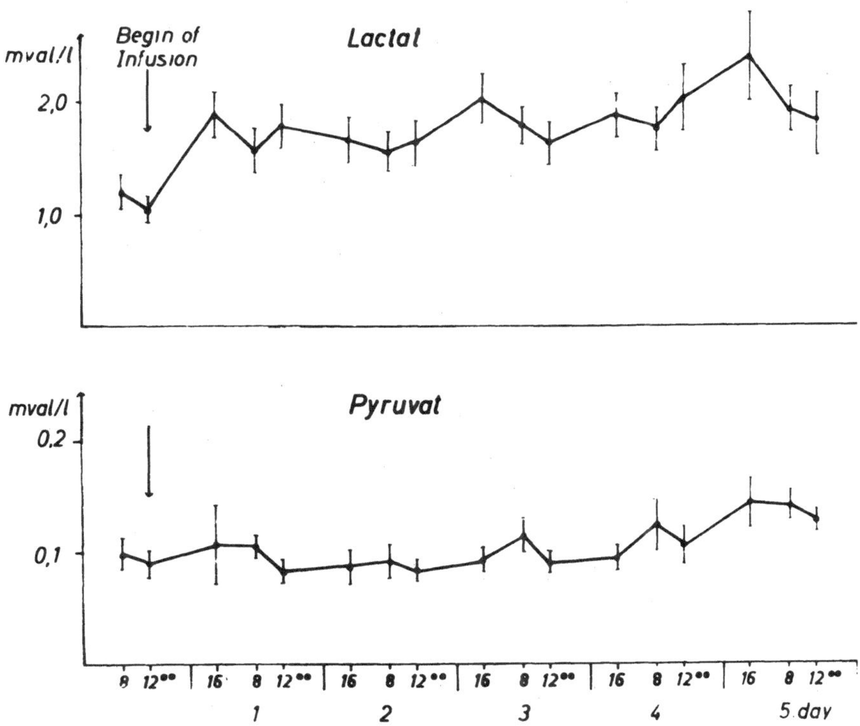

Figure 10. Concentrations of lactate and pyruvate in blood during the infusion of a carbohydrate mixture (0.5 g/kg/hour) for 5 days in severely traumatized patients).

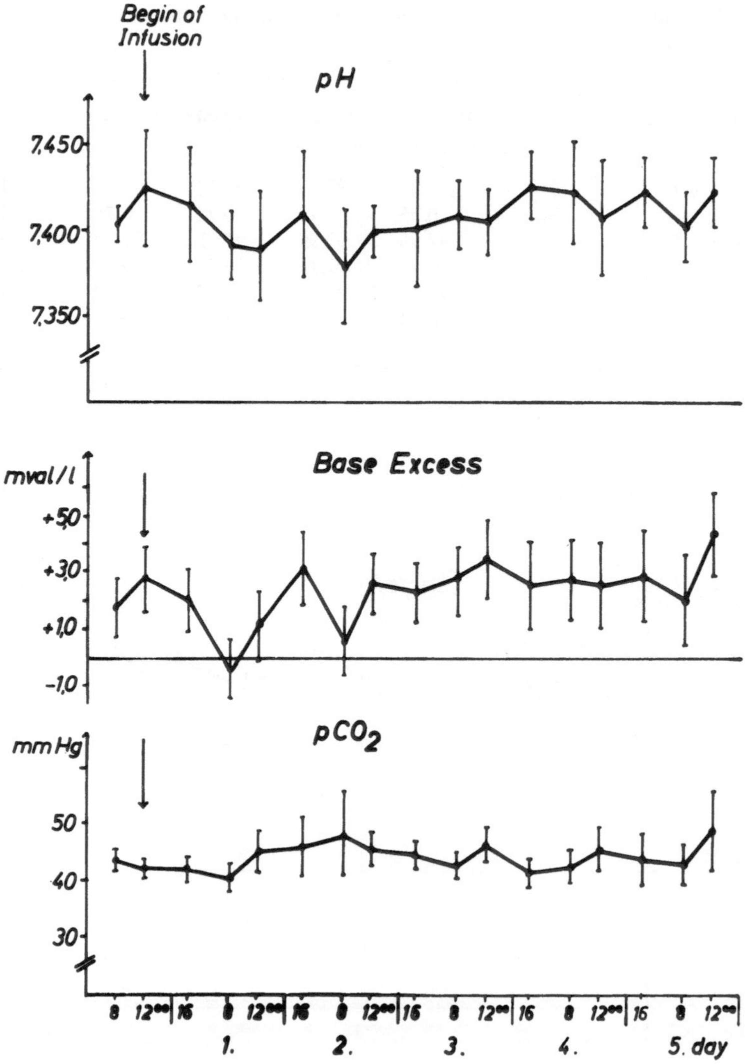

Figure 11. pH, base excess and P_{CO_2} values in blood during the infusion of a carbohydrate mixture (0.5 g/kg/hour) for 5 days in severely traumatized patients.

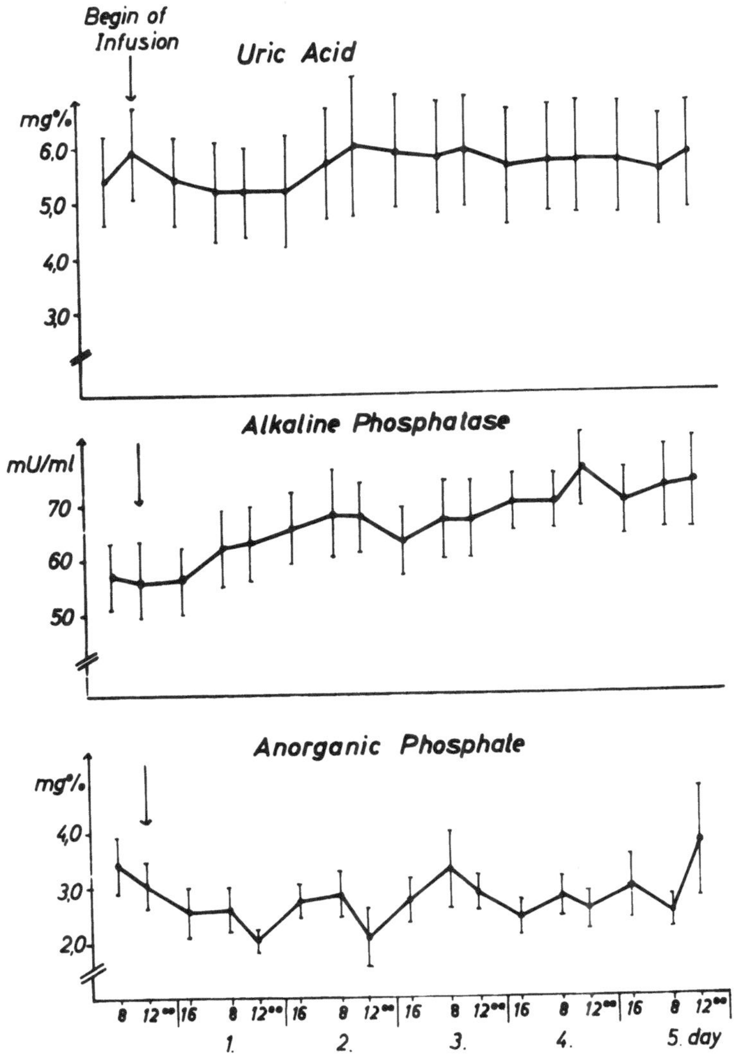

Figure 12. Concentrations of uric acid, alkaline phosphatase and anorganic phosphate during the infusion of a carbohydrate mixture (0.5 g/kg/hour) for 5 days in severely traumatized patients.

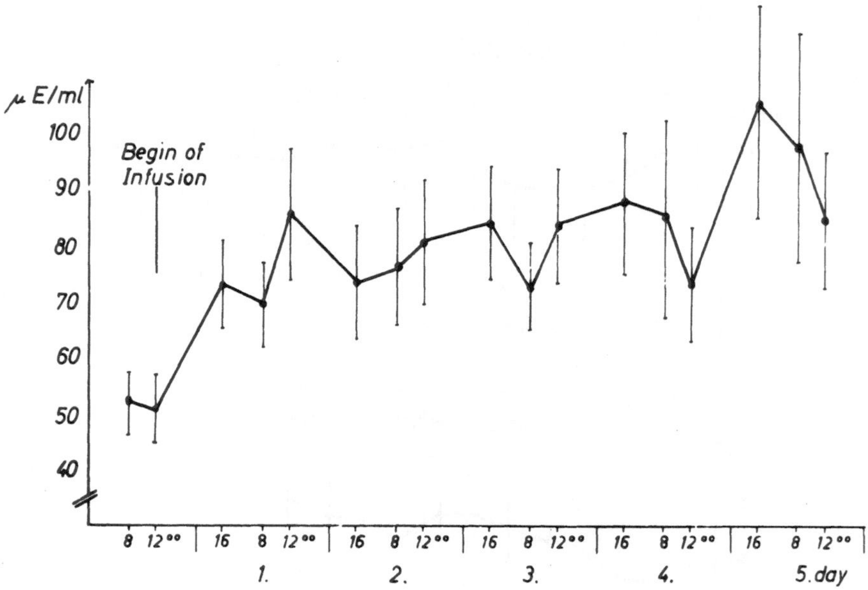

Figure 13. Insulin concentration during the infusion of a carbohydrate mixture (0.5 g/kg/hour) in severely traumatized patients.

In conclusion, it is clear that a normal healthy person can easily assimilate large amounts of glucose. However, severely traumatized patients are not able to metabolize glucose normally. Therefore, it can be dangerous to infuse large amounts of glucose. In these cases the advantage of a carbohydrate mixture over glucose is quite obvious. For these reasons our observations might suggest to use carbohydrate mixtures containing 50% fructose, 25% xylitol and 25% glucose to cover caloric needs in severely traumatized patients.

We recommend the use of amino acid solutions as a nitrogen source and fat-emulsion as a source of essential fatty acids. The nitrogen intake should be approximately 0.3 g nitrogen/kg body weight/day; the protein-free caloric intake of carbohydrates should reach 120% of a patient's basal metabolic rate; fat emulsions should be given at a rate of 500 cc of a 10% solution every second day after two weeks of intravenous nutrition. Water, electrolyte, calorie and nitrogen balances should be controlled in patients who are severely catabolic.

REFERENCES

1. Halmágyi, M. P. B. and Kilbinger, G., Clinical experimental study on the relationship between energy supply and nitrogen balance. In: Wilkinson, A. W. (ed.), Parenteral Nutrition. Churchill Livingstone, Edinburgh and London, 1972.
2. Collins, F. D., Sinclair, A. J., Royle, J. P., Coats, D. A., Maynard, A. T. and Leonard, R. F., 2nd Internat. Sympos. Atherosclerosis, Nov. 1969, Chicago, Ill. USA.
3. Zöllner, N. U., Berhenke und Heuckenkamp, P. U., Vergleich der Verwertung von Fruktose und Glukose beim Menschen bei langdauernder parenteraler Zufuhr. *Klin. Wschr. 45*- 848 (1967).
4. Weinstein, J. J. and Roe,'J. H., The utilization of dextrose, laevulose and invert sugar by normal and surgical patients. *The Am. J. of Proctology 4*: 117 (1963).
5. Bickel, H., Bünte, H., Coats, D. A., Misch, P., v. Rauffer, L., Scranowitz, P. und Wopfner, F., Die Verwertung parenteral verabreichter Kohlenhydrate in der postoperativen Phase. *Dtsch. med. Wschr. 98*: 809 (1973).
6. Müller, F., Zur Kinetik der Elimination aus dem Blut. *Acta biol. med. germ. 10*: 10 (1963).
7. Lotspeich, K., *J. Biol. Chem. 179*: 175 (1969).
8. Schuberth, IX. International Congress of Nutrition, Mexico, Sept. 1972.
9. Strauss, E. und Hiller, J., Die Leavuloseverwertung des Diabetes mellitus und ihre biochemischen Grundlagen. *Ärtzl. Forsch.* (Wörishofen) *4*: 326 (1952).
10. Stuhlfauth, K., Engelhardt-Gölkel, A., Plessner, K., Steinhuber, B., Wollheim, D., Struppler, V., Pirner, F., Netzer, C. D. und Tusban, L., Untersuchungen über die Störungen des Stoffwechsels nach Operationen und deren therapeutische Beeinflussung durch Kohlenhydrate. *Z. klin. Med. 153*: 287 (1955).
11. Carstensen, E., Infusionstherapie und parenterale Ernährung in der Chirurgie. Schattauer, Stuttgart 1964.
12. Schultis, K. and Geser, C. A., Observation on anticatabolic effect of xylitol in the posttraumatic phase. In: Horecker, B. L. et al. (ed.), Pentoses and Pentisols. Springer, Berlin-Heidelberg-New York, 1969.
13. Yoshikawa, K., Xylitol infusion related to pathophysiology in anesthesia. In: Horecker, B. L. et al. (ed.), Pentosis and Pentisols. Springer, Berlin-Heidelberg-New York, 1969.
14. Bässler, K. H., Die Rolle der Kohlenhydrate in der parenteralen Ernährung. In: Parenterale Ernährung, Springer, Berlin-Heidelberg-New York, 1966.

Parenteral nutrition for patients with severe cardiac illness

Ronald M. Abel, M.D.

In patients with compromised cardiac function, the regular use of intravenous solutions of any composition is a mainstay of modern patient care. The obvious hazard confronting physicians caring for this group of patients is the uncertainty regarding sodium and water metabolism which precludes a "laissez-faire" attitude when predicting the total fluid balance of these patients, since the onset of fluid overload and congestive heart failure can occur rapidly. When this major consideration is added to the difficulties in providing adequate nutritional substrate in the form of calories, nitrogen, minerals and electrolytes, it is obvious that to accept the challenge of providing total parenteral nutrition in such patients is to tackle a complex, but feasible therapeutic goal.

A GROWING PATIENT POPULATION

Cardiac disease is the leading cause of death in the United States in this decade. It is clear that an increasing percentage of older hospitalized patients will be encountered who have moderate to severe impairment of cardiac function. The most prevalent cause of cardiac disability is coronary artery disease which frequently results in an end-stage of poor left ventricular function accompanied by myocardial fibrosis and congestive heart failure. In the average group of hospitalized patients requiring total parenteral nutrition (TPN) over 60 years of age, it may be predicted that half of them will have moderate impairment of cardiac function. As aggressive treatment of chronic diseases in this age group becomes more successful, both surgically and medically, the need to provide adequate nutrition in this setting becomes paramount. The ability to maintain a man 80 years of age with end-state coronary disease in chronic congestive heart failure, who also requires a colonesophageal bypass to palliate an obstructing carcinoma, is the ability to provide total patient care.

The successful therapeutic application of TPN in patients severely restricted in water and sodium intake reflects the ultimate triumph of the discipline of parenteral nutrition. Applied understanding of the neuro-endocrine and renal aspects of congestive heart failure is mandatory. High concentrations of nutritional substances at low infusion rates is a partial solution to the problem of how to provide adequate nutrition in as small a volume of water as possible. The careful use of potent diuretics as an adjunct to intravenous feedings may permit the administration of an even greater number of calories with excretion of the excess free water. Many cardiac patients have required long-term chronic diuretic usage, and an increase in dosage or the addition of a second agent during TPN may be helpful in avoiding fluid overload. Specifically, patients who are not able to utilize their gastrointestinal tract even while receiving oral medicines can be given small increments of parenteral furosemide or ethacrynic acid thereby titrating the need for additional doses against the patient's weight change.

Interest in the management of the cardiac illness itself and the therapy directed toward dysfunction of the respiratory, renal, or central nervous system have taken a high priority in the overall consideration of these patients. The degree of inanition, fatigue, lack of strength and mental depression which are common among patients with chronic cardiac illness, is often quite remarkable and may well be related to poor nutrition. How significant improvement in calorie-nitrogen consumption under these circumstances might affect an overall improvement in the state of well-being is unknown, however. It seems logical to assume that improving a nutritional state which borders on protein-calorie malnutrition would bring some beneficial changes.

One of the advantages of parenteral, compared with oral feedings is the ability to administer a diet carefully controlled and independent of a patient's individual taste or ability to ingest specific amounts of food substances. Additionally, the lack of palatability of a typical "cardiac" diet frequently is the very reason for the poor caloric intake. For example, a diet limited in sodium to 500 mgs per day and in fluid to 1500 ml combined with the necessity of ingesting large quantities of potassium to cover losses that diuretic therapy frequently creates, is associated with a voluntary decrease of caloric intake of far less than 1,000 kilocalories per day in an average adult cardiac patient. In a similar condition, where there exists indications for TPN within the same limitations of fluid and sodium restriction, it is possible to nearly double the usual caloric and nitrogen intake with no dependence upon patient acceptance of a specific dietary regimen.

GENERAL MANAGEMENT CONSIDERATIONS IN PATIENTS WITH CARDIAC ILLNESS FLUID MANAGEMENT

The usual patient with mild congestive heart failure can be given from 1500 to 2500 ml per day with an appropriate sodium restriction. In patients who are unable to eat normally, similar guidelines for fluid administration should be followed carefully during parenteral nutrition. In patients with combined gastrointestinal and cardiac difficulties where intestinal fluid losses are also present (e.g. nasogastric drainage, bowel fistulae), the total "space" for fluid administration is increased. The loss of non-calorie containing endogenous fluids may be substituted by intravenous nutritional fluids on a millimeter per milliliter basis, thereby reaching an even greater caloric intake. Patients with respiratory failure, on the other hand, who require ventilatory support may tend to have altered fluid balances in the other direction because of the "imbibing" of free water which may take place while patients are on continuous positive pressure ventilation and the total amount of exogenous intravenous fluids must be decreased to prevent insidious fluid overloading (1).

ENDOCRINE AND METABOLIC CONSIDERATIONS

The effects of decreased renal perfusion and secondary hyperaldosteronism which occur in the setting of chronic congestive heart failure give rise to a tendency for the renal tubules to retain sodium tenaciously and to excrete potassium. Improvement in cardiac performance using positive inotropic agents such as digitalis, or by improvement in cardiac output which would occur following cardioversion from an atrial tachyarrhythmia to normal sinus rhythm can result in improved sodium and water excretion directly reflecting cardiac output. In patients with rheumatic heart disease, specifically involving the mitral valve, "normal" events which demand an increase in cardiac output, such as fever, general anesthesia, or trauma, are not met with the usual augmentation in cardiac output. Decreased blood pressure may occur because of an obligatory decrease in peripheral vascular resistance which may further decrease glomerular filtration rate and lead to an additional increase in water and sodium retension. It is likely that if these patients are to be fed parenterally under these conditions, they will be less able to tolerate a given volume and sodium load until additional metabolic stresses have been corrected.

Spironolactone is by itself, or in combination with one of the thiazide diuretics, a convenient drug used in reversing the abnormal sodium retention associated with hyperaldosteronism. The most frequently employed potent diuretics used in patients with acute and chronic cardiac decompensation are the tubular-active drugs, ethacrynic acid and furosemide. Potassium loss associated with diuretic therapy is compounded with the "usual" condition existing because of secondary hyperaldosteronism. Furthermore, once patients have improved metabolically because of TPN, the requirement for additonal amounts of exogenous potassium is generally increased (2).

Since many patients receiving diuretic therapy are also receiving digitalis glycosides for the treatment of congestive heart failure, the potential hazards of hypokalemia may become a serious management problem. Potassium salts in dosages from 40 to as high as 200 milliequivalents per 24 hours may be necessary to prevent significant hypokalemia which may result in caridac arrhythmias especially in the presence of digitalis therapy. It should be noted that with many of the potent diuretics, particularly furosemide, magnesium is lost via the renal tubules along with potassium. Although clinically-significant hypomagnesemia rarely becomes manifest in cardiac patients, this complication should be averted by monitoring serum magnesium concentrations and by appropriate replacement therapy.

As a general rule, there are no specific difficulties encountered with regard to calcium and phosphorus metabolism in patients with cardiac illness. Although total serum concentrations of calcium may be diminished in association with the hypoalbuminemia of inanition and chronic congestive heart failure, the ionized calcium concentration is usually normal. If phosphate-free solutions are utilized to provide TPN, however, resultant hypophosphatemia may result in clinically-significant proportionate increases in serum calcium concentrations.

GLUCOSE METABOLISM

Extremely low cardiac output states during which time alphadrenergic stimulation with peripheral vasoconstriction attempts to provide adequate blood flow to the coronary and cerebral circulations are associated with a marked diminution in splanchnic and skeletal muscle blood flow. This decrease in peripheral blood flow may be associated with diminished utilization of intravenous nutritional substrates. If a stable rate of intravenous carbohydrate infusion for a period of time suddenly becomes associated with glucose intolerance as reflected by hyperglycemia and glycosuria in the absence of the "usual" etiologic factors (sepsis, too rapid an infusion rate, pancreatitis, use of steroids, etc.), a high suspicion must be raised regarding a further decrement in cardiac output as an etiologic factor. Once this occurs, potassium utilization is also diminished so that a concomitant increase in serum potassium concentration may result if the infusion rate is not decreased appropriately. The use of additional amounts of exogenous insulin in this setting may be helpful. As a general rule, however, decrease in the infusion rate is the safest way to prevent serious complications of hyperglycemia.

Glucose intolerance may frequently be found in patients with coronary artery disease because of the obvious association of premature coronary artery disease with diabetes mellitus. Additionally, in patients with so-called "Type IV hyperlipoproteinemia" which may be also associated with adult-onset diabetes mellitus, the use of intravenous carbohydrate may provide a provocative test to make manifest latent a very mild diabetic patient with cardiac illness, this therapeutic modality must be employed with additional caution.

The adrenal response to cardiac emergencies may also result in a decrease in glucose tolerance. The stress of arrhythmias, acute myocardial infarction with or without cardiogenic shock, and the trauma of cardiac surgery itself may result in an increased secretion of catecholamines and glucorticoids which would tend to increase blood glucose concentrations even at a steady rate of intravenous glucose infusion (3).

MANAGEMENT CONSIDERATIONS IN CARDIAC SURGICAL PATIENTS

A basic difference between the cardiac "medical" and the cardiac "surgical" patient who may require TPN therapy is that in the former situation the degree of cardiac dysfunction is generally at a steady rate and few if any significant improvements in cardiac dysfunction can be expected over a long-term basis. In the surgical patient, however, the acute insult of cardiopulmonary bypass and its attendant decrement in cardiac function is usually reversed with the hemodynamic improvement seen following a corrective procedure. The cardiac surgical patient also reflects the "usual" metabolic and hormonal stress patterns so well known in the general surgical patient in the early postoperative period.

Fluids are usually restricted to no greater than 1500 ml/24 hrs in this early postoperative period. Since a certain amount of "allowable" water intake is required in the form of antibiotic infusion mixtures and cardiac pressor agents there is little "space" to indeed provide large quantities of nutritional solutions in this early postoperative period. By increasing the glucose concentration in the usual "keep open" intravenous infusions and by adding nitrogen-containing nutritional compounds, however, one can supply greater than the ordinary amounts of nutritionally-important substances compared to the "usual" 5% dextrose in water.

In an attempt to provide a more concentrated form of nutritional substrates, a highly concentrated parenteral nutrition formula was designed at the Massachusetts General Hospital in 1973. This so-called "cardiac hyperalimentation fluid" utilizes the mixed amino acid solution, Freamine, as the nitrogen source in a concentration of glucose approximating 43% (Table 1).

The hazards of this type of solution compared with the usual glucose-containing parenteral formulas which contain between 20%-25% glucose are obvious: unless low infusion rates are gradually advanced by small increments, problems of hyperglycemia and progressive glucose intolerance may become manifest. The specific metabolic problems peculiar to the postoperative cardiac surgical patient differ only quantitatively from those sus-

Table 1. Constituents of cardiac hyperalimentation solution used at Massachusetts General Hospital (1974).

Substance	Form	Amount	Volume (ml)	Kcal
Protein equivalent	FreAmine 8.5% (McGaw #50076)	28 gm	360	98
Dextrose	Dextrose 70% (McGaw #59185)	350 gm	500	1,190
Potassium	Potassium acetate 3 mEq/ml (McGaw # W-1110)	30 mEq	10	—
	Potassium phosphate 2 mEq/ml (McGaw # W-1140)	20 mEq	10	—
Sodium	—	3.6 mEq	—	—
Magnesium	Magnesium sulfate (Lilly #232)	4 mEq	5	—
Chloride	—	17 mEq	—	—
Ascorbic acid	—	500 mg	2	—
Multivitamins	Berocca C (Roche)	—	1.0	—
	M.V.I. concentrate (USV Pharmaceutical)*	—	2.5	—

* Used once weekly.

tained in the medical cardiac patient as outlined above. The management of electrolyte imbalances are similar, but may be merely more exaggerated during the acute postoperative stage when cardiac output remains variable and additional stresses such as hypo- or hyperthermia significantly effect substrate utilization in the peripheral tissues.

Table 2. Hemodynamic effects of intravenous amino acid infusion (FreAmine).

Time	Peak LVP (mm Hg)	LVEDP (mm Hg)	LV dp/dtmax (mm Hg/sec)	Peak force (GM-WTS)
Control	123	7	1471	50.9
30′ after amino acids	140	3	1833	61.1
Significance*	$p < 0.025$	$p < 0.0125$	$p < 0.025$	$p < 0.025$
Per cent change	+ 12.1	− 57.1	+ 19.7	+ 20.0

* One-tailed p-value.

INDICATIONS FOR TREATMENT

The application of TPN in patients with cardiac illness is quite similar to the general patient population.

Patients with severe protein-calorie malnutrition as a result of long-standing cardiac decompensation may manage to eke out a borderline existence in the absence of acutely stressful metabolic situations. If these patients develop acute illnesses which require the metabolic and nutritional support in order to heal surgical wounds, or to combat infection, for example, inadequate nutrition might potentially hold the balance between survival and death. Patients with long-standing rheumatic heart disease appear to have a higher incidence of malnutrition compared with patients with other forms of heart disease. The reasons for the prevalence of malnutrition in these patients may only be conjectured, but they probably include psychological depression, anorexia associated with chronic illness, lack of palatability of sodium-restricted diets, and poor cardiac output resulting in inadequate exercise. As cardiac reserve diminishes, the capacity to exercise skeletal muscles decreases and combined with inadequate nitrogen intake, peripheral muscle wasting increases.

TREATMENT REGIMEN

The most important aspect of the care of the cardiac surgical patient is scrupulous avoidance of bloodstream infection. Patients with valvular heart disease are not only highly susceptible to the development of bacterial endocarditis, but in low cardiac output states, the possible development of central venous thrombosis becomes more likely and could result in superior vena caval thrombosis with or without pulmonary emboli. In a large group of patients with prosthetic cardiovascular materials (heart valves and synthetic cloth materials such as used in replacement of the thoracic aorta or in patching the right ventricular outflow tract), the risk of established prosthetic endocarditis from "seeding" by a venous catheter is significant. Frequent changing of intravenous catheters used for TPN should follow any unexplained fever even at the great expense of obtaining new intravenous routes as often as every three to five days.

Other difficult problems of managing the care of the postoperative cardiac surgical patient includes care of the catheter entry site in patients with adjacent tracheostomy. Alternative technical approaches to the central veins may be attempted. By using a subcutaneous tunnel after subclavian or internal jugular venapuncture, the skin exit site of the catheter can be placed as far away from the supra-sternal notch as possible. The use of a completely water-tight dressing using an adhesive plastic sheeting (Steri-drape) has been helpful in these situations.

Following cardiac surgery, patients often have indwelling arterial, central venous, left atrial, and pulmonary arterial catheters for pressure monitoring and drug administration. One or two peripheral intravenous sites are additionally placed for colloid administration. The non-hyperalimentation central venous catheters are utilized for administration of hypertonic potassium solutions and for the infusion of cardioactive agents such as epinephrine, isoproterenol, norepinephrine and dopamine. Prophylactic antibiotics in high concentrations are also administered by bolus injection through these central venous catheters. When those patients require TPN, the identification and avoidance of catheter-related sepsis becomes difficult. In the absence of any obvious extra-vascular source of infection, it would be impossible to determine which of the intravascular materials may be responsible for bloodstream seeding and the production of a bacteremia. Furthermore, secondary seeding of intravascular catheters in any location might occur after a bacteremia arising in another anatomical focus, such as the lung, bladder or wound. Even if the primary infection site can be adequately treated with antibiotics and/or drainage, the possibility of a secondarily-infected catheter maintaining a locus of bacteria and fibrin within the bloodstream demands removal of all catheters and replacement of all required catheters at a suitable interval, preferably at least 12 hours if the general medical condition allows.

The management of glucose intolerance in these patients is analogous to general patients requiring TPN. The potential for "run-away" hyperglycemia is very real and may occur within a relatively short period of time. Monitoring of blood sugars as often as every four to six hours during an unstable period of stress (fever, peritoneal dialysis, arrhythmias, "low cardiac output syndrome") is mandatory. The use of increasingly large doses of exogenous insulin mixed directly in the hyperalimentation fluid containers is the preferential route for insulin administration in these patients. In addition, because of poor peripheral circulation, absorption of subcutaneous insulin from peripheral sites is inconstant to insulin ratio. Additional bolus quantities of crystalline zinc insulin should be given intravenously for threatening hyperglycemia.

In a retrospective review of 64 cardiac surgical patients at the Massachusetts General Hospital, (*vide supra*) the overall complication rate was low. Significant hyperglycemia occurred in only six instances and in no patient did hyperglycemic, nonketotic dehydration with coma occur. Those situations in which hyperglycemia occurred were very predictable: sepsis, peritoneal dialysis with glucose, or associated with high doses of gluco-corticoids. There were no instances of "clinical catheter sepsis" in this group of patients, but in one patient a culture of the catheter tip was positive although no blood cultures confirmed the presence of bacteremia. It is only with an extremely low complication rate that one could advocate intravenous feeding in this group of patients in which the complications of TPN could be devastating.

We have previously reported that although malnutrition is a significant negative risk factor in patients undergoing open-heart surgery (4), there was no apparent benefit in these patients of a brief course of "prophylactic" TPN in the early postoperative period.

In fact, the mortality of patients in a prospective study who received TPN using a mixture of crystalline l-amino acids and hypertonic dextrose by central venous catheter was somewhat higher than the matched controls. Although there appeared not to be a cause-and-effect relationship, it was necessary to examine any possible direct untoward cardiac effects of such a nutrient solution.

Although the positive inotropic effects of hypertonic dextrose have been well elucidated (5), no previous studies have reported the inotropic effects of the nitrogen sources commonly used in the commercially-available solutions for human parenteral nutritional use. Since protein hydrolysates are rapidly being supplanted by pure crystalline amino acid solutions, it seemed reasonable to examine the direct cardiac effects of such a latter solution on left ventricular performance (6) in the experimental animal.

In a series of laboratory experiments involving an isovolumetric left heart canine preparation on cardiopulmonary bypass, we examined the force-velocity, length tension, and diastolic compliance relations of the left ventricle prior to, and following administration of clinically-equivalent doses of carbohydrate-free amino acid solutions. Under these circumstances, the effects of such a solution resulted in slight, but statistically significant improvements in these precise indices of left ventricular performance (Table 2). No significant changes in the high energy phosphate stores in the myocardium following infusion of the amino acids was observed. These studies suggested that there was at least no consistent depletion of energy stores during mild, but positive inotropic effects seen of the amino acid infusion. Although we did not elucidate the mechanism of action, it is possible that some of the glucogenic amino acids, such as alanine, may have been directly converted by myocardium for immediate energy sources and the positive inotropic effect observed might have been analogous to that seen following carbohydrate administration itself. We can at least conclude, therefore, that parenteral nutritition is safe for patients with extreme cardiac decompensation.

SUMMARY

The application of TPN to patients with cardiac illness is feasible and is justifiable on many clinical grounds. The presence of cardiac dysfunction no longer serves as a contraindication to intravenous nutritional therapy, but in many instances may actually dictate the use of nutritionally-valuable intravenous fluids. The occurrence of major complications in patients undergoing cardiac surgical procedures provides an additional group of clinical indications for TPN. By careful clinical and biochemical monitoring, major complications of therapy can be avoided and salutory benefits obtained.

REFERENCES

1. Sladen, A., Laver, M. B. and Pontoppidan, H., Pulmonary complications associated with water retention during prolonged mechanical ventilation. *New Eng. J. Med. 279*: 448 (1968).
2. Dudrick, S. J., Wilmore, D. W., Vars, H. M. and Rhoads, J. E., Can intravenous feedings as the sole means of nutrition support growth in the child and restore weight loss in the adult – an affirmative answer. *Znn. Surg. 169*: 974 (1969)
3. Moore, F. D., *Metabolic care of the surgical patient*. Philadelphia: W. B. Saunders Company, 1960.

4. Abel, R. M., Fischer, J. E., Buckley, M. J., Barnett, G. O. and Austen, W. G., Malnutrition in cardiac surgical patients: results of a prospective, randomized evaluation of early postoperative parenteral nutrition. *Arch. Surg. 111*: 45 (1976).
5. Ko, K. K. and Paradise, R. R., The effects of substrates of contractility of rat atria depressed with halothane. *Anesthesiology 31*: 532 (1969).
6. Abel, R. M., Subramanian, V. A. and Gay, William, Jr., Effects of an intravenous amino acid nutrient solution on left ventricular contractility in dogs. *J. Surg. Res.*, in press, 1977.

Parenteral nutrition in hepatic failure

Peter B. Soeters

Patients with hepatic insufficiency tolerate protein poorly. Protein intolerance has been ascribed to the production of ammonia, but an increasing number of investigators has been dissatisfied with ammonia as the sole cause of protein intolerance. Recently, for example, Zieve and his co-workers postulated that interactions between ammonia, mercaptans and short-chain fatty acids may produce the observed mental changes (1).

At Dr. Joseph Fischer's laboratory in Boston, [where I worked for 18 months,] interest in the etiology of hepatic encephalopathy led to the documentation of the changes in the central neurotransmitter profile in experimental hepatic coma (2, 3, 4, 5). Notably, these included an increase in the beta-hydroxylated false neurotransmitters such as phenylethanolamine and octopamine, as well as an increase in serotonin and decrease in norepinephrine. Some of the factors which may influence the control and synthesis of central neurotransmitters are the plasma – and thus the brain concentrations of the neutral amino acids (NAA), including the aromatic amino acids (AAA), phenylalanine, tyrosine and tryptophan, and the branched chain amino acids (BCAA) leucine, valine and isoleucine (3, 4, 6, 7, 8). Phenylalanine and tyrosine are precursors of norepinephrine and dopamine, tryptophan is a precursor of serotonin. A characteristic amino acid pattern is seen in the plasma of patients (9, 10, 11, 12), dogs (13, 14) and rats (15) with chronic hepatic insufficiency or/and a portacaval shunt, including increased AAA levels and decreased BCAA levels. The decrease in plasma BCAA levels may be due to hyperinsulinism as has been suggested by Sherwin (16) and Munro (17). Hyperinsulinism is well-documented in humans (16, 18) and was confirmed by us in dogs (19) and rats (20) with experimental portacaval shunts (Figure 1).

Glucagon may also play a role since we found markedly elevated glucagon levels in dogs with hepatic insufficiency (19) (Figure 1). The observed pathological plasma amino acid pattern may at least in part be responsible for the changes noted in the central neurotransmitters and consequently may contribute to encephalopathy. It occurred to us that we might influence hepatic coma by manipulating this distorted plasma amino acid pattern. In this manner, we could test our hypothesis that a pathological amino acid pattern is related to hepatic encephalopathy and subsequently that normalization leads to an improvement in the mental state.

For this purpose (21), we infused a special glucose-amino acid formula calculated to normalize the plasma amino acid pattern in dogs; these animals had become encephalopathic spontaneously 4-5 weeks after introduction of a portacaval shunt. Notable are the markedly decreased AAA and the increased BCAA levels (Table 1). The controls received a commercially available glucose-amino acid mixture or glucose alone combined with plasma. The group on the specific amino acid solution survived in its entirety for 30 days (Table 2). The results for the other two groups were not as good, but it may be significant that the group which received exclusively glucose did better than the group on the commercial solution.

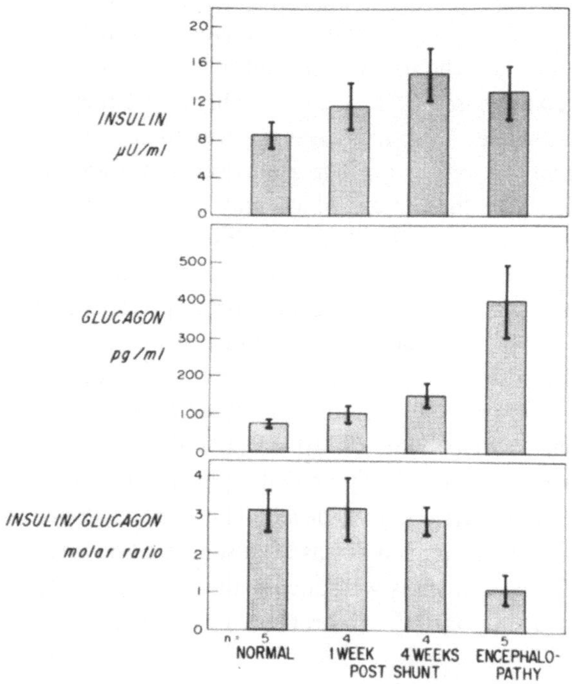

Figure 1. Serial measurement of insulin and glucagon following end-to-side portacaval shunt and in encephalopathy. Results are given as mean ± SME for groups of 5 animals.

Note that there is a modest rise in both insulin and glucagon after introduction of the end-to-side portacaval shunt. As the animal develops hepatic failure and encephalopathy, glucagon rises precipitously.

Table 1. Composition of amino acid mixtures

	Commercial solution gms/1000 ml	Hepatic failure solution gms/1000 ml
L-Essentials		
L-Isoleucine	2.95	4.50
L-Leucine	3.85	5.50
L-Lysine-HCl	3.85	3.80
L-Methionine	2.25	0.50
L-Phenylalanine	2.40	0.50
L-Threonine	1.70	2.25
L-Tryptophan	0.65	0.38
L-Valine	2.80	4.20
Non-Essentials		
L-Alanine	3.00	3.75
L-Arginine	1.55	3.00
L-Histidine	1.20	1.20
L-Proline	4.75	4.00
L-Serine	2.50	2.50
Glycine	9.00	4.50
L-Cysteine . HCl . H_2O	0.02	0.20
Glucose		
23%		
Electrolytes		

Composition of the special "hepatic failure solution" and the "commercial solution" used in these studies.

Table 2. Survival (dogs with portacaval shunts)

		Died in hepatic coma/Total
I.	23% Dextrose + Albumin	2/5
II.	Commercial glucose amino acid mixture	11/13
III.	Hepatic failure glucose amino acid mixture	0/8

Mortality in dogs with portacaval shunts, infused with three different types of solution. Note that none of the dogs that were infused with HFS died. Of the 13 dogs that were infused with a commercial solution 11 died within 30 days.

One might object to this protocol on the grounds that the large amount of protein given is not in agreement with the standard therapy for hepatic insufficiency and encephalopathy. To satisfy this objection and to discount a possible lucky randomization in the first group, we gave a second group either half the amount of amino acids of the commercial composition or a normal amount of specific solution. In addition, we did a cross-over trial using the dogs as their own control. The dogs were included only when they showed clear signs of encephalopathy. Stages of encephalopathy were assessed clinically according to a previously suggested scheme (21):

Stage O – Normal
Stage I – Delayed response, less lively, diminished appetite, but no obvious neurological symptoms.
Stage II – Unsteady gait, "blind" to obstacles (goes through them instead of around them), often profuse salivation.
Stage III – Sleeps most of the time, difficult to arouse, salivating in most cases.
Stage IV – Unresponsive coma.

Tables 3 and 4 show clearly that the mental state improved when the dogs were infused with hepatic failure solution and deteriorated when the dogs were infused with the commercial solution. An obvious explanation would

Table 3. 4 dogs started on hepatic failure solution (HFS)

	2 g protein/kg/hr
1 dog Stage III	– improved to Stage 0 (12 days) – died after 2 days on CS 2 g/kg/hr in Stage IV
1 dog Stage II-III	– improved to Stage 0-I (12 days) – died after 5 days on CS 2 g/kg/hr in Stage IV
1 dog Stage III	– improved to Stage I (12 days) – died after 8 days on CS 2 g/kg/hr in Stage IV
1 dog Stage III	– improved to Stage 0 (12 days) – deteriorated to Stage II after 8 days on CS 2 g/kg/hr and was sacrificed.

Mortality and Stage of Encephalopathy of dogs which were randomly infused with either a commercial solution (CS) (2 g protein/kg/24 hrs) or the hepatic failure solution (HFS) (4 g protein/kg/24 hrs). If the dog was still alive after 12 days, the dog was switched to the other solution.

Note that all dogs improved neurologically and survived with HFS. No dogs improved neurologically with CS and most of them died.

Table 4. 4 dogs started on commercial solution (CS)

	4 g protein/kg/24 hr
1 dog Stage IV	– died after 2 days in Stage IV
1 dog Stage III	– died after 2 days in Stage IV
1 dog Stage III	– stayed in Stage II (12 days)
	– improved to Stage 0 on HFS 4 g/kg/24 hr (8 days)
1 dog Stage III	– stayed in Stage III (4 days)
	– improved to Stage 0 on HFS 4 g/kg/24 hr (2 days)
	– died after another 10 days in Stage IV on CS 2g/kg/hr

Mortality and Stage of Encephalopathy of dogs which were randomly infused with either a commercial solution (CS) (2 g protein/kg/24 hrs) or the hepatic failure solution (HFS) 4 g protein/kg/24 hrs). If the dog was still alive after 12 days, the dog was switched to the other solution.

Note that all dogs improved neurologically and survived with HFS. No dogs improved neurologically with CS and most of them died.

be that prevention of the breakdown of endogenous protein stores clears the circulation of toxic nitrogen and improves the mental state. It should be realized however that a 20 kg dog with a high catabolic rate has to excrete a maximum of 10 gr of nitrogen per day. We gave the dogs approximately 13 gr of nitrogen per 20 kg per day and since they were in approximately 0 nitrogen balance, they still had to excrete 13 gr of nitrogen. The conclusion is, and this is new in hepatic failure treatment: while current management of patients with hepatic insufficiency consists of protein restriction, dogs – and as we will see later humans too (22) – tolerate large amounts of protein, provided AAA are almost excluded and extra BCAA are added. Apparently in a catabolic setting the breakdown of endogenous protein presents the liver with a substrate profile, specifically a nitrogen profile, which the liver can not handle. Tyrosine and phenylalanine are degraded almost exclusively in the liver and the K_m of tyrosine transaminase and phenylalanine hydroxylase are well above the plasma concentrations of their substrates, whereas BCAA are mainly degraded periferally.

Elevations of tyrosine and phenylalanine may reflect breakdown of body cell mass since muscle protein is relatively rich in AAA and because the dogs showed a very high catabolic rate. They were generally starved by the time they were encephalopathic since the fluid intake spontaneously decreased, but dogs and patients with marginal liver function do not appear to be able to adapt to starvation. Even small disturbances in metabolic balance elicit a high catabolic rate, higher than would be expected from the magnitude of the disturbance.

Another phenomenon presented itself in these experiments that may or may not be relevant to hepatic encephalopathy. Markedly elevated ammonia levels were observed in full blown hepatic encephalopathy (Figure 2), but these levels decreased very significantly within 24 hours after infusion of the hepatic failure solution. In most instances, they also decreased after infusion of the commercially available solution albeit to a lesser degree. We can only speculate on the mechanism. Is there an effect on the gut? Muscle and liver

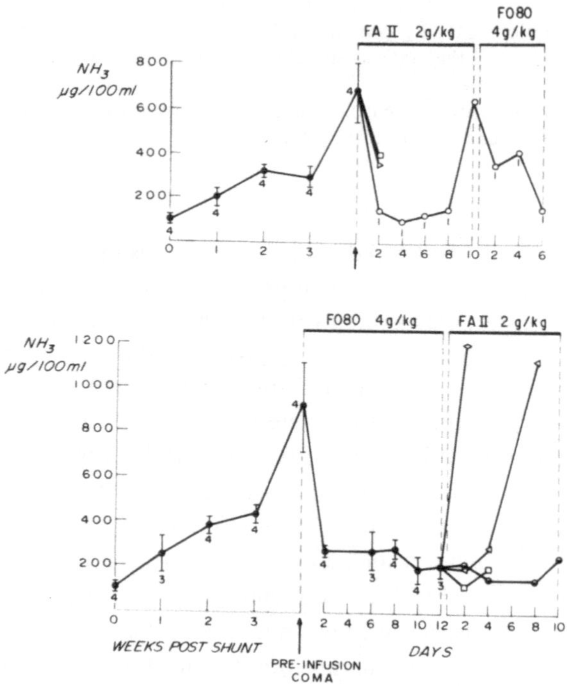

Figure 2. Serial measurement of NH_3 levels before and after introduction of end-to-side portacaval shunt, and during infusion of hepatic failure solution (F080) or a commercial solution (FA II). Results are given as mean ± SEM for groups of animals. The number of animals is depicted in the graph.

Note that NH_3 levels drop initially after infusion of either type of solution. Despite this drop 3 out of the 4 dogs infused with a commercial solution (FA II) died within 48 hrs. (No sample could be obtained from 1 dog). After an initial decrease in NH_3 levels the fourth dog showed a rapid increase. After switching to HFS NH_3 levels decreased again.

The group which was infused with hepatic failure solution (F 080) showed a persistent drop in NH_3 levels. After switching back to a commercial solution (FA II) 3 dogs died. Two had highly elevated NH_3 levels, one only slightly.

do not produce significant amounts of ammonia (23, 24, 25); on the contrary, they may even incorporate small amounts.

Is this ability enhanced by parenteral nutrition? The only organ which is able to produce significant amounts of ammonia apart from the gut is the kidney (24, 26), which is also involved in intermediary metabolism. It has been shown (27, 28, 29) that the kidney is able to produce considerable amounts of ammonia, especially in starvation (27). Maybe we are dealing with that situation since patients or animals in hepatic insufficiency are generally starving. If we feed the experimental animal or the patient parenterally, do we abolish ammonia production by the kidney?

Inclusion of extra BCAA may be crucial for different reasons:

1. Elevation of plasma BCAA may be beneficial at the level of the blood brain barrier, competing with toxic AAA for entry into the brain, resulting in an improved central neurotransmitter profile.
2. The BCAA (especially leucine) are among the more potent stimulators of insulin (30, 39). The insulin response elicited by infusion of a glucose-amino acid mixture may enhance liver regeneration, as recently described by Starzl in a different experimental setting (31).
3. Maria Buse recently proposed (32) that leucine might play a pivotal role in the protein sparing effect of amino acids.

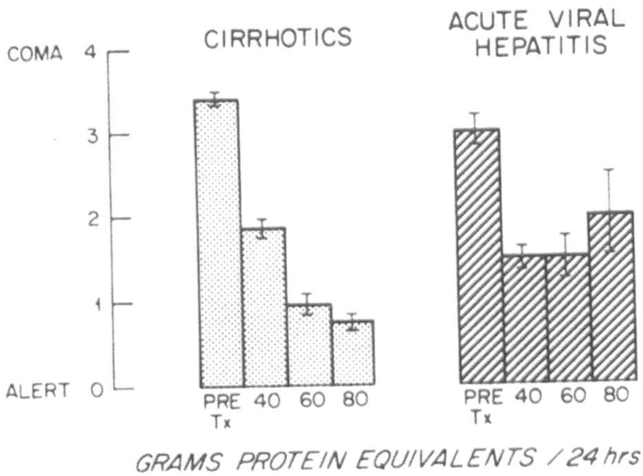

Figure 3. Mean encephalopathic scores vs. infusion of HFS (F080) in patients with two different types of hepatic insufficiency.

Note that in the patients with cirrhosis, there is a rapid return to near normal as the rate of 80 g of amino acids per 24 hrs is achieved.

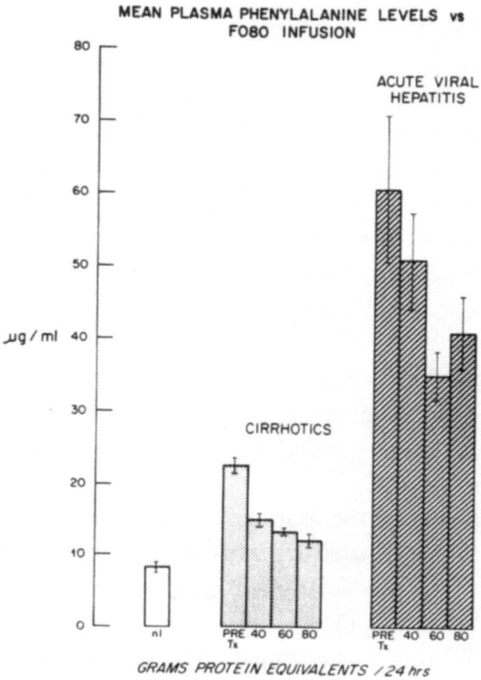

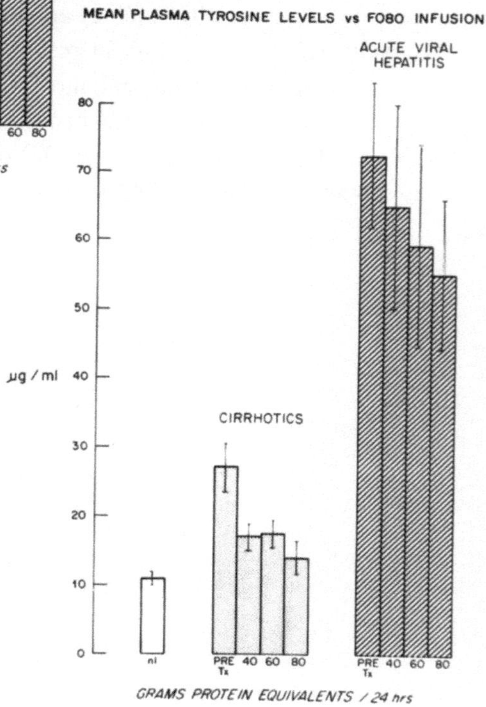

Figure 4, 5. Response of the aromatic amino acids phenylalanine and tyrosine in patients with two different types of hepatic insufficiency.

In the cirrhotics phenylalanine and tyrosine return to near normal with increased dosage.

It is surprising that AAA are elevated by any stimulus which is generally interpreted by the cirrhotic patient as being detrimental to his well-being. Thus, Schenker (33) has proposed the concept of increased cerebral sensitivity in patients with liver disease to explain why diffuse stimuli, such as diuresis, sepsis, gastro-intestinal bleeding, overdose of drugs or any stress situation, result in hepatic encephalopathy.

We proposed (34) that all these stimuli enhance catabolism. This is evident in bleeding with hypovolemia, sepsis, surgery etc. The well-documented reduction (35, 36, 37) in plasma insulin-like activity, elicited by diuretics, creates a diabetes-like state which is equally characterized by catabolism.

Finally, the hepatic failure solution was used in patients (22): all 8 patients with hepatic encephalopathy due to chronic cirrhosis improved neurologically within 24 hrs after starting the infusion of hepatic failure solution. The improvement seemed to be dose-related (Figure 3). In addition, a dose relationship with ammonia, tyrosine, phenylalanine and octopamine was observed (Figure 4, 5, 6, 7). Unfortunately, the multiplicity of problems encountered in these patients precluded a correlation of these parameters with nitrogen balance. Recently however a very significant correlation was found between brain tyrosine and brain phenylalanine and nitrogen balance in rats with experimental portacaval shunts (38).

In conclusion, hepatic encephalopathy appears to be associated with and perhaps caused by abnormalities in the plasma amino acid patterns in ex-

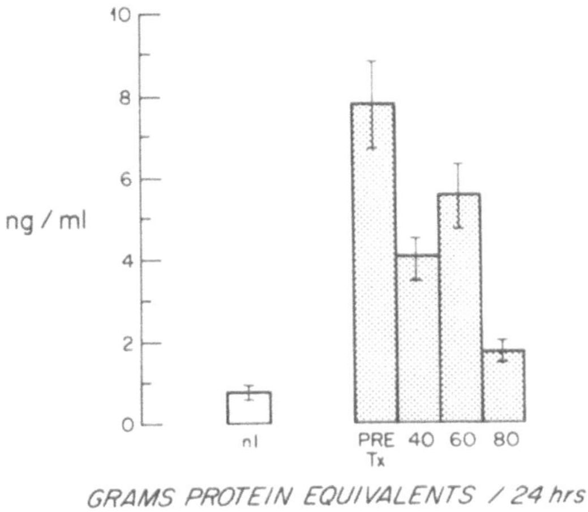

Figure 6. Mean plasma octopamine levels vs infusion of HFS (F 080) in cirrhotics. Plasma octopamine levels return to near normal at 80 gms of amino acids/24 hours.

perimental animals and man. The dominant plasma amino acid pattern appears to have at least two components, a decrease in BCAA and an increase in AAA. A variety of stimuli seems to be able to provoke encephalopathy. They seem to have one feature in common: eliciting catabolism or at least interfering with the metabolic economy of the body. Catabolism is associated with breakdown of endogenous protein from peripheral tissues like muscle and maybe from the liver itself.

Endogenous protein is relatively rich in AAA, which the failing liver is unable to catabolize; thus the AAA accumulate in the circulation, thereby allowing increased amounts of the toxic AAA to penetrate the blood brain barrier and encephalopathy to occur. Appropriate therapy for hepatic encephalopathy appears to consist of reversing the catabolic state by providing adequate amounts of BCAA and calories to decrease the flux of AAA from muscle and liver and maybe re-utilizing them in protein synthesis. Ammonia may or may not be a factor in the genesis of encephalopathy, but therapy via infusions decreases ammonia levels drastically. While our data may not exclude the validity of other hypotheses, they provide us with strong support for the false neurotransmitter hypothesis. The specific form of intravenous nutrition described provides the possibility of restoring nutritional status in patients with liver disease, at the same time improving their mental state. In addition, it may improve liver function by enhancing regeneration.

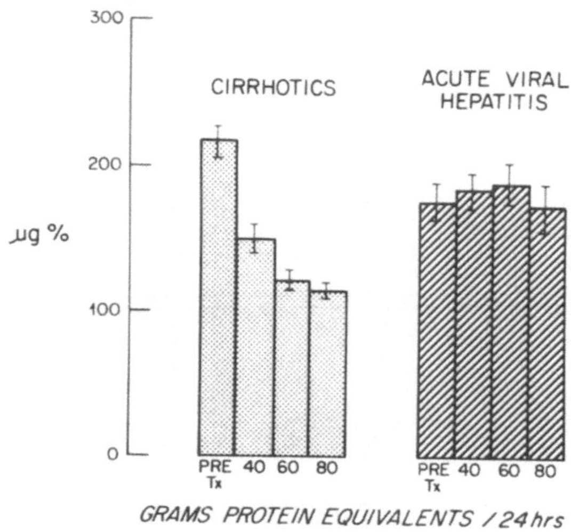

Figure 7. Mean serum NH_3 levels vs infusion of HFS (F 080). Note that in the patients with cirrhosis there is a return to near normal when 80 gms of amino acids per 24 hours is achieved.

REFERENCES

1. Zieve, F. J., Zieve, L., Doizaki, W. M. and Gilsdorf, R. B., *J. Pharmac. exp. Ther. 191*: 10 (1974).
2. Fischer, J. E. and Baldessarini, R. J., *Lancet 2*: 75 (1971).
3. Fischer, J. E. and Baldessarini, R. J. In: Progress in Liver Disease, Vol. 5 (edited by H. Popper and E. Schaffner), p. 363. New York, 1976.
4. Fischer, J. E., Res. Publs Ass. Res. nerv. ment. Dis. 1974, 53, 53.
5. Dodsworth, J. M., James, J. H., Cummings, M. G. and Fischer, J. E., *Surgery 75*: 811 St. Louis (1974).
6. Fischer, J. E. In: Artificial Liver Support (edited by R. Williams and I. Murray-Lyon), p. 31. London, 1975.
7. Wurtman, R. J., Larin, F., Mostafapour, S. and Fernstrom, J. D., *Science 185*: 183 (1971).
8. James, J. H., Hodgman. J. M., Funovics, J. M. and Fischer, J. E., *J. Neurochem. 27*: 233 (1976).
9. Iber, F. L., Rosen, H., Levenson, S. M. and Chalmers, T. C., *J. Lab. clin. Med. 50*: 417 (1957).
10. Richmond, J. and Girdwood, R. H., *Clin. Sci. 22*: 301 (1962).
11. Iob, V., Coon, W. W. and Sloan, M., *J. Surg. Res. 6*: 233 (1966).
12. Fischer, J. E., Yoshimura, N., Aguirre, A., Cummings, M. G., Abel, R. M. and Deindoerfer, E., *Am. J. Surg. 40*: 127 (1974).
13. Aguirre, A., Yoshimura, N., Westman, T. and Fischer, J. E., *J. Surg. Res. 16*: 339 (1974).
14. Iob, V., Mattson, W. J., Sloan, M., Turcotte, J. G. and Child, C. G., *Surgery Gynec. Obstet. 130*: 794 (1970).
15. James, J. H., Hodgman, J. M. Funovics, J. M., Yoshimura, N. and Fischer, J. E., *Metabolism 25*: 471 (1976).
16. Sherwin, R., Joshi, P., Hendler, R., Felig, P. and Conn, H. O., *New Engl. J. Med. 290*: 239 (1974).
17. Munro, H. N., Fernstrom, J. D. and Wurtman, R. J., *Lancet 1*: 722 (1975).
18. Marco, J., Diego, J., and Villanueva, M. L., *Ibid. 289*: 1197 (1973).
19. Soeters, P. B., Weir, G., Ebeid, A. M. and Fischer, J. E.*J. Surg. Research*. In press 1977.
20. Soeters, P. B., Keane, J., Escourrou, J. and Fischer, J. E., Unpublished results.
21. Fischer, J. E., Funovics, J. M., Aguirre, A., James, J. H., Keane, J. M., Wesdorp, R. I. C., Yoshimura, N. and Westman, T., *Surgery 78*: 276 St. Louis (1975).
22. Fischer, J. E., Rosen, H. M., Ebeid, A. M., James, J. H., Keane, J. M. and Soeters, P. B., *Ibid. 80*: 77 (1976).
23. Gauda, P. and Ruderman, N. B., *Metabolism 25*: 427 (1976).
24. Baertl, J. M., Sancetta, S. M. and Gabunda, G. J., *J. Clin. Invest. 42*: 696 (1963).
25. Bessman, S. P. and Bessman, A. N., *J. Clin. Invest. 34*: 622 (1955).
26. Owen, E. E., Tyor, M. P., Flanagan, J. F. and Berry, J. N., *J. Clin. Invest. 39*: 288 (1960).
27. Cahill, G. V., Jr., *N.E.J.M. 282*: 668 (1970).
28. Goodman, A. D., Fuisz, R. E. and Cahill, G. F., Jr., *J. Clin. Invest. 45*: 612 (1966).
29. Goorno, W. E., Rector, F. C., Jr. and Seldin, D. W., *Am. J. Phys. 213*: 969 (1967).
30. Floyd, J. C., Fajans, S. S., Conn, J. W., Knopf, R. F. and Rull, J., *J. Clin. Invest. 45*: 1487 (1966).
31. Starzl, T. E., Watanabe, K., Porter, K. A. and Putnam, C. W., *The Lancet 1*: 821-825 (1976).

32. Buse, M. G. and Reid, S. S., *J. Clin. Invest. 46*: 1250 (1975).
33. Schenker, S., *Viewpoints dig. Dis. 2*: 4 (1970).
34. Soeters, P. B. and Fischer, J. E., *Lancet 2*: 880 (1976).
35. Shapiro, A. P., Benedeck, T. G. and Small, J. L., *New Engl. J. med. 265*: 1028 (1961).
36. Chazan, J. A. and Boshell, B. R., *Diabetes 14*: 132 (1965).
37. Skulan, T. W. and Shideman, F. E., *J. Pharmac. exp. Ther. 148*: 356 (1965).
38. Rosen, H. M., Soeters, P. B., Keane, J. M., James, H. and Fischer, J. E., To be published.
39. Milner, R. D. G., *The Lancet 1*: 1075 (1969).

Complications of parenteral nutrition

Josef E. Fischer, M.D.

Complications of parenteral nutrition can generally be grouped under three headings. First, technical complications, those associated with access and with late thrombosis. The second and most dreaded complication is that of sepsis, both bacterial and fungal. Finally, metabolic complications.

1. TECHNICAL COMPLICATIONS

Most frequent technical complications are those of access. In a recently reported series (1), pneumothorax constituted approximately 4% of catheterizations performed by various house and visiting staff. Other technical complications of catheterization include arterial laceration requiring repair, which is rare, although arterial puncture is perhaps more common but generally subsides without difficulty. Although a number of arterial lacerations is perhaps more common than one might expect, AV fistulas are rare, although they have been reported. It is not clear why patients should sustain nerve injury during catheterization of the subclavian vein, although the phrenic nerve may be injured during an internal jugular approach. Nonetheless, nerve injury has been reported and we have seen this in our own personal experience in this institution. Malposition of the catheter tip in the neck, when a confirmatory x-ray is not taken, may result in thrombophlebitis. Thus, an x-ray is mandatory prior to beginning any hypertonic infusion. At times the catheter tip will have perforated the vein. This can easily be ascertained by lowering the bottle and watching blood flow back. Infusion of a glucose rich solution into the pleural space will result in prompt dyspnea, pleuritic pain, and shock. This can be confirmed by aspiration of a glucose rich solution from the pleural space. There is another form of pleural effusion whose cause is not known, but in whom a transudate appears within one of the pleural cavities, not a glucose rich infusion. The treatment of this involves removal of the catheter, as one of the causes may be mediastinal hematoma and bleeding.

Late complications include erosion to various structures and even erosion into bronchi has been reported.

A more distressing late complication is thrombosis (2). Thrombosis may be associated with sepsis, in which case patients become very ill, and long term treatment of antibiotics is necessary if a patient is to survive. On the other hand there is a disturbing frequency of nonseptic thrombosis or phlebothrombosis, in patients who do not get septic. In an autopsy report from this institution of 34 patients thus autopsied, 8 had thrombosis of the subclavian or superior vena cava. Casual clinical observations suggest that while this is not at all common, it does occur and sometimes one needs to see but a slightly swollen shoulder, side of the neck or face with an increased venous pattern to know that thrombosis has occurred. It seemingly has little to do with duration. Many of the catheters around which thrombosis was observed in the postmortem examination were in place for only 3-4 days and associated with low flow states. It can no longer be assumed that pulmonary emboli arise from the lower extremities as pulmonary emboli have arisen from thromboses of the superior vena cava. The material is perhaps at fault. Polyvinylchloride appears to be a more reactive material than, for example, silastic which appears in both animal and human experiments to have a much lower incidence of thrombosis.

2. SEPSIS

By far the most dreaded complication related to catheter sepsis. In examining this complication there are several possibilities as to its cause. First, the duration of catheterization and second, the technique of catheterization, the third the care of the dressings. Although other institutions have reported a higher incidence of sepsis following long term parenteral catheterization, i.e. after 30 days (3), this has not been the experience at this institution. In a study published in 1974 by Ryan, et al. (2), clinical catheter sepsis appeared to be correlated not with duration but with catheter care. In this study, the fates of 355 catheters in 200 patients were followed prospectively. In 275 patients whose catheters received good care and there were no violations reported, sepsis was approximately 3%, while a 20% incidence, 7 times higher, was reported in 80 patients whose catheter had been violated or whose protocol had not been exactly followed. This incidence is so high that one might consider pulling a catheter immediately after the protocol has been violated and replacing it rather than subjecting the patient to this risk of sepsis.

Bacteriological data gathered then and now supports the concept of sepsis by skin contamination. Hematogenous spread, while it must occur, is in our experience exceedingly rare, because of the predominance of skin organisms including staph epidermidis, now almost exclusively the cause of catheter bacteremias closely associated with violations in protocol. The particular strain of staph epidermidis that we are dealing with is a resistant one and often is only treatable with vancomycin once septicemia has been established.

Treatment of catheter sepsis depends on the organism. If a bacterium is involved removal of the catheter is often enough; antibiotics need not be started unless fever persists and blood cultures remain positive. If a bacteremia is of short duration the catheter may be replaced after an interval of 24 hours and one may expect no further difficulty. With fungal infections, however, occasional difficulties arise. In our experience catheters should not be

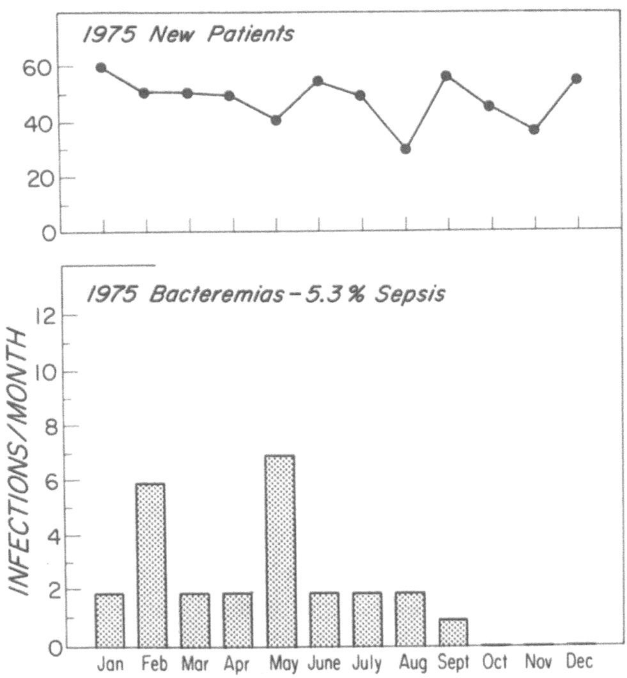

Figure 1. The sepsis rate in 1975 at the Massachusetts General Hospital. There are two peaks during which time a great deal of difficulty was experienced with filters and much manipulation of the lines. Note that the end of 1975 there is not a single bacteremia in three months in approximately 148 new patients added during that time. At the present time our sepsis rate is approximately one bacteremia every 380 patient days. It is not necessary to treat patients with bacteremias with antibiotics if the catheters are removed.

reinserted if the patient is suspected of having deep catheter sepsis or deep tissue invasion as evidenced by candida precipitins or positive crossed immunodiffusion electrophoresis (4). Under such circumstances blood cultures and immunologic tests should be drawn serially. Often, even with negative cultures, as soon as a high glucose solution is reinfused, blood cultures positive for fungi reappear.

Establishment of a parenteral nutrition unit enables one to monitor one's sepsis in collaboration with the infectious disease control group. Our group monitors the computer print out sheets of all bacteremias, (i.e. positive blood cultures) and catheter cultures in the hospital and identifies all patients on parenteral nutrition. Under such circumstances an accurate tabulation of catheter sepsis can be collected in an epidemiological fashion. In Figure 1 one sees the sepsis rate at our institution during 1975. The two spikes appear to have been associated with difficulties with filters in which we temporarily discontinued their use because of inability to get filters with sufficient quality control so that they did not crack and plug. It is our impression, but we have not been able to prove it, that the discontinuance of filters resulted in an increased incidence of sepsis as shown by the two spikes. At the present time our sepsis rate is approximately 1 bacteremia in every 380 catheter days, although it varies at different times of the year. In June and July, for example, with rapid personnel turnovers and large numbers of new house and nursing staff, the incidence increases. This perhaps is also associated with the hot weather and the fact the dressings tend to become saturated with perspiration. While this has not been a constant phenomenon (see Figure 1), it calls for increased vigilance for breaks in catheter technique at that time.

3. METABOLIC COMPLICATIONS

The metabolic complications may be prevented in part by identifying the groups at high risks. In general metabolic complications involve glucose or, what I would like to call the deficiency states. Taking the latter category first it is clear that the deficiency states or the complications such as hypophosphatemia (which have received somewhat lurid attention under the category of a mysterious complication) is nonetheless avoidable provided adequate amounts of ions are given with amino acids and glucose (Table 1). Thus, the requirements for phosphate and magnesium have increased with increased experience with parenteral nutrition. On the basis of four bottles of hypertonic glucose solution and amino acids containing approximately 30-40 gm

Table 1. Complications: Deficiency states

Hyponatremia
Hypokalemia
Hypophosphatemia
Hypomagnesemia
Zinc Deficiency
Copper Deficiency
Essential Fatty Acid Deficiency
Chromium Deficiency
? Other

of amino acid protein equivalent/liter, phosphate should be administered in patients with normal renal function to as much as 90-160 mEq potassium or higher, depending on renal function. It is my own personal experience that sodium is required up to 100 mEq/day to enable the excretion of the water load. This may seem paradoxical in patients with cardiac decompensation or a tendency to salt retention. On the other hand the withholding of salt generally results in dilutional hyponatremia and water retention.

Fatty acid deficiency tends to occur as a biochemical lesion approximately three days after the initiation of parenteral nutrition, particularly in depleted patients such as with regional enteritis (5). Although its exact contribution to healing or nonhealing is not known, it is presumably better to avoid since it is quite easy to do so. Intralipid in amounts of up to 200 cc/24 hours in a normal individual or one 500 cc bottle of 10% solution every 48 hours will easily prevent essential fatty acid deficiency. Any unsaturated oil, corn oil, even in the form of margarine (which some patients will take in preference to the unprocessed oil), safflower oil, or sunflower oil will prevent fatty acid deficiency.

Trace metals

We know little of trace metals. While it is clear that zinc deficiency occurs and is associated with a characteristic pustular rash and coloration in the skin creases, this appears to be rare in the United States and perhaps more common in other countries where the copper content is high (6, 7). Others have suggested that chromium deficiency is associated with development of a diabetic tendency in patients on long term parenteral nutrition (8), while copper deficiency may be associated with an anemia, although it clearly is not the anemia which most patients with parenteral nutrition develop (9, 10). In the incomplete state of our knowledge it seems most appropriate to use a trace metals additive solution such as has been proposed by many authorities.

It has been with glucose, however, that most of the severe metabolic complications of parenteral nutrition occur. Hyperosmolar, nonketotic coma may occur without warning and gives rise to nonspecific symptoms as fever, obtundation, and osmotic diuresis with a blood sugar often in the range of 700-1000. Its most frequent cause is that of too rapid initiation of an infusion, although it may supervene in a previously stable patient who becomes septic and sepsis is not promptly recognized. Under such circumstances it is necessary to stop the infusion, give no glucose, and give heroic amounts of insulin, up to 200 units/24 hours.

The predisposing causes of hyperglycemia are, of course, too rapid initiation of parenteral nutrition, as most common. Diabetes, particularly of the adult onset type, is not as much of a problem as one might expect since amino acid release of insulin occurs in diabetic patients in whom glucose does not appear to release adequate amounts of insulin. Indeed, we have had one juvenile diabetic whose blood sugar swings from 500 to less than 50 could only be controlled on parenteral nutrition with the addition of 2 units of pork insulin subcutaneously, and 15 units of crystalline zinc insulin to the bottle. In a recent survey at this institution of 200 patients, the incidence of a single blood sugar at some point in the course higher than 300 was 15%. Steroids, pancreatitis, pancreatic resection and liver disease all were prominent as causes of hyperglycemia. Surprisingly, diabetes played little role, only one patient out of the 30 was diabetic.There was no hyperosmolar coma and at no time was the infusion stopped in any patient. The absence of diabetes as a cause of hyperglcyemia may be due to the care exercised when starting a diabetic on parenteral nutrition (Table 2).

Additional complications are less common. Hyperammonemia may be seen in babies in a variety of solutions, particularly of those that are arginine deficient and may be corrected by the use of additional arginine. Ammonia in casein hydrolysates increases with shelf life although L-amino acid solutions appear free of this property. We have seen occasional hypercalcemia which we thought due to vitamin D toxicity. Since cutting down the amount of vitamin D added this complication has not been observed. When using casein hydrolysate peptide bound calcium is increased resulting in a higher blood calcium. Ionized calcium however, is normal.

Another rare complication which we have not seen since alcohol in parenteral nutrition was abandoned is pancreatitis. We have seen one fatal case of pancreatitis in a patient transferred to us from another institution following prolonged use of alcohol for home parenteral nutrition. Since there did not

Table 2. Common causes of hyperglycemia

1. Rapid Infusion
2. Decreased Insulin Output
   a. Diabetes
   b. Pancreatitis
   c. Pancreatic Resection
3. "Glucose Resistance"
   a. Sepsis
4. Hyperglycemic Factors
   a. Steroids
   b. Liver Disease (? Decreased Utilization)

appear to be any other reason for this patient, a 14 year old child, having pancreatitis, one assumes that infused alcohol may also cause pancreatitis.

In summary, the complications of parenteral nutrition are numerous and potentially dangerous. Prevention is the watchword. The groups at risk may be identified and various complications minimized by vigilance in patient care as well as by quality control by an established hyperalimentation team.

REFERENCES

1. Ryan, J. A., Jr., Complications of Total Parenteral Nutrition. In: Fischer, J. E. (ed.) *Total Parenteral Nutrition.* Boston: Little, Brown and Co., 1976, p. 55.
2. Ryan, J. A., Jr., Abel, R. M., Abbott, W. M., Hopkins, C. C., Chesney, T., Colley, R., Phillips, K. and Fischer, J. E., Complications of parenteral nutrition: A prospective study of two hundred consecutive patients. *New Engl. J. Med. 290*: 757 (1974).
3. Wilmore, D. W. and Dudrick, S. J., Safe long term venous catheterization. *Arch. Surg. 98*: 256 (1969).
4. Glew, R. H., Buckley, H. R., Rosen, H. M., Moellering, R. C. and Fischer, J. E., Value of prospective candida precipitins in fungemia in patients with hyperalimentation. *Surg. Forum 26*: 113 (1975).
5. Meng, H. C., Fat Emulsions in Parenteral Nutrition. In: Fischer, J. E. (ed.), *Total Parenteral Nutrition.* Boston: Little, Brown and Co., 1976, p. 305.
6. Takagi, Y., Itakura, T., Okada, et al., A clinical analysis of zinc deficiency during hyperalimentation. *Jap. J. Surgery 33*: 427 (1975).
7. Kay, R. G., Tasman-Jones, C., Pybus, J., et al., A syndrome of zinc deficiency during total parenteral alimentation in man. *Ann. Surg. 183*: 331 (1976).
8. Jeejeebhoy, K. N., Langer, B., Tsallas, G., et al., Total parenteral nutrition at home: Studies in patients surviving 4 months to 5 years. *Gastroenterology 71*: 943 (1976).
9. Palmisano, D. J., Nutrient deficiencies after intensive parenteral alimentation. *N. Engl. J. Med. 291*: 799 (1934).
10. Vilter, R. W., Bozian, R. C., Hess, E. V., Zellner, D. C. and Petering, H. G., Manifestations of copper deficiency in a patient with systemic sclerosis on intravenous hyperalimentation. *N. Engl. J. Med. 291*: 188 (1974).

Parenteral nutrition in obstetries and gynecology

L. Heller

In gynaecology the problems of parenteral nutrition have become increasingly important, especially in view of the advanced methods of radical surgery and the intensification of radiotherapy. Furthermore, more older patients in a poor state of health also undergo major surgery. In many of these patients food cannot be given by the oral route or can only be given inadequately. If this situation continues for any significant period, parenteral nutrition will be necessary. In gynaecology, long-term complete parenteral nutrition is seldom necessary; short-term complete parenteral nutrition, however, is required more often. Especially in ultraradical surgical procedures, an adequate metabolic control - and this means in many cases parenteral nutrition - is certainly necessary and decisive for therapeutic success.

In the Department of Obstetrics and Gynaecology at the University of Frankfurt/Main, about 4.500 women receive clinical treatment every year. On the average, about 150 to 200 of these women receive parenteral nutrition for short or long periods.

INDICATIONS

Complete parenteral nutrition becomes necessary in almost every case of radical and ultraradical surgery in gynaecology. After ultraradical operations and frequently also second-look operations, short-term or long-term parenteral nutrition is one of the most essential conditions for any success. After radical operations for cancer of the cervix uteri, we generally give short-term parenteral nutrition for four or five days. If, however, complications such as infections, ileus or renal failure occur, complete parenteral nutrition becomes necessary for a longer period. Further indications for total parenteral nutrition in gynaecology are cancerous cachexia, patients undergoing chemotherapy and anorexia nervosa.

In obstetrics, parenteral nutrition is seldom indicated. It becomes necessary in cases of severe eclampsia with acute renal failure, in cases of septic shock and finally in some cases of puerperal psychosis. In almost every case, these women have already delivered or the fetus has already died as in septic shock. Special problems arise for parenteral nutrition in those cases when the fetus is still alive. This is valid above all in hyperemesis gravidarum. In these cases, the particularities of the pregnancies have to be taken into account.

ULTRARADICAL SURGERY

Generally, postoperative water and electrolyte substitution no longer present any difficulties. However, for routine gynaecological operations the minimum requirements of calories, structural proteins and vitamins should be covered in the immediate post-operative phase. The number of complications is then markedly diminished and the convalescent period is shorter. An ample protein and energy turnover benefits to the healing processes at the site of the wound. Poorly nourished and previously stressed women tend, however, to develop more complications. The clinical picture includes adynamia, anemia, retarded wound healing, susceptibility to infections, tendency towards a circulatory collapse as well as lack of ferments, and disturbances of the hormone synthesis.

Parenteral nutrition is of the utmost importance for ultraradical operations (anterior, posterior or total pelvic exenteration), particularly the surgical treatment of progressive as well as x-ray-resistant genital cancer in women. These surgical procedures can heal about 30% of the women who would otherwise have died inevitably within a short time from their disease (1-5). As a rule, these women must receive complete parenteral nutrition for some time; this must be followed by partial parenteral nutrition over a longer period (6, 7). Today, these patients hardly ever die from blood losses, surgical shock or anesthesia, but from biochemical effects.

Covering of the nitrogen losses is of prime importance in parenteral nutrition in ultraradical surgery (7, 8, 9). During routine gynaecological operations, nitrogen losses amount to 5 to 15 g per day (7). In ultraradical surgery, however, nitrogen losses of up to 32 g per day were observed. These excessive nitrogen losses must be corrected as soon as possible after the operation or should at least be kept within tolerable limits.

In contrast to the general opinion, the nitrogen losses during surgery and in the postoperative phase do not consist only of losses due to bleeding, tissue destruction or lymphorrhea into the tissues of the surgical site (9). The catabolic stage which means the protein degradation during the postoperative phase, is even more important. Since the carbohydrate reserves of the organism are quickly exhausted, fats and proteins are used to meet the increased energy requirements.

Analysis of the urinary nitrogen excretion shows that real protein degradation is present and that this protein degradation serves to cover the increased energy requirements. The excretions of urea nitrogen and total nitrogen are nearly parallel. The relative increase in the nonurea portion arises from the increased excretion of peptides and amino acids.

The excretion of potassium, phosphorus and sulphur proves the protein degradation. The excretion of these substrates runs nearly parallel to the nitrogen excretion. It is true that the potassium values are regularly higher than expected from calculations. This is, however, observed for all operations. Therefore it is necessary to administer sufficient potassium in addition to nitrogen.

To administer parenteral nutrition after lutraradical operations, a knowledge of the status of the renal function is of prime importance. These women quite often have a developing or even chronic pyelonephritis, which can be recognized postoperatively by an isotonic urine with a low potassium and nitrogen content. In the first two postoperative days, the administration of amino acids and potassium has to be restricted. The calorie requirements of the basal turnover, however, must at any rate be met in this phase. If the renal function is adequate, the administration of amino acids is considerably increased. If after 4 or 5 days oral food cannot be tolerated, total parenteral nutrition is compulsory.

To cover the requirements of components, the minimum requirements are usually taken as a basis. For short-term parenteral nutrition this is sufficient in most cases. After ultraradical surgery, however, these quantities do not suffice. The calorie supply should be between 2500 and 3000 kcal per day. Nitrogen substitution should largely be conform to the nitrogen losses, which have to be determined daily. We administer at least 100 g of amino acids daily. The supply of energy carriers is, however, just as important. The carbohydrates in particular have a protein-sparing effect as the following investigations will show.

PATIENTS AND METHODS

After 38 abdominal hysterectomies, nitrogen balances were carried out for the first three postoperative days. 10 women received water and electrolytes exclusively. 9 women received in addition 50 g of amino acids per day, and 19 women received in addition 1,000 kcal per day in the form of carbohydrates and fat emulsions. In group 1, the mean nitrogen losses for all 3 days amounted to 8 g of nitrogen. For group 2, however, we found a mean loss of only 5 g of nitrogen and for group 3 only 2.5 g of nitrogen per day. From this, the protein-sparing effect of the pure calorie carriers becomes evident.

After major surgery we proceed as follows:
During the first two postoperative days, we are cautious with amino acids and potassium. If the renal function is adequate during these two days, large amounts of amino acids and potassium have to be given starting on the third day to compensate for the excessive nitrogen losses. During the initial postoperative days, the calorie supply should – if possible – cover the basal metabolic requirement. If after 5 or 6 days oral nutrition is still not feasible, the parenteral supply of nutrients must be increased considerably. Hereby, the physiological proportions between the main nutritive components fat, carbohydrates and amino acids should be maintained, but the proportion of amino acids to the total calorie supply should be slightly increased according to the nitrogen losses.

Following these principles, long-term parenteral nutrition has been carried out in 32 women. The longest period was 67 days. In one case, pelvic exenteration had been carried out because of a progressive ovarian cancer.

The patient was given in addition to 4 liters of blood, 150 g carbohydrates intravenously on the day of the operation and on the following day. On the second, third and fourth postoperative days, she received 200 g of carbohydrates and 100 g of amino acids per day. Afterwards, a subileus developed which lasted several weeks and was probably due to her previous intensive x-ray-therapy. Therefore, complete parenteral nutrition was necessary. Up to the 67th postoperative day, complete food intake was given via a subclavian catheter. The daily intake was 275 g of carbohydrates, 150 g of amino acids and 90 g of fat, with a total of 2,580 kcal.

This balanced parenteral nutrition was supplied exclusively for a period of 60 days. If the initial period of 7 days is included, the patient was given a total of 16.5 kg of carbohydrates, 9.0 kg of amino acids and 5.5 kg of fat intravenously. The weight of the patient was 48.5 kg before surgery and 50.2 kg at the end of the period of total parenteral nutrition.

In total, we have given complete parenteral nutrition to 32 women following ultraradical surgery, which lasted from 5 to 67 days. For the 32 women, this amounted to a total of 331 days. 13 women died in the first year after the operation, another one after 4 years. 19 women are still alive, 9 of them more than 5 years after surgery and one even 11 years after surgery.

Major surgery has been rendered possible only by the advances in balanced parenteral nutrition. Postoperatively, these patients are threatened by a biochemical death. The most important aspect of postoperative metabolic treatment and thus of balanced parenteral nutrition is to avoid this high risk.

PATIENTS UNDERGOING RADIOTHERAPY AND/OR CHEMOTHERAPY

With respect to the interrelationships between the main components of nutrition, our animal experiments have shown (8) that under the conditions of complete parenteral nutrition the best nitrogen balances are achieved when 20% of the calories are derived from amino acids, 30% from fat and 50% from carbohydrates. Under the same conditions, at least a nitrogen equilibrium can also be achieved in the healthy adult. This, however, cannot be applied with the same degree of certainty to sick patients, especially patients who have undergone radiotherapy because of cancer. These patients are generally in an exceedingly poor state of health. Therefore the calorie requirements of these patients are somewhat greater than those of healthy adults of the same age and sex (10). In these cases, the nitrogen balance often remains negative when 3,000 kcal are administered per day.

We measured the nitrogen balances under various conditions in 12 women who were irradiated because of advanced genital cancer and for clinical reasons received total parenteral nutrition. All women received 2,700 kcal daily.

As you can see:

Group 1 received 20% of the calories in the form of amino acids, 50% in the form of fat and 30% in the form of carbohydrates.

Group 2 again received 20% of the calories in the form of amino acids, 30% of the calories as fat and 50% as carbohydrates.

Group 3 received 20% of the calories in the form of amino acids, 20% as fat and 60% as carbohydrates. The infusion solutions were administered in 24 h per day through a subclavian catheter.

Group 1 included 3 women with a total of 27 parenteral nutrition days. At no time was a nitrogen equilibrium observed. The nitrogen loss ranged between 1.2 and 5.6 g of N per day. The average nitrogen loss for all 27 balance days was 4.2 g per day.

Group 2 comprised 5 women and 48 days studied. Here, too, the nitrogen balance stayed negative during the whole period. The nitrogen losses averaged 2.6 g per day, while the values ranged between +0.3 and −4.4 g of N per day.

Group 3 included 4 women and 36 days studies. In this group, who received 20% of the calories in the form of fat and 60% in the form of carbohydrates, the nitrogen balances ranged within relatively narrow limits between +0.3 and −1.3 g of N per day. The mean value for 36 days was 0.2 g of N per day; so, the balance was almost in equilibrium.

Under the conditions of group 3, the nitrogen balances were measured in 3 women undergoing chemotherapy.

Here, especially high nitrogen losses were observed. The chemotherapy, however, was tolerated much better than by patients on oral nutrition. Patients, who received an additional 2,000 kcal of a balanced diet via the intravenous route, tolerated far higher dosages of cyclophosphamide or methotrexate than patients who were only nourished by the oral route.

It is not possible to answer clearly the question of why women suffering from cancer and having to undergo radiotherapy or chemotherapy show greater nitrogen losses on normal or higher parenteral fat intake than on lower fat intake. The protein-sparing effect of fats is certainly only slight in severely ill patients, especially in patients undergoing radiotherapy.

The importance of the parenteral fat supply is to be found in the intake of the essential fatty acids.

The energy requirements of these patients may be met almost completely by carbohydrates.

SOME SPECIFIC PROBLEMS OF PARENTERAL NUTRITION IN OBSTETRICS

In obstetrics, it becomes far more important to cover the calorie requirements. As long as the fetus is alive, the infusion of fat emulsions is contraindicated. There are several reasons for this.

1. A physiological hyperlipemia exists during pregnancy. Even fat which is given by the oral route is poorly metabolized, especially in the second half of pregnancy. If pregnant women receive fat emulsions an excessive increase in the serum triglycerides results, often with simultaneous temporary ketonemia which is harmful to the fetus.

2. Intravenously administered fat emulsions may induce labor. The occurrence of labor is much more certain when the rate of infusion of the fat

emulsion is high. This effect of intravenously administered fat emulsions on the myometrium has been confirmed repeatedly (11, 12). During the early stages of pregnancy, contractions may also occur during fat infusion but not as in the late stages of pregnancy.

3. After the infusion of fat emulsions abundant fat deposits are found in the placentas of rats and dogs. Similar observations have yet not been made in humans. Infarctions of the placenta maybe due to fat emboli, however, are frequent in humans. Therefore it is possible that the infusion of fat emulsions induces a placental insufficiency. For all of these reasons we do not administer fat to pregnant women.

The energy requirements during pregnancy must therefore be covered with carbohydrates. During pregnancy, however, glucose on its own is just as inappropriate as in the postoperative phase. The fetus utilizes only glucose and therefore needs a steady and constant glucose supply. However since the renal threshold for glucose is lowered in pregnancy and infused glucose is lost via the kidneys, complete parenteral nutrition of pregnant women is inevitably dependent on fructose and polyalcohols. The great advantage of fructose, sorbitol and xylitol in parenteral nutrition when compared with glucose is that glucose is slowly formed from these substrates. In addition, xylitol has a nitrogen-sparing and an antiketogenic effect which are superior to those of glucose. Both of these properties are desirable during pregnancy. Therefore our energy source is almost exclusively the so-called "three sugar solution" composed of fructose, glucose and xylitol in the proportions 2:1:1.

Today, parenteral nutrition has an established place in obstetrics and gynaecology. Some major surgical interventions would not be possible without complete pre- and postoperative parenteral nutrition. Parenteral nutrition therefore means decisive and lifesaving progress for surgical gynaecology.

REFERENCES

1. Brunschwig, H., What are the indications and results of pelvic exenteration? *J. Am. Med. Ass. 194*: 480 (1963).
2. Barber, H. R. and Brunschwig, A., Treatment and results of recurrent cancer of corpus uteri in patients receiving anterior and total pelvic exenteration, 1947-1963. *Cancer 22*: 949 (1968).
3. Bricker, E. M., Die radikale Evisceration des Beckens für fortgeschrittene und rezidivierende Karzinome. *Arch. Gyn. 204*: 1 (1967).
4. Rutledge, F. N. and Burns, B. C., Pelvic exenteration. *Am. J. Obstetr. Gynec. 91*: 692 (1965).
5. Uhlfelder, H., Extended radical surgery of recurrent and advanced cervical cancer. *Clin. Obstetr. Gynec. 10*: 922 (1967).

6. Heller, L., Stoffwechseluntersuchungen bei ultraradikalen Operationen. *Arch. Gyn. 204*: 27 (1967).
7. Heller, L., Die parenterale Ernährung in der Frauenheilkunde. *Geburtsh. Frauenheilk. 28*: 848 (1968).
8. Heller, L., Clinical and experimental studies of complete parenteral nutrition. *Scand. J. Gastroenterol. 4*: Suppl. 4, 7 (1968).
9. Moore, F. D., Metabolism in the posttraumatic state. Grune and Stratton, New York, 1960.
10. Berg, G. und Fackler, R., Parenterale Ernährung Karzinomkranker. *Fortschr. Med. 86*: 246 (1968).
11. Luukainen, T. U. and Csapo, A. J., Induction of premature labor in the rabbit pretreatment with phospholipids. *Fert. Steri. 14*: 65 (1963).
12. Järvinen, P. A., Luukainen, T., Short, R. V., Adlerkreutz, H., Pesonen, S., and Huhmar, E., The effect of an infusion of phospholipid on the human myometrium. *Ann. Med. exp. Biol. Fenn. 42*: 21 (1963).

The nutritional care of the cancer patient

Stanley J. Dudrick, M.D.
Edward M. Copeland, M.D.
Bruce V. MacFadyen, Jr., M.D.

Nutrient substrates are needed in the human body in sufficient quantities to supply basal requirements and to support a state of nitrogen and nutritional equilibrium under a wide variety of conditions associated with catabolism. Ordinary requirements can be accentuated by trauma, sepsis, metabolic disorders and possibly malignancies. Increased metabolic demands have been postulated to occur in patients with malignant neoplasms for many years but have never been documented clearly. When cancer is diagnosed initially in today's health environment, the patient is usually adequately nourished. However, the use of the various antineoplastic therapies often results in severe caloric deficits and produces marked weight loss and inanition. On the other hand, loss of body mass can be the initial clinical sign in patients with specific malignancies such as leukemia, lymphoma and oat-cell carcinoma of the lung. Tumor bulk in patients with these malignant disorders is often quite large before any symptoms are produced, and weight loss, in part, may reflect the increased nutritional demand imposed upon the patient by this tumor mass. In contradistinction, malignant melanoma, breast cancer, most soft tissue sarcomas and most gastrointestinal malignancies produce early signs and symptoms, such as a palpable mass or bleeding, while the tumor is relatively small and before any weight loss secondary to the caloric demands of the malignancy can be identified. Specific gastrointestinal (GI) tract malignancies, particularly those of the oropharynx and esophagus, produce weight loss because of reduced oral intake secondary to pain on deglutition or GI obstruction. Similarly, lymphoma of the small intestine and certain gastrointestinal hormone secreting tumors such as carcinoma of the pancreatic islet cells can result in malnutrition secondary to malabsorption. Nevertheless, the majority of cases of inanition seen in a categorical cancer institution are initially iatrogenic and the result of oncologic therapy, unless the patient has neglected his symptoms for several months and has become malnourished secondary to diminished oral caloric intake and increased tumor bulk.

Inanition during oncologic therapy can be prevented or corrected by the appropriate use of available intravenous and oral nutrient regimens. When possible, the gastrointestinal tract should be utilized for delivery, absorption and assimilation of nutrients. The easiest method of food ingestion is by mouth and the next simplest method of food delivery is by GI tract intubation with nasogastric feeding tubes. However, insertion of a gastrostomy or jejunostomy tube may become necessary for long-term nutritional maintenance when the oral route is unavailable. Unfortunately, nutritional rehabilitation via the GI tract can be time consuming, and oncologic therapy cannot always be deferred until protein and energy stores have been replaced adequately via this route.

Within the last 10 years, intravenous hyperalimentation (IVH) and chemically defined (elemental) diets, two new methods of nutritional rehabilitation, have become available to the oncologist. The concept of concentrating intravenous nutriments in order to meet the high caloric requirements of critically ill individuals was originally tested by Dudrick, Rhoads and Vars in 1966 (11). These investigators initially fed beagle puppies exclusively by infusing a 30% nutrient solution, primarily glucose with protein hydrolysates, via the superior vena cava. These animals grew and developed normally for periods exceeding 200 days. It was from this experience that the technique of intravenous hyperalimentation was adapted for use in human beings (12).

The extensive application of intravenous hyperalimentation to the nutritional rehabilitation of the cancer patients was pioneered at the M.D. Anderson Hospital (4). Since the hyperalimentation team was established 5 years ago, 2000 patients have received IVH as a means of nutritional replenishment or maintenance prior to, during and/or following treatment by surgery, chemotherapy, or radiotherapy. Utilizing IVH, the gastrointestinal tract is bypassed and positive nitrogen balance, anabolism and nutritional equilibrium can be attained within 7-10 days. The technique is safe (5), and stimulation of tumor growth has not occurred.

Chemically defined diets have become widely available for clinical use. These diets are of known qualitative and quantitative composition and contain simple sugars, L-amino acids, electrolytes, minerals, trace elements and sometimes fatty acids in amounts sufficient for daily human nutritional maintenance if 1800-2000 calories of the diet are consumed daily. These diets are low in residue, absorbed primarily in the upper gastrointestinal tract, and produce minimal stool output. Use of the gastrointestinal tract for alimentation is the primary advantage of these diets and overcomes the two major disadvantages of IVH, which are potential sepsis from the indwelling venous catheter and the necessity for hospitalizing most patients. Two major disadvantages of chemically defined diets are monotony of taste and consistency and the necessity of ingesting at least 2 liters of the solution in order to achieve nutritional equilibrium in the basal state. The motivation to drink the diet is difficult to maintain because patients are often anorectic secondary to their malignant disorders or to the oncologic treatment modalities employed. This motivational component can be overcome to some extent by gastric intubation with a nasogastric feeding tube through which the diet can be administered by bolus injection or constant infusion. If nasogastric intubation is to be employed, however, hospitalization is usually necessary, and one of the advantages of chemically defined diets over intravenous hyperalimentation is lost.

When mixed at "full" strength, chemically defined diets provide one calorie per ml, and the osmolality is approximately 800 to 1200 mOsm per liter depending upon the flavoring agent that is used to disguise the amino acid taste of the diet. Nausea, bloating and diarrhea can result because of high osmolarity of these diets, and this further limits the patient's desire to ingest them. Nevertheless, chemically defined diets are increasing in importance in our nutritional armamentarium.

An intelligent approach to the nutritional rehabilitation of the cancer patient is to rapidly replenish him using intravenous hyperalimentation until the gastrointestinal tract becomes suitable for use and then maintain him with a chemically defined diet until ingestion, absorption and assimilation of adequate normal foodstuffs is possible enterally.

For the purposes of this chapter, 183 consecutive patients with a wide variety of malignant diseases were reviewed. Each patient received intravenous hyperalimentation as nutritional support during his oncologic therapy. The technique of subclavian vein catheter insertion and maintenance, administration of the nutrient solutions, indications for IVH, results of nutritional replenishment, diagnosis and management of complications incurred during IVH and the potential use of chemically defined intravenous and oral diets in the future treatment of cancer patients will be discussed.

PREPARATION AND COMPOSITION OF THE NUTRIENT SOLUTION

Intravenous hyperalimentation solutions are hypertonic and exert between 1800 and 2400 mOsm per liter. They may be constituted by mixing 350 ml of 50% glucose with 750 ml of 5% protein hydrolysate in 5% dextrose, or by mixing 500 ml of 50% glucose with 500 ml of an 8.5% amino acid solution. Such solutions contain approximately 1000 calories per liter and provide between 5.25 and 6.25 gm of nitrogen per liter. To these base solutions must be added daily maintenance electrolytes and vitamins. Although the protein hydrolysate solutions (casein or fibrin) contain various trace elements virtually as contaminants of their processing and storage in glass containers, the major electrolytes must be added to them prior to infusion. The usual electrolyte additives to hypertonic nutrient mixtures derived from the hydrolysate solutions are approximately 40-50 mEq sodium chloride, 20-40 mEq potassium chloride, 10-15 mEq magnesium chloride and 15-20 mEq potassium acid phosphate per liter. Even though the casein hydrolysates, which are prepared by the enzymatic hydrolysis of the phosphoprotein casein, contain large amounts of phosphorus (20-40 mmoles/liter), the phosphorus is apparently bound to the peptides and/or amino acids in such a manner as not to be effective in maintaining normal serum phosphorus concentrations. Indeed, the first reported occurrence of hypophosphatemia during hyperalimentation was in a patient receiving casein hydrolysate. Fibrin hydrolysate, prepared by the acid hydrolysis of beef or porcine fibrin, contains no significant amounts of phosphorus, and additives of this crucial intracellular element must be made to solutions using this nitrogen source.

The amino acids within the commercially available amino acid products currently available in this country are present as the acetate and chloride or hydrochloride salts; nevertheless, these preparations are acidic, and the addition of inordinate amounts of sodium and/or potassium chloride can result in hyperchloremic metabolic acidosis in some patients, particularly those in the pediatric and geriatric age groups. Consequently, sodium and potassium should be added as the chloride, lactate, acetate, bicarbonate or acid phosphate salt as dictated by the patient's acid-base status and serum electrolytes. Although phosphate has been added to some commercially prepared amino acid solutions in relatively small quantities, our experience has indicated that between 15 and 25 mEq of phosphate per liter, added as the potassium acid phosphate salt, is necessary to maintain phosphate equilibrium. Hypomagnesemia will often occur within 10 days of intravenous hyperalimentation if sufficient quantities of magnesium are not added. Similarly, hypocalcemia will result if adequate quantities of calcium are not provided, usually in dosages of 4 to 9 mEq daily. Both the fat and water soluble vitamins must be added to one liter of IVH solution per day, and folic acid, vitamin K and vitamin B_{12} must be administered regularly as necessary. Serum albumin concentrations below 3.0 gm% should be corrected to at least 3.5 gm% by the daily administration of 12.5-50 gm of albumin, which can be added directly to the IVH solution. Thereby, colloid osmotic pressure will be restored, and protein nutrition will be supplemented. In most patients, serum albumin synthesis will be restored to normal within 7-10 days of IVH administration, and exogenous serum albumin administration may be discontinued. The formulation of the IVH solutions for daily infusion to a patient with normal serum electrolytes, magnesium, phosphorus and calcium is depicted in Table 1.

The minimum daily energy expenditure necessary to maintain an adult patient in the basal metabolic state is approximately 1500 calories per day. In the absence of adequate exogenous calories, energy is derived by lipolysis and the conversion of tissue protein into glucose through gluconeogenesis. Cuthbertson's earlier work on negative nitrogen balance in post-traumatic human beings showed that the infusion of 150 gm of dextrose solution per day would result in a significant nitrogen-sparing effect (9). These data have been confirmed and extended to show that infusions of greater quantities of glucose or of fat-containing solutions will result primarily in fat deposition with little or no further protein sparing, unless nitrogen sources (amino acids or protein hydrolysates) are administered simultaneously (10, 15). If amino acids are administered together with the concentrated glucose solutions (as in IVH) gluconeogenesis is minimized, and lean tissue synthesis is augmented. Protein synthesis depends somewhat on the activity of the patient, and for adequate replacement of skeletal muscle protein, physical exercise is necessary. For this reason, we recommend a daily program of physical rehabilitation for patients receiving IVH as early as their clinical conditions allow.

Potassium and nitrogen deficits often coexist during periods of catabolism, in part because the muscle mass contains 75% of the body's total potassium,

Table 1. Amino acid substrate solution

500 ml 50% Dextrose plus
500 ml 8.5% Amino acid solution
Additives:
40-50 mEq Sodium Chloride
20 mEq Potassium Acetate
15 mEq Potassium Acid Phosphate
15 mEq Magnesium Sulfate
5 ml Multivitamins* (M.V.I.)**
1 gm Calcium Gluconate*

* Added to only one unit of solution daily.
** M.V.I. - USV Pharmaceutical Corp., Tuckahoe, N.Y.

and as muscle is catabolized during gluconeogenesis, potassium is released to the extracellular fluid compartment and is excreted by the kidneys. If a mixture of protein hydrolysates and hypertonic glucose is given to a potassium-depleted animal, growth and positive nitrogen balance will not occur (3). In order to achieve positive nitrogen balance and tissue synthesis, the intracellular requirements of potassium must be met without producing excessive extracellular hypokalemia. Indeed, failure to do so may result in the catastrophic myocardial dysfunction which accompanies serum potassium concentrations below 2.0 mEq per liter. To meet this requirement, approximately 40 mEq of potassium per 1000 calories administered is usually necessary. The degree of potassium depletion parallels the extent of protein-calorie malnutrition but is *not* reflected accurately by the serum potassium concentration in malnourished patients. Not until adequate intravenous nutritional replacement is begun does hypokalemia and a better idea of the true magnitude of the total body deficit of potassium becomes manifest. Consequently, the severely malnourished patient may need as much as 60-100 mEq of potassium per 1000 calories administered initially in order to maintain potassium equilibrium. As anabolism progresses and protein synthesis returns to normal, potassium requirements will be reduced commensurately.

Phosphorus and magnesium depletion parallel potassium and protein depletion in the catabolic patient. The exact reason for depletion of these elements is unknown, but it is hypothesized that the mechanism for their loss is similar to that for potassium. Magnesium concentration is much higher in the intracellular than in the extracellular compartment, and loss of body mass probably results in a relative tissue magnesium deficiency. The body stores energy within the high energy phosphate bonds of adenosine triphosphate. Although phosphate is found in high concentrations within bone, it is not sufficiently labile or available for general body use because hypophosphatemia will regularly result if adequate quantities of phosphorus are not administered within the IVH solutions. As glucose and amino acids are infused to provide adequate calorie and nitrogen sources, high energy phosphate bonds probably are replenished by the utilization of extraosseous as well as osseous phosphorus. If exogenous phosphorus is not given during IVH therapy, severe, symptomatic hypophosphatemia may result.

As anabolism is promoted by IVH administration, an increased daily intake of calcium becomes necessary. This calcium requirement is even greater in a phosphate depleted patient. Calcium and phosphate are in solution as a salt with a constant solubility coefficient. Consequently, as phosphate is infused, the serum concentration of calcium will be depressed, and vice-versa. Thus, when hypophosphatemia occurs during hyperalimentation, adequate calcium must be supplied along with the phosphorus, or reciprocal hypokalemia will result.

Sterility is of utmost importance in the preparation of intravenous nutrient solutions. Aseptic mixing of the various additives under a laminar-flow filtered air hood is essential for optimal safety. Electrolytes should be added to the hyperalimentation solutions in the pharmacy immediately prior to infusion in order to satisfy the current electrolyte requirements of the patient. After the solutions are prepared, they should be refrigerated and infused within 24 hr. Periodic aliquots of IVH solutions should be removed and cultured for bacteria and fungi in order to provide quality control over the aseptic mixing of the solutions.

Catheter insertion

Thrombophlebitis will regularly result if the hypertonic nutritional solutions are infused through a peripheral vein. For safe delivery of the solutions, accurate catheterization of a large-diameter vein is essential. Our hyperalimentation team has used the superior vena cava exclusively for infusion into the bloodstream. Access to this vessel is obtained preferably by infraclavicular percutaneous catheterization of the subclavian vein. Superior vena caval catheterization via the external or internal jugular vein is acceptable, but the catheter dressing is cumbersome because it interferes with freedom of neck motion, it is uncomfortable, and it is difficult to anchor the delivery tubing to the patient's neck or to the side of the face. Catheter dressings are easiest to apply, most secure, and most comfortable for the patient when they lie on the upper thorax.

Successful subclavian venipuncture is dependent upon the physician's knowledge of the anatomy of the subclavian vein and its related structures as well as adequate filling and dilatation of this vein. The latter requirement is fulfilled by positioning the supine patient in the Trendelenburg position. A rolled sheet is placed under the spine between the shoulders to facilitate hyperextension of the shoulders. The head is turned away from the side of catheter insertion. The skin is prepared by shaving all of the hair from the upper thorax, neck and shoulder on the side of catheter insertion. This area is then defatted with ether or acetone and prepped for three minutes with povidone iodine or a 2% tincture of thimerosol. The surgeon puts on sterile gloves and places sterile towels around the prepared field as in any other surgical procedure.

Essential items of equipment at this point are sterile scissors and hemostats, local anesthetic, a 2 or 3 ml syringe, a 2-inch long #14 needle through which a #16 radiopaque catheter will pass, and a 3-0 silk or nylon suture on a straight skin needle. A wheal is raised using 1% lidocaine at the inferior border of the middle of the clavicle, and the anesthetic is injected into the deeper tissues to the periosteum of the clavicle. A 5% dextrose solution with a microdrip infusion attachment and a 30-inch long extension tubing is assembled by the nurse. The #14 needle is attached to the 2 ml syringe, and the appropriate catheter length is measured by approximating the course of the catheter from the skin-entrance site under the clavicle to the middle of the superior vena cava. The total length of the catheter is about 8 inches in the average adult, with $5\frac{1}{2}$ to 6 inches lying deep to the skin and 2 to $2\frac{1}{2}$ inches lying external to the puncture site. This is particularly important because the catheter tip should not lie within the right atrium or close to the tricuspid valve, for if it does, fibrin is more likely to be deposited on these structures and may become infected by hematogenously-borne micro-organisms. Moreover, the catheter itself may traumatize directly and even puncture these cardiac structures with potentially disastrous consequences.

A fingertip is pressed firmly into the suprasternal notch as a guidepoint. The needle is inserted through the skin, and the inferior surface of the clavicle is identified. The needle is then directed in a frontal (coronal) plane immediately beneath the medial one-third of the clavicle and toward the finger in the suprasternal notch. If gentle suction is created within the syringe as the needle is advanced, a flash-back of blood will be obtained when the needle is within the subclavian vein. The entire one cm long beveled tip of the needle should be within the vein, and the patient is asked to hold his breath in deep inspiration or to perform a Valsalva maneuver to prevent air embolism when the hub of the inserted needle is opened to the air. The syringe is detached from the needle, and a #16 radiopaque polyvinyl catheter is inserted through the needle and threaded into the superior vena cava. When the hub of the catheter has reached the hub of the needle and has interlocked, the catheter and needle are withdrawn as a unit so that approximately 2 cm of catheter is free between the skin and needle tip. If difficulty in advancing the catheter through the needle is encountered during any portion of this procedure, further manipulation should be terminated, and the catheter and needle should be withdrawn as a unit to avoid shearing off a portion of the catheter. The catheter must never be withdrawn after it has been inserted more than two inches for this important reason. Once accurately in place, the catheter is sewn to the skin using a 3-0 silk or nylon suture, and a plastic clip is placed around the sharp point of the needle to prevent inadvertent severance of the catheter. Antimicrobial ointment is placed around the catheter exit site, a small sterile dressing is applied, tincture of benzoin is painted or sprayed on the skin, and water-repellent adhesive tape secures the dressing. All tubing and catheter connections are taped to prevent inadvertent disconnections with resultant contamination of the hyperalimentation delivery system and possible air embolization. A chest roentgenogram is obtained to confirm the proper position of the indwelling catheter within the central venous system in the middle of the superior vena cava. If the catheter has been directed into an internal mammary vein or internal or external jugular vein, or if it is otherwise malpositioned, it should be removed and replaced. Otherwise, thrombophlebitis will usually ensue promptly. Following confirmation of correct catheter placement, infusion of the concentrated nutrient solution can begin.

Any use of the catheter and delivery system other than to supply intravenous nutriments should be disallowed or discouraged. At least three times a week, the dressing should be dismantled, the skin around the catheter should be reprepared with defatting agent and antiseptic solution, and antimicrobial ointment should be reapplied and a new sterile dressing should be placed over the catheter exit site. Aseptic technique is used throughout the dressing change procedure. The hyperalimentation delivery system should not be used for infusion of blood or blood products, for intermittent or regular injection of bolus medication or for central venous pressure monitoring unless an absolute emergency arises. It must be considered the patient's nutritional lifeline and regarded accordingly with due respect.

The hyperalimentation delivery system consists of the IVH bottle or bag connected to a pediatric microdrip set and a 30-inch extension tubing which inserts directly into the catheter hub. Administration of other intravenous solutions simultaneously with IVH should be accomplished preferably through a peripheral venous site if possible. If necessary, however, simultaneous intravenous solutions may occasionally be administered through the "side arm" adaptor of the delivery tubing, provided that the connection is made via male to female fittings, is covered with antiseptic ointment and is secured with tape. This method is particularly applicable to the administration of intermittent chemotherapy or antibiotics. The IVH delivery system, including the tubing of any simultaneous intravenous infusions, is changed routinely every Monday, Wednesday and Friday by a nursing member of the hyperalimentation team. At the termination of the course of hyperalimentation, each catheter is removed aseptically, and the most distal 2-inch long segment of the catheter is transected and immediately cultured for aerobic and anaerobic bacteria and fungi. If the patient is febrile at the time of catheter removal, a blood culture sample is first withdrawn through the subclavian catheter.

Central venous feeding catheters are removed if the patient becomes febrile and no obvious source of sepsis other than the catheter can be identified. Fever, per se, is not an absolute indication for discontinuing IVH. The febrile patient should first be evaluated thoroughly in an attempt to discover the etiology of the fever. If a source of infection is discovered elsewhere, it can be treated appropriately and the hyperalimentation catheter may remain in place. Frequent blood cultures, however, should be done routinely in any febrile patient who has a central venous feeding catheter. Regardless of the source of infection, the feeding catheter must be removed if a positive blood culture is obtained. The catheter should not be reinserted until the blood cultures are negative and at least 48 hours have elapsed following the return of temperature to normal. If the catheter was the source of the septic episode, temperature will return to normal within 48 hours after the catheter is removed, without the use of antibiotics. Routine catheter changes have not been necessary, and the longest time that a single catheter has remained in place is 96 days. Nine percent of the patients have required catheter changes during the course of hyperalimentation, usually because of an unexplained fever or mechanical problem with the delivery system.

Administration of the hyperalimentation solutions and metabolic monitoring
The hypertonic IVH solutions must be delivered at a constant rate throughout each 24-hr period in order to allow optimal assimilation of glucose, amino acids and the other nutrients by the body cell mass. Pancreatic insulin output increases gradually throughout the 24-hr period following the initiation of hyperalimentation, and blood sugar concentrations will gradually fall to normal levels during this time. Although 2000 or 3000 ml of IVH can be given to some patients during the first day of nutritional repletion, such glucose dosages may result in hyperglycemia and excessive glycosuria in other patients because of insufficient circulating insulin. Our recommendation is to administer 1000 ml of IVH during the first 24-hr period, followed by 1000 ml every 12 hr for the next 48 hr. This schedule will avoid problems with hyperosmolarity and hyperglycemia because the pancreatic islet cells have the opportunity to adapt to increased insulin output in response to the continuous glucose infusion. Within the first three to five days of nutritional rehabilitation, the average adult will tolerate a daily ration of 3000 ml of IVH. This may not be the case, however, with the severely cachetic cancer patient. Until glucose and water tolerances are established, only 2000 ml of IVH per

day should be administered to the cancer patient who has lost 20% or more of his usual body weight.

Fractional urine sugars are checked every 6 hours in order to monitor glycosuria. Regulation of the pediatric microdrip system is satisfactory for maintenance of a fairly constant infusion rate, and pumps are not absolutely necessary when treating an adult patient. A widely fluctuating rate of delivery or bolus infusion of IVH will be signalled by glycosuria. The staff nurses on each floor must be informed of the necessity for constant infusion of IVH solutions, and if glycosuria usually occurs only during one shift, then further nursing instruction for this group is necessary. Prolonged glycosuria can result in an excessive osmotic diuresis and resultant hypertonic dehydration. If constant glycosuria is encountered in the patient with normal blood sugar concentrations, then the rate of delivery should be slowed until the glycosuria becomes minimal. If constant glycosuria is encountered in the patient with elevated blood sugar concentrations, then the patient's capacity for metabolizing the administered glucose has been overcome, and either the glucose delivery rate must be reduced or exogenous insulin must be supplied. An isolated 4+ urine sugar determination does not require insulin administration because it often reflects only a brief bolus administration of several milliliters of IVH solution.

When additional insulin is necessary, our experience has indicated that it be added directly to the IVH solutions rather than given subcutaneously. A minimum of 2000 ml of IVH should be administered to virtually all malnourished adult patients. If pancreatic insulin output is not adequate for cellular incorporation of this administered glucose ration, then crystalline insulin should be added to the hyperalimentation solutions initially in dosages of 5 to 10 units per 1000 ml, and the amount gradually increased until blood sugar levels return to normal range. It is recognized that some of the crystalline insulin adheres to the bottle and the administration tubing; however, the quantity of insulin lost in this manner is insignificant, and sufficient insulin is added to achieve the desired metabolic effect. If the insulin is within the IVH bottle, and the infusion stops, then insulin administration also ceases. If insulin has been administered subcutaneously however, and the infusion stops, marked hypoglycemia with catastrophic clinical results might occur.

Since the pancreatic islet cells produce insulin virtually to maximum capacity in response to the continuous glucose load during hyperalimentation, the abrupt cessation of IVH lead to "rebound" insulin shock. Although the abrupt cessation of IVH can be accomplished without incident in most patients, a few will have profound reactive hypoglycemia. For this reason,

IVH should be tapered over a 24-48 hr period prior to completely discontinuing it. Rapid tapering can be accomplished safely over a 4-6 hr period if a 10% glucose infusion is administered through a peripheral vein when the IVH is stopped. Hyperalimentation should be tapered and discontinued prior to any general anesthetic, for if insulin hypoglycemia occurs while the patient is asleep, it may go unrecognized and permanent brain damage may result.

Serum electrolyte, blood urea nitrogen and blood sugar concentrations are determined each Monday, Wednesday and Friday. Liver function tests, serum albumin, magnesium, calcium, phosphorus and creatinine concentrations are determined each Monday. A complete blood count and limited coagulation profile are also obtained once weekly.

A metabolic scale is used to determine the patient's weight each morning. In a severely depleted patient, an initial 3 to 4 lb weight gain is expected during the first 48 to 72 hr of treatment because of rehydration. Following this time period, accumulation of lean body mass will not exceed one-half pound per day, and if daily weight gain exceeds one pound per day, fluid retention must be presumed to have occurred, and the delivery rate of the IVH must be reduced and/or diuretics administered.

THE HYPERALIMENTATION TEAM

At our institution, an average of 27 patients have been receiving IVH at any one time. To properly care for this number of patients, the team approach is necessary. The hyperalimentation team consists of an attending physician, his house officers and fellows, two registered nurses, and a research technician. The attending physician is responsible for evaluating each patient's nutritional status and candidacy for IVH. Nutritional depletion is defined as a recent uninrentional weight loss of 10 lb or more of body weight, a serum albumin level of less than 3.4 gm%, and/or energy to a battery of recall skin test antigens. Nutritional depletion, however, is not the only indication for IVH in the cancer patient. Often the nutritionally intact patient's treatment plan will indicate multiple courses of chemotherapy, possibly combined with surgery or radiation therapy. For the patient to remain an adequate treatment candidate, he should maintain a certain body mass throughout therapy or treatment might necessarily be curtailed or abandoned because of secondary malnutrition. Since most chemotherapeutic drugs and radiation therapy to the gastrointestinal tract produce anorexia, nausea and often diarrhea, with resultant reduced oral intake and weight loss, previously adequately nourished patients who will receive intensive anti-cancer treatment become hyperalimentation candidates in order to maintain them nutritionally throughout therapy.

An IVH manual is issued to the fellows and residents as they rotate onto the hyperalimentation team at 3 to 4-month intervals. Although most physicians in training today are familiar with a technique of subclavian vein catheterization and some have used IVH, we insist that there be uniformity of patient management by the team members. Consequently, during the first few days of the rotation, the house staff is taught the principles and practice of IVH used at our institution. The nurses are familiar with our method, and variance from it can be confusing to them, and detrimental to patient care.

The two registered nurses assigned to the team have the responsibility for daily catheter care. They change the catheter dressings and IVH delivery tubing on Monday, Wednesday and Friday and inspect the system for leaks or other mechanical failures. The nurses provide "in-service" instruction to the floor nurses regarding the administration of the IVH fluids and are readily available throughout the day to answer questions about IVH. The team nurses provide quality-control over catheter insertion because they are present to aid the physician with each catheter inserted, and the nurses are asked to insure that the established team technique is followed specifically. Since the hyperalimentation nurses see the patients regularly, they provide psychological support for the patients as they interrelate with them professionally throughout the day.

The research technician is responsible for maintenance of a daily flow sheet which lists weight, caloric intake, serum electrolyte, magnesium, calcium, phosphorus and albumin concentrations, leukocyte count, temperature, chemotherapy or other treatment and tumor response. The research technician is also responsible for maintenance of the technical aspects of the various active research protocols and their quality control.

Although no specific pharmacist or rehabilitation therapist is a member of the team, the safety and outcome of intravenous nutritional repletion depends, in large part, on these people. In our institution, all pharmacy personnel are familiar with the formulation of hyperalimentation solutions, and frequent communication between the pharmacy and the rest of the team is necessary. For example, IVH solutions are mixed up to 24 hr in advance of administration; consequently, a minor change in electrolyte concentration which is not critical for patient health could await the mixing of the bottles for the next 24 hr rather than requiring that all current bottles be discarded at a financial expense to the hospital and the patient.

Since a proper program of active physical exercise is important for optimal nutrition and for rehabilitation of the musculo-skeletal system, the rehabilitation service is consulted on each IVH patient. A patient who remains inactive during IVH is more likely to lay down fat and less likely to synthesize lean tissue than is a patient who is exercising his skeletal musculature. Quarterly seminars are presented to the rehabilitation personnel to outline potential hazards they might encounter when working with an IVH patient.

Temperature, weight gain, electrolyte balance, adequacy of glucose metabolism, quality and quantity of fluid intake and important physical findings are evaluated at the bedside daily as the hyperalimentation team visits each patient receiving IVH.

CLINICAL MATERIAL

Table 2 lists the indications for IVH in 183 consecutive patients evaluated and treated during a one year interval at The M. D. Anderson Hospital. Each of these patients either had inadvertently lost at least 10 pounds of usual body weight, had a serum albumin concentration of less than 3.4 gms%, were negative to a battery of recall skin test antigens or were to receive multiple "back-to-back" courses of oncologic therapy which would restrict oral intake and result in weight loss. These patients would not have been candidates for adequate ocnologic therapy without some form of nutritional repletion, and in most instances, rapid nutritional replenishment or nutritional maintenance via the gastrointestinal tract had failed prior to the institution of IVH.

Table 2. Indications for intravenous hyperalimentation

Indications	# Patients
Chemotherapy	58
General surgical support	48
Head and neck surgery	23
Radiotherapy	14
Fistulas	13
General support	13
Leukemia	10
Renal failure	3
Scleroderma	1
	183

Throughout this study, doses of radiation therapy were those recommended by the Radiation Therapy Department of the M. D. Anderson Hospital, and chemotherapeutic drugs and dose schedules were those recommended by the medical oncology services at our institution. With the exception of those patients with cancer of the colon who received high doses of 5-fluorouracil (5-FU), no attempt was made to administer the maximum tolerated doses of chemotherapeutic agents. Response to chemotherapy or radiation therapy was considered to be a 50% or greater reduction in measurable tumor volume, and no patient was accepted for IVH unless the tumor was potentially responsive to antineoplastic treatment.

In our experience, the terminal patient who has previously received the indicated drugs, failed to respond and has little else to be offered in the form of definitive therapy against his cancer should not, in general, receive IVH because in many instances weight gain will result, and the patient will feel better; however, when IVH is discontinued, rapid weight loss, inanition and death will occur. When outpatient intravenous nutritional maintenance becomes widely available and affordable, then treatment with IVH in the terminal patient may be justified, and we predict that IVH will provide short term improvement in quality of remaining life. At the present time, quality of life for these patients might be improved if they could be motivated to ingest an elemental diet. Most terminal patients, however, have lost all desire to ingest food orally and regardless of palatability or texture of the foodstuffs, they will not eat adequately. Thus, the primary indication for intravenous hyperalimentation in the 183 patients to be discussed was to prepare and maintain them nutritionally and metabolically so that either chemotherapy, surgery, radiation therapy or immunotherapy could be undertaken and completed with maximum safety and efficacy.

CHEMOTHERAPY

Intravenous hyperalimentation was used as an adjunct to chemotherapy in 58 patients (6). Hyperalimentation was administered for an average of 25.9 days and the patients gained an average of 6.8 lb during this period. Intravenous nutritional repletion was usually begun 3-7 days prior to instituting chemotherapy and was continued until the patient could nourish himself adequately by oral food ingestion. Anorexia, nausea, vomiting and diarrhea produced by chemotherapeutic drugs were generally better tolerated while the patient attempted to eat, and since eating was unnecessary during IVH, these symptoms were minimized. Whether or not nausea, stomatitis and general malaise were reduced in response to IVH administration depended upon the chemotherapeutic regimens employed. For example, the gastrointestinal toxic side effects of vinblastine and bleomycin were not reduced by IVH, whereas nausea, vomiting and stomatitis secondary to 5-FU administration were reduced.

Leukocyte depression below 2,500 cells/mm^3 occurred in 48% of the patients and lasted for an average of 7.2 days. No effect of IVH on the nadir or duration of leukocyte depression was apparent when these effects were compared in patients who were not receiving IVH. The average weight gained during IVH by patients who had leukocyte depression was the same as the average weight gained in those individuals who experienced no leukocyte depression.

No episodes of catheter related sepsis occurred in these 58 patients. Sixty-seven subclavian vein catheters were utilized, and all were cultured. Only three catheters were contaminated, and in each instance the organism was *Staphylococcus epidermidis*, probably a skin contaminant. Catheters were considered contaminated when organisms were grown from their tips, but unassociated with positive blood cultures or clinical evidence of sepsis.

Thirty-six per cent (21 patients) had a greater than 50% reduction in measurable malignant disease when treated with chemotherapy and concomitant IVH (Table 3). Although no randomization of patients was done in this series because it would have been unethical to treat most of these patients with chemotherapy without nutritional replenishment, the response rates were similar to those obtained in healthier patients with similar metas-

Table 3. Chemotherapy responses among intravenous hyperalimentation patients

Disease	Number of patients	Responders (> 50%)
Carcinoma of the Lung		
Squamous	10	5
Adenocarcinoma	5	2
Small Cell	5	2
Sarcoma	11	2
Carcinoma of the Colon	10	4
Carcinoma of the Testicle	5	3
Miscellaneous	12	3
Total	58	21

(Adapted from Copeland, 1975)

tatic patterns who did not receive IVH. Patients in the miscellaneous category in Table 3 either had transitional cell carcinoma of the kidney, metastatic melanoma or metastatic adenocarcinoma from an unknown primary site. Two patients with carcinoma of the kidney and one patient with an adenocarcinoma from an unknown primary site responded to chemotherapy. Five patients died either during or within 30 days of completion of IVH. The causes of death were gastrointestinal hemorrhage in one patient and pneumonia in the other 4 patients. The average duration of IVH was 26 days, and each patient gained in strength prior to death from complications secondary to toxic side effects of the administered chemotherapeutic drugs.

There may be a positive correlation between good nutritional status and potential for response to chemotherapy (14). Thirty patients with non-oat cell carcinoma of the lung, evaluable for chemotherapeutic response, have afforded partial control of variables by sharing a similar diagnosis, extensive disease category (Veterans' Administration Cooperative Study Criteria) and identical treatment (bleomycin, cyclophosphamide, vincristine, methotrexate and 5-FU). Ten of these patients were candidates for IVH and received a minimum of 2,000 kcal/day for an average of 22 days before, during and immediately following the administration of chemotherapy. All of these patients had lost 6% or more of their usual body weight before beginning therapy. Twenty patients did not receive hyperalimentation, although 12 of these patients also had lost more than 6% of their usual body weight.

Five of 10 patients in the IVH group responded to chemotherapy, and the magnitude of prior weight loss appeared to have no adverse effect on response. For example, 2 responding patients had a recent weight loss of greater than 20% of the usual body weight (Table 4). There were no responses in the non-IVH patient group if recent weight loss had been greater than 6% of the usual body weight; however, 6 of 8 patients who had lost less than 6% of their usual body weight responded to chemotherapy (Table 4). The response advantages for the nutritionally intact patients were not explained on the basis of number of courses or doses of chemotherapy, or by distribution of histologic types, age, symptom status, prior treatment or metastatic site. Certainly, the response rate for the IVH patients was no worse than for the non-IVH group, and the data would imply that, in general, response rate was improved in patients who weie adequately nourished at the outset of chemotherapy, a parameter which can be controlled, in part, by the administration of IVH.

The effect of "bowel rest" and nutritional maintenance on control of toxicity from 5-FU administration was investigated initially in Sprague-Dawley rats (20). If rats were allowed to nourish themselves ad libitum with ordinary rat chow, an intraperitoneal dose of 5-FU (15 mg/kg/day for 7 days) resulted in death of 80% of the animals by the tenth day. Only 30% of the rats treated with the same dose of 5-FU, allowed nothing by mouth and nourished entirely by IVH perished during the 10 day interval. This experience was extrapolated to human beings, and 10 patients with metastatic colon carcinoma, evaluable for chemotherapeutic response, were placed on IVH (average 2,500 kcal/day) for 7 days before beginning treatment with 5-FU (15 mg/kg/day diluted in 50

Table 4. Thirty patients with lung cancer evaluable for chemotherapeutic response

Treatment group	Patient number	Histology	Weight loss (%)	Chemotherapy response
IVH	1	Undifferentiated	6.5	Yes
	2	Adeno	8.2	No
	3	Adeno	10.7	No
	4	Adeno	13.3	Yes
	5	Undifferentiated	17.2	Yes
	6	Adeno	18.6	No
	7	Adeno	19.4	No
	8	Adeno	19.6	Yes
	9	Squamous	21.7	Yes
	10	Squamous	23.3	No
Non-IVH	11	Squamous	0.0	Yes
	12	Adeno	0.3	Yes
	13	Adeno	0.8	Yes
	14	Squamous	1.8	Yes
	15	Squamous	1.9	Yes
	16	Undifferentiated	2.7	No
	17	Adeno	3.7	No
	18	Undifferentiated	5.7	Yes
	19	Adeno	6.5	No
	20	Squamous	7.3	No
	21	Squamous	8.1	No
	22	Adeno	9.1	No
	23	Undifferentiated	9.9	No
	24	Squamous	12.8	No
	25	Adeno	13.0	No
	26	Squamous	13.8	No
	27	Squamous	14.2	No
	28	Squamous	14.7	No
	29	Adeno	16.1	No
	30	Undifferentiated	16.8	No

(Adapted from Lanzotti, 1975).

ml of 5% dextrose and water and delivered intravenously over a one hour interval). In each instance, drug toxicity initially was manifested by mild stomatitis, nausea or diarrhea, which cleared within 24 hr of discontinuing the drug. Four of the patients responded with greater than 50% reduction in either perineal, sacral, intra-abdominal or pulmonary metastases. Responding patients received an average dose of 8.1 gm of 5-FU administered over an average period of 10 days, whereas non-responding patients tolerated only an average dose of 6.0 gm of 5-FU administered over an average period of 7.3 days. Control patients who did not receive IVH tolerated only 3.8 gm of 5-FU given in an average period of 4.4 days. Control patients routinely lost weight during chemotherapy, whereas the IVH patients gained an average weight of 8.7 lb in an average period of 24.8 days of IVH. Responding patients survived an average interval of 12 months following administration of IVH and 5-FU, whereas non-responding patients were all dead 6 months following treatment. One patient who had intra-abdominal metastases and was not considered evaluable for response to therapy remains alive 2 years later.

The administration of 5-FU had no effect upon positive nitrogen balance after it was established. Vincristine administration, however, did depress nitrogen balance regularly. Excretion of increased nitrogen in the urine following chemotherapy administration may reflect a deleterious effect of the drug upon the cancer cell (or the normal cell) with subsequent elimination of cytotoxic by-products in the urine. For example, an aminoaciduria during treatment of leukemia has been reported (21).

By utilizing IVH prophylactically, more intensive chemotherapeutic treatment of the initially well-nourished patient has been undertaken. Often multiple courses of cytotoxic drugs may be given during the same hospitalization because the patient does not need to go home between courses of chemotherapy in order to recover nutritionally. For example, the young adult male with metastatic testicular carcinoma is usually healthy before his initial treatment with chemotherapy. If intensive therapy with vinblastine and bleomycin is utilized, weight loss of 20 to 30 pounds will often occur. Since the ultimate objective of treatment is complete remission, multiple courses of chemotherapy are usually necessary, and the next course of chemotherapy cannot be initiated safely until the patient has regained some of the weight lost during his previous chemotherapy course. The use of intravenous hyperalimentation during treatment with vinblastine and bleomycin has prevented weight loss and, in fact, usually has resulted in weight gain during therapy; thus, subsequent courses of chemotherapy can be initiated immediately upon return of bone marrow elements to normal.

The majority of patients who were treated with IVH and chemotherapy gained weight. If the malignant process responded by a greater than 50% reduction in size, weight gain was maintained after adequate oral intake was established and IVH was discontinued. If there had been no tumor regression, however, weight gained during hyperalimentation was lost usually within two to three weeks of discontinuing IVH. Because weight was lost so rapidly in the non-responding patient after IVH was discontinued, only those patients whose tumors have a good chance of responding to a chemotherapeutic drug regimen have been chosen for intravenous nutritional replacement, and the obviously terminal patient is not considered a candidate for intravenous hyperalimentation.

Leukemia has not been a contraindication to intravenous hyperalimentation. Ten patients with acute leukemia have been maintained nutritionally with IVH for an average of 21.2 days. Weight gain in these patients has been minimal (average 1.2 lb); however, an increase in strength and general well-being has occurred. There were no hemorrhagic or septic complications secondary to insertion or maintenance of the subclavian vein catheters. If the platelet count at the time of catheter insertion was below 30,000/mm^3, 6 units of platelets were given immediately prior to catheter insertion, and another 6 units of platelets were given immediately following the insertion of the subclavian vein catheter. Otherwise, maintenance of the IVH delivery system was not altered from the routine care given to other patients. Thus, IVH can be used safely in these patients, but the efficacy of intravenous nutritional replenishment in leukemic patients has not been established because of our limited experience in the treatment of these patients to date.

SURGERY

The efficacy of intravenous hyperalimentation in preoperative nutritional repletion of surgical patients has been demonstrated previously. A prospective randomized study of malnourished patients with resectable upper gastrointestinal tract malignancies was carried out by Heatly and his group in England (13). The data that they presented at the XIth International Cancer Congress revealed that those patients who were randomized to IVH for 10 days prior to operation had minimal postoperative morbidity and mortality. Anastomotic problems, wound infections, wound dehiscence and postoperative pneumonia were significantly less in the group receiving IVH. Moreover, the group receiving IVH had a shorter hospital stay than the group which did not receive intravenous nutritional support. Although our team has not done such a randomized prospective study, we have made similar observations.

In our series, 48 patients received IVH as nutrient support for general or thoracic surgical procedures. Without intravenous nutritional replenishment, recovery from the extensive surgical procedures performed would have been questionable in each instance. Sixty per cent of patients underwent curative operations which included esophagectomies, total gastrectomies and abdominal-perineal resections. The remaining 40% of the patients underwent major palliative procedures which required laparotomy. The average age of the patients was 54.8 years, the average duration of IVH was 20.6 days, and the average weight gained was 5.8 lb. Only two patients expired postoperatively, and catheter-related sepsis occurred in one patient.

In 24 patients, IVH was used for an average period of 11.5 days preoperatively and for an average period of 12.8 days postoperatively. In 15 patients, IVH was used only postoperatively for an average of 18 days, and in 9 patients, IVH was used only preoperatively for an average of 19 days.

If a malnourished patient requires a surgical procedure, we strongly recommend that he be nutritionally prepared preoperatively rather than waiting until the postoperative period to institute intravenous nutritional therapy. In this series, those individuals who received IVH only postoperatively usually had virtually no postoperative complications and often were eating adeparalytic ileus, wound infection, decubitus ulcer or wound dehiscence) before IVH was instituted, whereas the patients who received IVH preoperatively had virtually no postoperative complications and often were eating adequately within four to five days after bowel resection.

More recently, IVH has been a particularly impressive adjunct to the surgical management of patients with obstructing carcinomas of the esophagus treated by radiation therapy and/or esophagectomy combined with colon interposition. Of 10 severely malnourished patients treated to date, only one patient has expired postoperatively, and there has been no morbidity secondary to anastomotic failure.

Patients with oropharyngeal malignancies often present weight loss because the lesion either obstructs the gastrointestinal lumen or produces pain on deglutition. Moreover, these patients often have a history of heavy alcohol intake, smoking and dietary indiscretions. Nasogastric intubation and appropriate tube feeding will suffice to nutritionally replete most of these patients, but sometimes these feedings are not tolerated because of regurgitation or malabsorption, and weight gain either is not achieved or is minimal. Intravenous hyperalimentation has been used in 23 such patients who did not tolerate nasogastric tube feedings (7). Prompt nutritional repletion and weight gain were achieved in each patient.

Fifteen patients with large resectable lesions of the head and neck were candidates for IVH. Twelve patients required laryngopharyngectomy, 9 with concurrent radical neck dissection and thoracoacromial flap reconstruction. The average age of the patients was 64.3 years; IVH was utilized for an average of 44.2 days; and average weight gain was 13.5 lb. Wound healing was complete in all patients with the exception of the three who expired. Two patients died from aspiration pneumonia and one from a ruptured carotic artery. The resected specimen exceeded the limits of wound healing in each of these 3 patients. Good surgical judgment is necessary when choosing methods for treatment of squamous cell carcinoma of the head and neck because these lesions often grow to relatively large size before distant metastases occur and often are resectable anatomically, but for reasons of malnutrition and poor wound healing, are not resectable physiologically.

Six patients received IVH as nutritional supportive care within 24 months after major operation or irradiation therapy for head and neck cancer. Intravenous nutritional support was utilized for an average period of 26.6 days and the average weight gain was 10.5 lb. Four of these patients were discharged from the hospital after their tolerance to nasogastric tube feedings improved, and two patients required gastrostomy feeding tube insertion for long term ambulatory nutritional maintenance.

To date, 6 patients with pharyngocutaneous fistulas have been treated. Two of the fistulas closed spontaneously after 17 and 20 days of IVH, and the remaining four fistulas required surgical closure after 21 to 47 days of IVH. Previous attempts at surgical closure had failed in three of these patients. More recently, three additional patients have received IVH because of postoperative pharyngeal incompetence. Concomitant with return of general body muscle strength and tone, swallowing function also returned between 18 and 48 days of intravenous nutritional support.

Catheter-related sepsis is the most common complication resulting from the use of IVH in patients with head and neck cancer. Five positive catheter cultures were obtained from the tips of the subclavian vein catheters removed from these 23 patients. *Candida tropicalis* was grown from 2 catheters, and *Candida albicans* was grown from another catheter. In 2 patients, Candida was grown from both the catheter and the blood stream. Each patient with a positive catheter-culture had undergone major surgery and had a pharyngocutaneous or tracheostomy stoma which allowed secretions to frequently contaminate the subclavian vein catheter dressing. Consequently, maintenance of hyperalimentation delivery systems and catheter dressings must be particularly meticulous in this patient group. Often catheter dressings must be changed on a daily basis, and routinely, a water repellent plastic sheet is placed over the catheter dressing in order to minimize contamination. It was only in the head and neck cancer patient group that catheter-related sepsis was a problem. Nevertheless, realization of this potential risk allowed physicians to properly care for patients and minimize the incidence of catheter-related sepsis. To date, no deaths secondary to catheter-related sepsis have occurred.

FISTULAS

Gastrointestinal external fistulas may be treated adequately by "bowel rest" and intravenous hyperalimentation. Patients who have had a resection of a portion of the GI tract for cure or long term palliation and have developed an external fistula present no insurmountable problem and may be managed as if they had benign intra-abdominal disease. Often, however, when a gastrointestinal fistula develops in a patient who was explored surgically and was found to have mutiple intra-abdominal metastases, how aggressive should the physician be in attempting to heal these fistulas? Thirteen such patients were treated in this series (Table 5), and the fistulas in 11 patients closed spontaneously in an average period of 32 days of IVH. Two of these patients expired before discharge from the hospital; otherwise, the patients returned home, later underwent appropriate antineoplastic therapy and lived useful lives until their demise.

Spontaneous closure of fistulas involving radiated bowel or the abdominal wall was difficult to obtain. Six patients with radiation fistulas of this type

Table 5. Gastrointestinal external fistulas

Site of origin	# patients		
Esophagus	3	Spontaneous closure	85%
Stomach	3	IVH days	32
Duodenum	1	Operative closure	15%
Ileum	4	Deaths on IVH	15%
Cecum	2		
Total	13		

have been treated to date. Two ileocutaneous fistulas and one duodenocutaneous fistula closed spontaneously between 22 and 102 days of IVH. The remaining 3 fistulas required operative closure, and 2 of these patients expired one week postoperatively. All 6 patients were dead within 9 months of fistula closure. Thus, our results with radiation-induced fistulas were dismal when compared with the results obtained with fistulas involving non-radiated bowel. We currently recommend that patients with fistulas involving radiated bowel be prepared for surgery by preoperative intravenous nutritional support. Following the initiation of anabolism and positive nitrogen balance, a long intestinal tube such as a Miller-Abbott or Cantor tube is inserted into the small bowel. At exploratory laparotomy, proximal small bowel is easy to identify from distal small bowel because it contains the tube. As much of the proximal small bowel as can be retained is anastomosed end-to-side to the colon in a non-radiated area. The distal small bowel is oversewn, and the fistula tract is left within the defunctionalized distal bowel to serve as a vent. This method of treating small bowel fistulas is most applicable to patients who are expected to have dense adhesions within the abdominal cavity and it has been more successful than resection of the fistula with reanastomosis of the bowel.

RADIATION THERAPY

Radiation treatment of the gastrointestinal tract produces mucositis with resultant pain, nausea, vomiting, anorexia and diarrhea. The patient ingests less food and is less able to absorb those nutrients which reach the gastrointestinal lumen. The reparative phase of mucosal injury is delayed, and prolonged mucositis may result in fibrosis and stricture of the gastrointestinal tract. Usually some degree of radiation stomatitis or enteritis must be accepted in order to allow delivery of an adequate tumor dose of irradiation to a malignancy which lies within or next to the gastrointestinal tract. If, however, radiation enteritis becomes disabling, therapy must often be discontinued before an adequate tumor dose has been administered. We have treated 14 such patients by "bowel rest" and hyperalimentation. Anorexia, nausea and vomiting disappeared unless the patient attempted to eat, in which case all symptoms recurred. These patients received IVH for an average period of 34 days, gained an average weight of 5.4 lb and completed their planned courses of radiation therapy. Eight patients had good tumor responses to therapy, maintained their gained weight after IVH was discontinued and had no disabling sequelae as a result of radiation enteritis.

NUTRITIONAL MAINTENANCE

Often palliative or potentially curative chemotherapy or radiation therapy is administered to the patient as an outpatient. Nevertheless, limited anorexia and gastroenteritis occur and may result in marked weight loss. These patients have little desire to eat, although their gastrointestinal tracts are functional. This problem can be solved partially by short term intravenous nutritional repletion. Thirteen such patients have been treated with IVH for an average period of 14.5 days, and during this time, food was offered to them by mouth. Appetite gradually improved as the patients gained strength. By the time of discharge, they could ingest adequate calories orally and continue chemotherapy or begin radiation therapy on an outpatient basis.

COMPLICATIONS

Catheter-related clinical sepsis is the most feared complication of intravenous hyperalimentation. For example, one group of investigators reported that 61.4% of the subclavian vein catheters in their series grew organisms upon removal (1). The incidence of catheter-related sepsis in the initial 93 patients who underwent hyperalimentation for 10 days or longer at our institution was 2.2% (5). We have continued to culture all catheters upon removal, and our rate of catheter-related sepsis has remained approximately 2.2% during the treatment of more than 2000 subsequent patients. As in other published reports, *Candida albicans* was the organism most frequently grown from the catheters; nevertheless, amphotericin flush of the IVH delivery tubing as advocated by Brennan and his co-workers has not been necessary (2).

Thrombogenesis is increased in cancer patients, but evidence of subclavian vein thrombosis occurred in only 3 patients in our series. In each patient, the ipsilateral arm became edematous, but the edema resolved spontaneously within one week of removing the subclavian vein catheter. Heparin was not utilized and no documented episodes of pulmonary emboli occurred. Two other patients did have a proven pulmonary embolus while receiving IVH, and the clots were demonstrated to originate in the pelvis in each instance.

Hyperchloremic metabolic acidosis occurred in one patient. This complication resolved 48 hr after reduction of the administered chloride in the IVH solution. Symptomatic hypophosphatemia occurred in one patient who was recovering from a head and neck surgical procedure. His only symptom was abnormal behavior which resolved after the serum phosphate level was restored to normal by the infusion of phosphate. Two patients developed transient pulmonary edema because of fluid overload. Often the medical oncologist infuses chemotherapeutic drugs through a peripheral intravenous site. If the peripherally administered water volume is not coordinated with the volume of centrally administered IVH nutrients, fluid overload can occur. For this reason, members of the IVH team should be responsible for the total water and electrolyte content of all parenteral and enteral fluid intake.

INTRAVENOUS HYPERALIMENTATION – FUTURE CONSIDERATIONS

Nutritional support of patients receiving oncologic therapy has proved effective in allowing adequate treatment programs to be carried out in a series of patients who otherwise would not be candidates for any antineoplastic therapy. Tumor growth has not been measurably enhanced and septic complications have been minimal. It would appear that there is a correlation between adequate nutrition and the potential for tumor response to chemotherapy. Moreover, it would appear that there is an increased tolerance for certain chemotherapeutic drugs, particularly 5-FU, and that the tumor response to these drugs may be improved because more drug can be delivered per unit time. Whether these latter impressions are true, false, related or unrelated will require further investigation, probably with randomized prospective trials, because the results have not been clear-cut. Initially, we postulated that malignant cell replication might be stimulated by IVH and that cell cycle specific chemotherapeutic drugs might be more effective under these circumstances. This theory has neither been proved nor disproved; however, we have shown that patients who were too malnourished and cachectic to receive any form of anti-cancer therapy, have not only tolerated a complete course of treatment after intravenous nutritional preparation, but have frequently experienced a positive therapeutic effect.

With current emphasis on immunotherapy, interrelationships between the body's immune mechanisms and nutritional status should be explored. The combination of nutrition and chemotherapy, radiation therapy or surgery may render the patient immunologically incompetent. The most potent of these factors in eradicating established delayed hypersensitivity is probably malnutrition. Bacillus Calumet Guerin (BCG) is a non-specific immune stimulant administered, in part, to boost established cell-mediated immunity, but if this system is depressed by malnutrition, BCG will be minimally effective.

Recently, we have completed a study of 47 cancer patients who received IVH in preparation for and during treatment with either chemotherapy, radiation therapy or surgery (8). Each patient received selected recall skin test antigens intradermally in the forearm at the initiation of IVH and at 7 day intervals throughout antineoplastic treatment.

Seventeen of 23 patients receiving chemotherapy were initially skin test negative. Thirteen of these patients converted their skin tests to positive during an average of 11.4 days of IVH. Four patients responded to chemotherapy, and each converted skin tests to positive before much regression in tumor volume had occurred. No patient whose skin tests remained negative or converted to negative during treatment had a response to chemotherapy.

No septic complications were encountered in patients with positive skin tests. Short term chemotherapy frequently suppresses primary delayed hypersensitivity but has little effect on established immunity. Thus, the adequately nourished patient receiving chemotherapy still has potentially intact immunological defense mechanisms against some viruses and most fungi. Malnourished patients receiving chemotherapy, however, may be virtually defenseless against microorganisms because both primary and established delayed hypersensitivity are suppressed, and total circulating leukocytes often are depressed markedly. In this series of 47 patients, death occurred in only those patients with negative skin tests, and pneumonia was the cause of death in 3 of the 4 patients who expired.

Although the number of patients in this series was too small to warrant definite conclusions, three important observations were made: a) only patients with positive skin tests responded to chemotherapy; b) during radiation therapy, skin tests remained negative even though nutritional repletion was considered adequate; and c) those surgical patients who developed or retained positive skin tests preoperatively had an uncomplicated postoperative recovery, whereas those patients with negative tests either expired or had a prolonged, complicated period of recovery.

From the clinical observations made with the use of IVH as adjunctive treatment for cancer patients and from previous research conducted on the mechanisms of cancer cell metabolism, several potential avenues for investigation are apparent. For example, amino acid, glucose, vitamin and electrolyte manipulations as specific treatment for cancer have been attempted both in man and animals, but success with these maneuvers has been limited because the administered diets were cumbersome and the method of delivery of these diets was ineffective and inaccurate. Intravenous hyperalimentation now gives the clinical scientist total control over patient intake, and specific dietary deletions or additions can be made while the host is maintained in nutritional equilibrium. More specifically, an amino acid mixture might be formulated which is deficient in an amino acid necessary for tumor metabolism but relatively less necessary for maintenance of host nutrition. Research of this nature will not be easy because such a diet probably will have to be administered over a long period of time before any deleterious effect on tumor growth can be documented. Amino acid profiles of various tumors might be different, and the choice of which amino acids to manipulate will be difficult.

Increasing evidence indicates that cancer cells have a greater dependence upon anaerobic glucose consumption as an energy source than do normal cells. Lactic acid is the end product of glycolysis, and concentrations of this compound within the tumor environment probably increase as more glucose is made available for tumor metabolism. Meyer has data to suggest that methotrexate may have a higher cell penetrance in an acid environment and a consequent better cancericidal effect (16). This postulate should be examined in the patient receiving IVH because glucose is thereby administered at an average rate of 25 grams per hour. Tumor pH should theoretically fall and, if Meyer's theory is correct, the uptake of methotrexate by the tumor should be facilitated.

The major metabolic pathway for glucose utilization in the gastrointestinal mucosal cell is aerobic. Thus, there is an apparent dislocation in glucose metabolism between the more rapidly growing cancer and the mucosal cells, both of which are affected adversely by chemotherapy. Possibly, this differential effect upon glucose metabolism could be exploited by the infusion of large concentrations of glucose during chemotherapy administration. We have shown that intravenous hyperalimentation protects the gastro-intestinal tract from the toxic side-effects of 5-FU while a somewhat better than expected tumor response to 5-FU was promoted.

The effect of most hormones on tumor growth is poorly understood. For example, growth hormone increases amino acid uptake in rapidly multiplying cells (17), and also is elevated in malnourished patients (18). Does the elevated growth hormone in malnourished cancer patients potentiate growth of tumor because of the stimulated amino acid uptake? Our group has demonstrated diabetic glucose tolerance curves, depressed serum insulin levels, and increased levels of serum growth hormone in 8 malnourished patients with metastatic cancer (19). Following 10 days of intravenous hyperalimentation and induced positive nitrogen balance, serum levels of growth hormone were reduced to almost normal. No effect on tumor growth was identified in this small series of patients secondary to this growth hormone reduction; nevertheless, the concept that growth hormone has an effect on the tumor-host relationship merits further investigation. Certainly, if growth hormone facilitated tumor growth, then lowering growth hormone levels by nutritional repletion in malnourished patients would be desirable.

With proper patient selection for study in a controlled environment such as in a metabolic unit, many of the above suggested hormonal, biochemical and epidemiological parameters could be studied within the same patient group. This modality of research offers potentially major exciting breakthroughs in the management and treatment of cancer patients.

ACKNOWLEDGEMENTS

The authors gratefully acknowledge the expert nursing assistance of Mary Ann Rapp, R.N. and Sandra Norman, R.N. and the technical assistance of Ms. Jerry Brown.

This work was supported in part by Grant CA-05831 and CA-16672 from the National Institutes of Health, U.S. Public Health Service.

ABBREVIATIONS

BCG – Bacillus Calmette-Guerin
GI – gastrointestinal
IVH – intravenous hyperalimentation
5-FU – 5-fluorouracil

REFERENCES

1. Bernard, R. W., Stahl, W. M. and Chase, R. M., Subclavian vein catheterization: a prospective study. II. Infectious complications. *Annals of Surgery 173*: 191-200 (1971).
2. Brennan, M. F., Goldman, M. H., O'Connell, R. C., Kundsin, R. B. and Moore, F. O., Prolonged parenteral alimentation: Candida growth and the prevention of candidemia by amphotericin instillation. *Annals of Surgery 175*: 265-272 (1972).
3. Cannon, P. R., Frazier, L. E. and Hughes, R. H., Influence of potassium on tissue protein synthesis. *Metabolism 1*: 49-57 (1952).
4. Copeland, E. M., MacFadyen, B. V., Jr. and Dudrick, S. J., Intravenous hyperalimentation in cancer patients. *Journal of Surgical Research 16*: 241-247 (1974).
5. Copeland, E. M., MacFadyen, B. V., Jr. and Dudrick, S. J., The use of hyperalimentation in patients with potential sepsis. *Surgery, Gynecology and Obstetrics 138*: 377-380 (1974).
6. Copeland, E. M., MacFadyen, B. V., Jr., Lanzotti, V. J. and Dudrick, S. J., Intravenous hyperalimentation as an adjunct to cancer chemotherapy. *American Journal of Surgery 129*: 166-173 (1975).

7. Copeland, E. M., MacFadyen, B. V., Jr., MacComb, W. S., Guillamondegui, O., Jesse, R. H. and Dudrick, S. J., Intravenous hyperalimentation in patients with head and neck cancer. *Cancer 35*: 606-611 (1975).
8. Copeland, E. M., MacFadyen, B. V., Jr., Rapp, M. A. and Dudrick, S. J., Hyperalimentation and immune competence in cancer. In: *Surgical Forum* (Proceedings of the 31st Annual Session of the Forum on Fundamental Surgical Problems, 61st Clinical Congress of the American College of Surgeons). Chicago, Illinois, American College of Surgeons, 1975, Vol. XXVI, pp. 138-140.
9. Cuthbertson, D. P., Further observations on the disturbance of metabolism caused by injury, with particular reference to dietary requirements of fracture cases. *British Journal of Surgery 23*: 505-520 (1936).
10. Daly, J. M., Steiger, E., Vars, H. M. and Dudrick, S. J., Postoperative oral and intravenous nutrition. *Annals of Surgery 180*: 709-715 (1974).
11. Dudrick, S. J., Vars, H. M. and Rhoads, J. E., Growth of puppies receiving all nutritional requirements by vein. *Fortschritte der Parenteralen Ernährung*. Symposium of the International Society of Parenteral Nutrition in 1966. Lochham bei Munchen, West Germany, Pallas Verlag, 1967, pp. 2-4.
12. Dudrick, S. J., Wilmore, D. W., Vars, H. M. and Rhoads, J. E., Long-term total parenteral nutrition with growth, development and positive nitrogen balance. *Surgery 64*: 134-142 (1968).
13. Heatly, R. V. and Hughes, L. E., Preoperative intravenous nutrition in cancer patients (Abstract). Proceedings of the XIth International Cancer Congress *4*: 874 (1975).
14. Lanzotti, V. C., Copeland, E. M., George, S. L., Dudrick, S. J. and Samuels, M. L., Cancer chemotherapeutic response and intravenous hyperalimentation. *Cancer Chemotherapy Reports 59*: 437-439 (1975).
15. Long, J. M., Wilmore, D. W. and Pruitt, B. A., Comparison of carbohydrate and fat as caloric sources. In: *Surgical Forum* (Proceedings of the 31st Annual Session of the Forum on Fundamental Surgical Problems, 61st Clinical Congress of the American College of Surgeons). Chicago, Illinois, College of Surgeons, 1975, Vol. XXVI, pp. 108-110.
16. Meyer, J. A., Potentiation of solid-tumor chemotherapy by metabolic alteration. *Annals of Surgery 179*: 88-93 (1974).
17. Noall, M. W., Riggs, T. R., Walker, L. M. and Christensen, H. N., Endocrine control of amino acid transfer. *Science 126*: 1002-1005 (1957).
18. Pimstone, B. L., Wittmann, W., Hansen, J. D. L. and Murray, P., Growth hormone and kwashiorkor. *The Lancet 2*: 779-780 (1966).
19. Solomon, N., Copeland, E. M., MacFadyen, B. V., Jr., Dudrick, S. J. and Samaan, N. A., Intravenous hyperalimentation and growth hormone in cancer patients. In: *Surgical Forum* (Proceedings of the 30th Annual Session of the Forum on Fundamental Surgical Problems, 60th Clinical Congress of the American College of Surgeons). Chicago, Illinois, American College of Surgeons, 1974, Vol. XXV, pp. 59-60.
20. Souchon, E. A., Copeland, E. M., Watson, P. and Dudrick, S. J., Intravenous hyperalimentation as an adjunct to cancer chemotherapy with 5-fluorouracil. *Journal of Surgical Research 18*: 451-454 (1975).
21. Wiseman, C., McGregor, R. F. and McCredie, K. B., Urinary amino-acid excretion in acute leukemia. *Cancer* 38: 219-224, 1976

The application of parenteral nutrition to renal failure patients

H. A. Lee, B.Sc., M.B., B.S., F.R.C.P.

The metabolic response to trauma in patients with acute renal failure is no different from that which occurs in patients with normal renal function (1, 2). Thus, in both situations the metabolic response is characterised by a breakdown of the muscle cell mass, associated with the release of potassium, phosphate and hydrogen ions into the extracellular fluid and increased ureagenesis. The essential difference is that whereas patients with normal renal function can excrete all the excess products of this metabolic response into the urine, renal failure patients cannot do so adequately and thus hyperkalaemia, metabolic acidosis and uraemia occur. Furthermore, if the catabolic patients with renal failure are not treated they, like their normal renal function counterparts, will show evidence of negative nitrogen balance characterised by loss of body weight, impaired immunocompetence, decreased ability to heal wounds and hypoproteinaemic oedema resulting in increased morbidity and mortality.

Therefore, any attempt to practice parenteral nutrition in acute renal failure patients who have associated gastro-intestinal failure, must take into account (a) the effects of the uraemic environment upon substrate utilisation and (b) volume constraints for intravenous administration. Even in patients with normal gastro-intestinal function, ward surveys have shown how they often cannot take the full recommended oral intakes, this as a result of apathy, nausea or pain which decrease appetite. In such patients parenteral nutrition may play a complete or supplementary role.

In spite of the enormous advances made in the management of chronic renal failure over the past twenty years, it is disappointing to note the persistent high mortality of acute renal failure (3), particularly in the age group above 50 years, where mortality still exceeds 50% and is most commonly associated with infection (4). It has long been recognised that malnutrition and infection go hand in hand. It may be equally well relevant to note that acute renal failure patients often become severely malnourished which may lead to their increased susceptibility to infection. Thus, it seems pertinent to recommend aggressive nutritional management of these patients which in turn may improve their immunocompetence both at humoral and cellular levels and, thereby, their survival.

Any consideration of parenteral nutrition in renal failure patients must take into account the increased nutritional losses imposed by the very dialysis procedures used. During peritoneal dialysis up to 20-30 g of protein (5) and 13-15 g of amino acids may be lost per 40 litre exchange (6). During haemodialysis although protein losses do not occur between 2-3 g of amino acids are lost per hour (7).

The question of how best to assess the nutritional status in these patients is a more difficult problem. Some of the indices normally used to assess nutritional status are shown in Table 1. Body weight is of little value in acute renal failure patients because of fluid retention and likewise measurement of body potassium not so readily performed. Skin fold thickness and mid-arm circumference measurements may be a useful guide in long-term management problems but not for the immediate assessment of acute renal failure. Serum albumin is of limited value and serum pro-albumin less easily measured. The short half-life proteins serum transferrin and C3 complement are easily measured and useful indices of the hepatic protein synthesis rate and hence nutritional equilibrium (7). Measurement of the serum 3-methylhistidine is a good marker of muscle protein catabolism since this metabolite represents the breakdown of muscle actinomycin and is nonrecyclable (8). However, few laboratories are currently equipped to measure this metabolite. Serum amino acid profiles may also be a valuable index through perhaps more useful in chronic renal failure patients.

The consideration of intravenous energy substrates for parenteral nutrition in renal failure must take into account whether normal metabolism may

Table 1. Some indices to measure nutritional status

1. Body weight
2. Clinical assessment of patient well-being
3. Skin fold thickness (energy reserves)
4. Mid arm circumference (protein reserves)
5. Urine urea nitrogen (guide to catabolic rate, assuming minimal extra renal losses)
6. Serum transferrin, complement C3
7. Serum albumin
8. Total body potassium
9. Serum amino acid profiles
10. Urine 3-methyl histidine levels
11. Skin anergy e.g. to candida antigen
12. Peripheral lymphocyte count

be anticipated in the uraemic environment, the consequences of fluid constraint, whether the energy substrates interfere with the normal performance of dialysis membranes and whether there may be any increased metabolic risk from using these substrates in a uraemic individual. In the author's opinion the only two intravenous energy substrates that need be considered are (a) glucose and (b) a fat emulsion, soya bean oil ("Intralipid"). Although there is a glucose intolerance during uraemia (9), glucose-insulin regimes can circumvent this problem. There is no indication for using fructose with its greater risk of producing lactic acidaemia and even lactic acidosis. In chronic renal failure patients it has been shown that one-third of such patients have a pre-existing lactic acidaemia (10).

Although lipid metabolism is abnormal during uraemia, it has been clearly shown that post-dialysis normal triglyceride clearance (11) and postheparin lipolytic activity return (12). There is no indication for xylitol or sorbitol or combinations of these two energy substrates with ethanol.

As for the amino acid profile to be used in acute renal failure, it appears that provided the profile is balanced and complete i.e. essential and non-essential amino acids, as opposed to using a casein hydrolysate, then this is satisfactory.

There are special problems with intravenous nutrition in acute renal failure. These are (a) increased insulin resistance (b) possible amino acid toxicity (c) dialysis-related nutrient losses (d) the relevance of phosphate magnesium and potassium provision (e) the requirements of essential biological elements e.g. zinc and copper and (f) substrate tolerances.

During intravenous nutrition for non renal failure patients it has been shown that 45 kcals and 0.22 g of nitrogen/kg body weight are optimal for achieving nitrogen balance (13). In chronic renal failure patients the optimal oral caloric intake has been shown to be greater at 55 kcals/kg body weight (14). Whether the same is true for intravenous nutrition in such patients is debatable. The possibility that renal failure patients require a greater energy intake to induce nitrogen-adaptive metabolic pathways is a possibility. In oral feeding experiments it has been shown that manipulation of the carbohydrate versus fat intake between 35 and 65% does not adversely affect nitrogen balance (15). It is the author's practice to supply calories on a nearly 50% basis from carbohydrate (glucose) and fat (16). Such a regime provides a large number of calories in a relatively small fluid volume, decreases insulin requirements, reduces osmotic load and provides the essential fatty acid requirement (see table 8, p. 268).

It has been postulated that the amino acid nitrogen used for the management of acute renal failure patients need provide only the essential amino acids since urea nitrogen can be recycled for provision of non-essential nitrogen (17). However, this premise may be mistaken since there is little evidence to support that urea nitrogen recycling has any nutritional value in acute renal failure patients and only contributes up to 6% for albumin synthesis in chronic renal failure (18). It is important not to confuse the question of urea nitrogen recycling with the nutritional value of urea nitrogen. It seems reasonable to assume that in acute renal failure there is a requirement for a given amount of nitrogen of which a certain percentage e.g. 50% may be represented by essential amino acids. There can be no virtue in providing an excess of essential amino acids at the expense of non-essential ones. The concept that only essential amino acids should be given so as to reduce the rate of urea production or indeed actually cause diminution of the blood urea level is not the only aim of intravenous nutrition in acute renal failure patients. However, it is true that such treatment may not only reduce the blood urea production rate, but also reduce the rate of increment in respect of hyperkalaemia and hyperphosphataemia and diminish the incidence of metabolic acidosis by reducing tissue catabolism (17) (Table 2).

Early research into the effects of fat emulsions on the dialysis characteristics of artificial kidney membranes showed that these were not adversely affected (19). It has also been previously pointed out that amino acids should not be infused during haemodialysis as these will be rapidly lost (their mean molecular weight is 200).They are preferably infused evenly over the last 2-3 hours of haemodialysis. This infusion time is particularly important with any amino acid solution that has a high content of glutamic acid, otherwise

Table 2. Advantages of TPN in acute renal failure*

1. Maintenance of nutritional equilibrium
2. Decreased catabolism with:
   (i) Diminished ureagenesis
   (ii) Diminished hyperkalaemia
   (iii) Decreased metabolic acidosis
3. Decreased dialysis requirement [in non hypercatabolic (> 20 g N/day) patients]
4. Improved patient well being
5. Less susceptible to infections
6. Improved survival
7. Less "toxic" problems e.g. myocardial
8. Decreased duration of acute renal failure

* For patients who cannot, will not or must not take food orally.

an intravenous "Chinese restaurant syndrome" results. It is our practice to add amino acids routinely to our peritoneal dialysate. For this purpose we add 10 ml per litre of peritoneal dialysate of a Vamin-N solution which provides 94 mg of amino acid nitrogen per litre of dialysate. A further practical point concerns the addition of heparin with intravenous lipid administration. It should be noted that normal post heparin lipolytic activity is inhibited in uraemic patients and only returns to normal once the metabolic environment approaches normality after dialysis. Thus there can be little rationale for the addition of heparin for increasing the rate of triglyceride clearance from the bloodstream.

The advantages of parenteral nutrition in acute renal failure associated with gastro-intestinal failure are: (a) maintenance of adequate nutrition (b) possible decreased frequency of dialysis (c) decreased incidence of metabolic toxic effects (d) a decrease in the rate of rise of blood urea (e) an improved survival (f) a decreased tendency towards hyperkalaemia, metabolic acidosis and hyperphosphataemia (g) increased patient well-being (h) improved immunocompetence and decreased susceptibility to infection and (i) a possible reduction in the duration of acute renal failure. The latter suggestion arises from the observations of Abel et al. (17) who have shown that the provision of amino acids may actually accelerate the regenerative processes in the acutely damaged kidney. The discussion as to the appropriateness of a full amino acid profile or simply an essential amino acid profile as the nitrogen source for parenteral nutrition in acute renal failure should not detract in any way from the undoubted value of this therapeutic approach in such patients. Equally, it has been shown that beneficial effects are obtained when all the energy is either derived from a glucose-insulin regime or a glucose-fat energy substrate regime. When glucose only is used it can be anticipated that the insulin requirement will be higher and may amount to 200-300 units per day. Also, the insulin requirements are likely to be higher at the start of such treatment when the patient is particularly hypercatabolic and then stabilise after three or four days. Thus over the first 48 hours it is most important that blood sugar estimations are done every 6 hours so that blood sugar is kept at around 10 mmol/l. It appears that the amount of nitrogen required at least for the non-catabolic acute renal failure patient may be as little as 0.07 g of nitrogen/kg body weight compared to the normal values referred to earlier (Table 3). This decreased nitrogen figure requirement may reflect some adaptive process in nitrogen economy which is not related to urea nitrogen recycling.

Unless the patient has some inherent bleeding tendency then there is little merit in necessarily trying to reduce the dialysis frequency and thus having to modify an intravenous complete nutritional regime. It is more important to feed the patient as required and adapt dialysis requirements (2) to keep the metabolic environment as near normal as possible. By so doing, substrate utilisation at maximum efficiency will be ensured (11). The infraclavicular percutaneous subclavian vein access route is the one ideally used for such patients particularly those receiving hypertonic nutritional regimes. Although a peripheral route for the less hypertonic infusion regimes may be used, these are usually less satisfactory.

Table 3. Total parenteral nutrition regimes in acute renal failure (Non hypercatabolic)

Vol	Source	Energy CH_2O	Fat	Nitrogen g(AAg)	Na+ mmol	K+ mmol	mOSm	Comments
0.5L	Vamin-Glu	50 g (200)	–	4.7 (35)	25	10	637	No essential fatty acids
1.0L	50% Glucose	500 g (2000)	–	–	–	–	3800	Must give insulin
1.5L		2200		4.7 (35)	25	10	4437	
0.5L	Vamin-Glu	50 g (200)	–	4.7 (35)	25	20	637	May require insulin
0.5L	20% Intralipid	–	100 g (1000)	–	–	–	175	
0.5L	50% Glucose	250 g (1000)	–	–	–	–	1900	
1.5L		2200		4.7 (35)	25	10	2712	
0.5L	Vamin-N	–	–	4.7 (35)	25	10	526	Least hypertonic
0.5L	20% Intralipid	–	100 g (1000)	–	–	–	175	
0.5L	50% Glucose	250 g (1000)	–	–	–	–	1900	
1.5L		2000		4.7 (35)	25	10	2601	

All regimes need addition of water soluble vitamins and essential biological elements for completeness. All may need addition of phosphorus, potassium and magnesium dependent upon degree of anabolism. For hypercatabolic acute renal failure patients use normal regimes and dialyse accordingly.

The post-operative intravenous nutritional requirements for renal transplanted patients are no different from those for normal patients if renal function has been established. If renal function has not been established and there is a need to avoid immediate haemodialysis in the post-operative period even when there is adequate gastro-intestinal function either (a) because of a bleeding diathesis or (b) potential inadequacy of extracorporeal heparinisation, then the introduction of a parenteral nutrition regime (Table 2) can delay haemodialysis for 2 or 3 days so that the risk of bleeding around the graft site is minimised. With the modern immunosuppressive regimes used, including methyl prednisolone pulse therapy, there is no need to allow for an excessive load of urea nitrogen as a result of prolonged high steroid dosage. As for normal patients, so in acute renal failure patients requiring intravenous nutrition, where the serum oncotic pressure needs to be rapidly corrected, plasma or human plasma protein fraction should be used and not amino acids. It is just as inappropriate here to use amino acids for immediate restoration of normal serum albumin levels as it is to use serum albumin as the source of immediately available intravenous amino acids.

The application of parenteral nutrition in chronic renal failure is of more limited impact. Nevertheless, occasional patients with established chronic renal failure become emaciated as a result of intercurrent infection or intractable hypertension due to a hyper-renin state. These patients become anorexic and grossly emaciated. Often the only way to treat both groups is by bilateral nephrectomy which in the one case eradicates the source of infection and in the other removes the cause of the hyper-renin state. Full parenteral nutrition can be practised on these patients by adopting a total parenteral nutrition regime which provides energy, amino acids, essential biological elements, water soluble vitamins and other appropriate electrolyte requirements. Thrice weekly haemodialysis can be adopted allowing for an adequate intravenous fluid volume. Advantage can be taken of the actual dialysis time to improve the nutritional status by priming the coil with albumin or human plasma fraction and infusing a litre of 20% fat emulsion ("Intralipid") providing 2,000 kcals during the dialysis period. Over the last 3 hours of each haemodialysis 0.5 litres of Vamin-N or Vamin-glucose (4.7 g of nitrogen) can be slowly infused. By such practice thrice weekly haemodialysis allows for provision of 6,000 additional calories and 14.1 g of nitrogen per week in addition to a daily intravenous nutritional regime. An intravenous daily nutritional regime supplying between 7-10 g of nitrogen and 2,000 calories with other nutrients can be designed (see Table 4) and can dramatically improve a patient's well-being.

Table 4. Daily TPN regime for regular dialysis patient having three dialyses per week

Vol	Source	Energy CH_2O	Fat	Nitrogen g (AAg)	Na+ mmol	K+ mmol
1.0L	Vamin-Glu	400	–	9.4 (70)	50	20
0.5L	20% Intralipid	–	1000	–	–	–
0.5L	50% Glucose	1000	–	–	–	–
2.0L		2400	–	9.4	50	20

- Will usually need to add phosphorus (neutral phosphate solution) up to 0.5 mmol/kg body weight as patient becomes anabolic.
- Similarly, potassium additions become necessary.
- Usual additions of water soluble vitamins and essential biological element (Addam solution, Sweden); also vit. K.
- This regime is in addition to nutrition given across haemodialysis.

Thus parenteral nutrition can be the difference between death and survival in acute renal failure and chronic renal failure patients. The intravenous energy substrates required are no different from normal although the amount of energy needed may be higher than normal. The nitrogen provision, preferably a complete amino acid profile (essential and non-essential amino acids) is probably less than in normal because of possible induction of adaptive metabolic pathways.

Finally a brief mention of the application of parenteral nutrition to uraemic patients, acute or chronic, with incipient coma or rather neurological sequelae. In hepatic coma it has been suggested that a specific alteration in the amino acid profile may be instrumental in the induction of coma (20). Animal studies in that setting have shown that the brain energy substrate levels are unchanged (21). It has been shown that in hepatic coma there is a diminution of the serum levels of branched chain amino acids (leucine, isoleucine and valine) with an increase in the aromatic amino acids phenylalanine and tyrosine while tryptophan levels remain unchanged and likewise many of the straight chain amino acids. In view of the known differences between plasma amino acid profiles and intracellular amino acid profiles in both postoperative patients and renal failure patients (22) a cautious interpretation must be given with respect to alterations seen in plasma amino acid profiles and possible brain cell changes. Nevertheless, it has been postulated that the brain synthesis of serotonin, a neurodepressant is enhanced whilst noradrenaline is depressed with the suppression of the neuro-activator system. Preliminary re-

Table 5. Changes in serum amino acid profiles in chronic renal failure and uraemic coma patients*

Essential amino acids reduced	≏ 30%
Relative increase in non-essential amino acids	≏ 15%
Branched chain amino acids reduced	≏ 25%
Phenylalanine, proline levels raised	
Phenylalanine/tyrosine ratio greatly increased	
Tyrosine levels considerably reduced	
$\frac{\text{Valine + Leucine + Isoleucine}}{\text{Phenylalanine + Methionine}}$	= 2.6-3.4
$\frac{\text{Valine + Leucine + Isoleucine}}{\text{Phenylalanine + Methionine + Lysine}}$	= 2.4-2.6

Consideration of varying levels and proportions may point the way to more appropriate amino acid solution profiles for treating certain types of renal failure patients.

* Reviewed from literature and personal observations.

sults from this laboratory suggest that a similar alteration in amino acid profile may occur in patients with uraemic coma. Thus there may be a case made for extending the work of Fischer with respect to hepatic failure patients (23) to renal failure patients. His preliminary work in animals has shown that an amino acid solution with emphasis on increased branched chain amino acids and decreased aromatic content can have a beneficial effect. Some of the changes seen in the amino acid patterns in chronic renal failure patients or acute renal failure patients going into coma are shown in the accompanying table 5.

One final area of application for partial parenteral nutrition in chronic renal failure patients may be in regular dialysis patients. Some studies have shown that patients receiving thrice weekly haemodialysis, who also have restricted protein intakes develop biochemical evidence of malnutrition with a tendency for an absolute fall in the serum essential amino acid levels, a lowering of the branched chain amino acids and an increase in the serum levels of 3-methylhistidine. Associated with these changes were decreases of serum transferrin and C3 levels which are thought to be good indicators of malnutrition. In one study it was found that by infusing 14 g of amino acid as a washback over the last half hour of haemodialysis all the biochemical evidence of nutritional deficiencies could be corrected (24). It might be argued therefore that where doubts exist about a patient's ability to take at least 1 g of protein/kg body weight and who is having thrice weekly haemodialysis then a washback procedure of 13-18 g of essential amino acids at the end of each haemodialysis might be of nutritional benefit. In our own Unit where all patients take at least 1 g of protein/kg.body but not more than 1.2 g no evidence of malnutrition has been seen.

REFERENCES

1. Moore, F. D., *Metabolic Care of the Surgical Patient*. Saunders, London (1959).
2. Lee, H. A., *S. African Med. J.50*: 1703 (1976).
3. Lindsay, R. M., in: *Acute Renal Failure*, p. 103. ed. Flynn, C. T., M.T.P. Co. Ltd., Lancaster, U.K. (1974).
4. Montgomerie, J. Z., Kalmanson, G. M. and Guze, L. B., *Medicine* (Baltimore) *47*:1 (1968).
5. Berlyne, G. M., Jones, J. H., Hewitt, V. and Nilwarangkur, S., *Lancet 1*: 738 (1964).
6. Berlyne, G. M., Lee, H. A., Giordano, D., De Pascale, C. and Esposito, R., *Lancet 1*: 1339 (1967).
7. Schaeffer, G., Heinze. V.. Jontofsohn, R., Katz, N., Rippich, Th., Schafer, B., Sudhoff, B., Zimmermann, W. and Kluthe, R., *Clin. Nephrol. 3*: 228 (1975).
8. Long, C. L., Haverberg, L. N., Young, V. R., Kinney, J. M., Munro, H. N. and Geifer, J. W., *Metabolism 24*: 929 (1975).
9. Spitz, I. M., Rubenstein, A. H., Bersohn, I. and Abrahams, C., *Quart. J. Med.* (N.S.), *39*: 201 (1970).
10. Lee, H. A., Hill, L. F., Hewitt, V., Ralston, A. J. and Berlyne, G. M., *Proc. Europ. Dial. Trans. Ass. 4*: 150 (1967).
11. Lee, H. A., Ginks, W., Hill, L. F. and Pohl, J. E. F. In: *Nutrition in Renal Disease*, p. 216. Ed. Berlyne, G. M. E. and S. Livingstone Ltd. (1968).
12. Gutman, R. A., Uy, A., Shalhoub, R. J., Wade, A. D., O'Connell, J. M. B. and Recant, L., *Am. J. Clin. Nutr. 26*: 165 (1973).
13. Hartley, T. F. and Lee, H. A., *Nutr. Metabol. 19*: 201 (1975).
14. Hyne, B. E. H., Fowell, E. and Lee, H. A., *Clin. Sci. 43*: 679 (1972).
15. Fowell, E., *M. Phil. Thesis*. University of Surrey, U.K. (1974).
16. Lee, H. A. and Wretlind, A., *Acta Scand. Suppl. 466*: 6 (1976).
17. Abel, R. M., Beck, C. H., Abbott, W. M., Ryan, J. A., Barnett, G. O. and Fischer, J. E., *New Engl. J. Med. 288*: 695 (1973).
18. Varcoe, R., Halliday, D., Carson, E. R., Richards, P. and Tavill, A. S., *Clin. Sci. Molecular Med. 48*: 379 (1975).
19. Lee, H. A., Sharpstone, P. and Ames, A. C., *Postgrad. Med. J. 43*: 81 (1967).
20. Munro, H. N., Fernstrom, J. D. and Wurtman, R. J., *Lancet 1*: 722 (1975).
21. Biebuyck, J. F., Dedrick, D. F. and Scherer, Y. D. In: *Molecular Mechanisms of Anaesthesia*, p. 451. Ed. Fink, B. R., *Progress in Anesthesiology*, Vol. 1. Raven Press, New York (1975).
22. Bergstrom, J. and Furst, P., *Proc. Europ. Dial. Trans. Ass. 9*: 393 (1972)
23. Aguirre, A., Funovics, J., Wesdorp, R. I. C. and Fischer, J. E. In: *Parenteral Nutrition*, p. 219. Ed. Fischer, J. E., Little, Brown and Company (Inc.) U.S.A. (1976).
24. Heidland, A. and Kult, J., *Clin. Nephrol. 3*: 234 (1975).
25. Lee, H. A. and Hartley, T. F., *Postgrad. Med. J. 51*: 9 (1975).

Parenteral nutrition in burn patients

Douglas W. Wilmore, M.D.

Modification of the accelerated rate of tissue breakdown and loss of protoplasmic mass is a major priority following extensive injury. This chapter reviews the role of nutritional support following major injury, and emphasizes those factors which have maintained or improved organ system function during the hypercatabolic state.

THE LOSS OF BODY WEIGHT

Most easily recognized and readily documented is the loss of body weight which occurs following injury. Like other metabolic responses, weight loss is related to the extent of injury – the greater the burn, the greater the weight loss. Patients with injuries greater than 40% of the total body surface predictably lose more than 20% of the initial body weight if vigorous nutritional support is not instituted. Soroff and associates demonstrated that body weight changes were an accurate reflection of loss of protoplasm only after the first several weeks postburn (1). Moore interpreted studies of body composition as indicating that cellular loss was approximately half fat and half lean body mass following severe surgical stress (2). Kinney noted that the ratio of fuel burned in stressed patients was remarkably constant, with fat contributing from 80-85% of the calories utilized, and the remaining energy originating from body protein. In addition, a large component of weight loss is water, and weight stabilization in the surgical patient is often a reflection of loss or gain in total body water (3).

Maintenance of protein mass appears critical to survival. Loss of one-fourth to one-third of protein mass from the body is predictably fatal, and this degree of negative nitrogen balance in man is associated with a 40-50% weight loss. Weight loss in excess of 10% of the body mass results in rapid deterioration of maximal work performance. Subjects evaluated in semi-starvation studies for 10 days, with weight loss of less than 10%, demonstrated no impairment in physical performance (4). At some point then, between 10% and 40% body weight loss, malnutrition contributes to the disability of previously healthy patients who had normal body composition before injury. Controlling the rate of weight loss and accepting more than 10% of body weight loss in patients with normal body composition only if successful coverage of the burn wound can be assured in the immediate future, is an important guideline for the nutritional care of individuals with small thermal injuries.

However, patients with burns greater than 40% of the body surface demonstrate a near maximal stress response with predictable erosion of body mass. In these individuals, providing early protein and caloric support of at least predictable basal energy requirements is necessary for optimal care and may be essential for survival. The importance of nutritional support to a successful outcome following major burn injury has been emphasized by several authors. Sutherland fed thermally injured children their necessary requirements, frequently employing tube feeding techniques, and achieved nitrogen balance and maintained their body weight in spite of hypermetabolism, extrarenal nitrogen losses, and septic episodes which added to the catabolic response (5). Liljedahl and associates have studied a group of patients with burns of more than 75% of the total body surface (6). Several of their patients, who were treated in an environment of warm dry air, received early homograft coverage of the burn wound, and were maintained by forced feeding (using combined enteral-parenteral feeding techniques), lost only 5-7% of initial body weight during their entire postinjury course. Hinton and associates have administered large quantities of insulin (between 200 and 600 units/day) and 50% dextrose to burn patients to decrease loss of urinary nitrogen and potassium and increase excretion of urinary sodium (7).

Combined enteral and parenteral diets containing up to 4,350 kilocalories were administered to 14 burn patients during the first 30 days postburn (8). Those patients with an average burn size of 56% of the total body surface (range 32-72%) who received an average of 3,320; kcal/day for from 3-8 days (average duration 7 days) maintained their body weight at a time when weight loss was anticipated. In the more recent study of parenteral nutrition, using a 10% intravenous fat emulsion which contributed an average of 38% of the average total 3,770 calories per day, 10 critically ill burn patients showed nitrogen sparing manifested by nitrogen retention of a variable magnitude depending on extent of burn and level of nutritional support (9).

Curreri et al. identified in 20 patients, with burns averaging 61.7% of the body surface who received an average of only 1,609 kcal/ day, a significant elevation of erythrocyte sodium concentration (10). Seven patients with burns of similar extent given a minimum of 3,000 kcal/day and up to 6,000 kcal/day had red cell sodium concentrations statistically indistinguishable from those of unburned controls. Four of the former patients given the "supranormal" intake of calories sufficient to meet predicted energy requirements showed return of erythrocyte sodium concentration to normal levels within 3-5 days. This return of intra-erythrocytic sodium to normal levels may be an objective index with which to assess effectiveness of alimentation regimens.

Weight loss following injury is not an obligatory component of the response to trauma, but rather reflects the difference between the total energy requirements of the patient and the ability to provide these requirements in the form of adequate calories. Recent developments in feeding techniques allow vigorous enteral-parenteral nutritional support following thermal injury to meet or exceed calorie and nitrogen requirements in the hypermetabolic patient. Weight loss can be prevented only if energy support provided by these means equals energy demand.

In order to evaluate the effect of exogenous caloric administration on metabolic activity of thermally injured patients, six adult males with extensive injuries (ranging from 17.5-72% of the body surface area) were studied; two of the patients with smaller burn injuries had associated soft tissue trauma and multiple fractures (8). Each patient was studied while receiving three different dietary regimens which included 600 calories per day administered as 5% dextrose and water, 2,000 calories per day administered as flavored milk shakes or tube feedings, and 6,000 calories per day, 3,000 of which were administered by oral or tube feeding, and an additional 3,000 calories of hypertonic dextrose and amino acid administered intravenously through a large catheter placed in a large bore vein. Each of the three diets were administered to each patient for 48 hours, and resting oxygen consumptions were measured during the second 24-hour period for each of the three diets.

In all cases, energy production, as determined by oxygen consumption, did not change while the composition of the metabolic fuel utilized was reflected in the increased production of carbon dioxide, which accompanied the increase in carbohydrate administration (Table 1). There was a significant shift in RQ from a mean of 0.80 to a mean of 1.01, representing a shift in metabolic substrate utilization from body fat stores and oxidation of dietary carbohydrates. Additional studies demonstrated that "supranormal" caloric diets maintained energy requirements and reversed the progressive and ongoing weight loss which heretofore has characterized the metabolic response to severe injury.

Table 1. Mean respiratory gas measurements during three levels of feeding in six thermally injured patients

Caloric intake (kcal/day)	600	3,000	6,000
VCO_2 (ml/min)	259	302	345
VO_2 (ml/min)	325	337	341
RQ	0.80	0.89	1.01

DETERMINANTS OF NUTRITIONAL AND HORMONAL FACTORS AFFECTING POSITIVE NITROGEN BALANCE

The effect of nutritional support on metabolic rate and nitrogen loss was evaluated in 43 studies in normal and injured man (11). Patients with a mean burn size of 53% of the total body surface received a wide variety of nutritional support, administered by the enteral, parenteral, or enteral-parenteral routes. Normal individuals were studied while on a fixed caloric and nitrogen intake, following a period of equilibration. Resting metabolic rate was determined in all subjects between 6 and 8:00 A.M., following at least three hours of restricted, ad libitum, oral-caloric intake. However, calories and nitrogen administered by the intravenous route were continued at a constant infusion rate during the measurement period. Blood was obtained for determination of glucose, urea, free fatty acid, insulin, human growth hormone, glucagon, cortisone, and catecholamine. A timed urine specimen was obtained for catecholamine determination. Calorie and nitrogen intake for the accompanying 24-hour period was determined from the composition of intravenous nutrients as listed by the manufacturer, and food intake was determined by the dietitian from known lots of food prepared in the research metabolic kitchen. Urine was collected in 24-hour pools for determination of urine urea nitrogen and total nitrogen. Insulin was administered as required to those patients with elevated blood or urine glucose levels. Human growth hormone, 10 International Units, was given daily by intramuscular injection to nine subjects to evaluate the effect of endogenous reset of insulin on nitrogen excretion. Mean values of all measurements obtained over 3-7 days in the patients were computer processed with control data to determine the interaction effect of calorie and nitrogen support and the metabolic rate on nitrogen excretion.

Increased nitrogen excretion was associated with hypermetabolism and/or with increased dietary protein intake (Table 2). Nitrogen excretion decreased

Table 2. Mathematical relationships between nitrogen balance, energy production, food intake, and basal insulin

N_{IN}	=	Nitrogen Intake (kcal/m²/day)
N_{BAL}	=	Nitrogen Balance [N_{IN} − N] (kcal/m²/day)
MR	=	Metabolic Rate (kcal/m²/day)
NPC	=	Non-Protein Caloric Intake (kcal/m²/day)
BI	=	Basal Insulin (μU/ml)
		$p < 0.05$, Factors listed in order of F-ratio
N_{BAL}	=	$3.830 + 0.6072\, N_{IN} - 0.006599\, MR + 0.004376\, NPC + 0.05570\, BI$
N	=	43 (Normal men and burn patients fed enterally, parenterally and by the combined routes)
r^2	=	0.9001

with administration of nonprotein calories and/or an increase in plasma insulin. Metabolic rate was related to urinary catecholamines, as previously described, and a positive correlation existed between glucagon levels and catecholamine excretion. Each of the three variables relate in a similar fashion to protein metabolism, with a positive correlation existing between urinary catecholamines, metabolic rate, or glucagon and nitrogen excretion. Metabolic rate and catechol excretion were not reduced by caloric and nitrogen administration, confirming the previous studies reported. Protein wasting, resulting from the hypermetabolism, was diminished or reversed by nonprotein caloric intake, nitrogen administration, and/or maneuvers which increased basal insulin levels.

To further evaluate the nutritional efficacy of high carbohydrate insulin-stimulating diets, isonitrogenous oral diets containing 15 g of nitrogen/m²/day were fed to 14 severely injured burn patients (mean burn size 44% total body surface) and seven normal volunteers (12). Thirty-seven study periods of 5-25 days duration were evaluated with the average length of study equalling 8 days. Each diet contained known doses of carbohydrate (0-1,768 kcal/m²/day) and fat (0-1,488 kcal/m²/day). Urinary nitrogen was measured daily, and metabolic rate was determined from oxygen consumption and carbon dioxide production in each subject.

Nitrogen excretion was inversely related to carbohydrate intake and directly related to metabolic rate. Over the broad range of carbohydrate dosages, nitrogen excretion consistently decreased more than 50%. Fat calories did not appear to affect nitrogen excretion.

To evaluate the effect of hypocaloric intravenous nutrition in burn patients, crystalline amino acids were infused at varying doses (0-150 g/m^2/day) with or without glucose (60 or 120 g/m^2/day) for 3-7 days following successful resuscitation with glucose-free solutions in 35 thermally injured patients matched for burn size (mean 55% total body surface). Increasing glucose or amino acid dose improved nitrogen balance. The effect of the two substrates was equal and additive on a gram for gram basis. Renal sodium and amino acid per cent fractional excretions were increased, and the disappearance constant for hepatic extraction of indocyanine green dye decreased in all patients deprived of glucose. Glucose addition returned all indices of organ function toward normal. Near isotonic hypocaloric diets containing glucose and amino acids significantly diminish nitrogen loss in severely burned patients, and are the most efficacious hypocaloric diet for short-term alimentation in the critically ill patient.

FEEDING THE BURN PATIENT

Protein catabolism and mobilization of body fat depend upon hormonal signals which summon these substrates, apparently for wound healing and energy utilization following injury. The signal for substrate mobilization or storage appears in part to be an interrelationship between insulin elaboration which favors protein biosynthesis and glycogen storage and the catabolic effects of increased sympathetic nervous activity.

Because the burn patient is hypermetabolic following injury, energy and protein requirements for equilibrium are increased. Most individuals with burns ranging from 30-60% total body surface can achieve caloric equilibrium following the first week or 10 days of injury by receiving 2,000 to 2,200 calories and 15 g of nitrogen per square meter body surface per day (13). These requirements can usually be met by administering high carbohydrate, high protein enteral feedings. In addition, some polyunsaturated fat is necessary to prevent essential fatty acid deficiency, which may occur during the catabolic phase of trauma (9). Multivitamins are administered daily, along with supplemental Vitamin C, which has increased requirements following burn injury (14). Trace elements and electrolytes are present in the standard hospital diet, but increased potassium supplements may be required to maintain normal serum concentrations of this electrolyte. Although the need for zinc has been demonstrated experimentally, clinical reports of zinc replacement therapy in burn patients provide no clear-cut answers as to the benefit of this supplement following injury (15). Zinc supplementation may be administered to the severely malnourished or markedly catabolic patient who cannot take a balanced diet.

Enteral feedings

The priorities of care of the injured patient suggest that other factors such as adequate fluid resuscitation, fluid and electrolyte balance, and optimal cardiopulmonary function are more important in the first week postinjury than achieving nutritional balance. Patients are supported in the early postburn period with 5 or 10% dextrose and amino acids containing solutions until resolution of the post-traumatic ileus when oral fluids and a hospital diet, modified by the nutritional history and food preferences of the patient, can be started. The hospital diet usually provides more than adequate calories but is slightly low in nitrogen. However, a burn patient will seldom consume more food from his three meals a day than he did before injury; yet his requirements are twice as great. Additional calories and protein can be provided by liquid beverage supplements fed at intervals throughout the day and night to provide additional nutrient intake and achieve caloric and nitrogen equilibrium. In the first several weeks following injury, calorie-containing beverages usually supply the major portion of the nutritional intake, but, with time, appetite improves and increased intake from the food tray may decrease the need for frequent between meal liquid supplements. However, it is important to establish minimal caloric and protein requirements so that the entire staff work diligently, on all shifts if necessary, to satisfy these needs. After calorie and protein requirements for equilibrium have been satisfied, additional nitrogen, not calories, is needed to achieve positive protein balance.

Tube feeding

In some patients, enteral feeding through a small soft pliable feeding tube is the only method of providing sufficient round-the-clock intake. This technique is quite successful in infants, small children, and patients with tracheostomies or associated injuries of the head and neck. A blenderized or commercially available nutritional solution, containing about a calorie per ml, may be used but protein fortification is necessary to meet the nitrogen requirements. No clear-cut benefits have been noted with the use of elemental or synthetic diets when compared with blenderized or commercially available tube feedings, although individual situations may occur which favor the use of one particular preparation. All tube feedings usually produce some diarrhea, which may be diminished by the addition of Kaopectate or paregoric to the nutrient mixture. It is an exception, however, to provide more than 2,500 to 3,000 calories each day by tube feeding alone, and most adults with extensive burns who require tube feeding will also need parenteral nutritional supplementation.

Parenteral feedings

In some patients, however, enteral feedings may be inadequate or impossible and intravenous nutritional support is indicated. This is particularly true in individuals whose weight loss exceeds 10% of body weight, nutritional intake remains inadequate, and wound closure is not immediately anticipated. Parenteral nutrition is also indicated following resuscitation in debilitated or malnourished patients who have limited body fuel stores. Because of the tremendous energy requirements of burned individuals, combined enteral-parenteral feedings allow delivery of sufficient calories and nitrogen to prevent negative energy and nitrogen balance following even the most severe injury. Efficient use of the gastrointestinal tract can be achieved in the critically injured or obtunded patient by using liquid tube feedings as outlined above. However, it is rare that more than 2,500-3,000 calories can be provided by tube feedings, and supplemental feedings are necessary in patients with burns of more than 40% of the body surface if caloric equilibrium is to be achieved. If the patients receive enteral feedings, vitamins and trace elements are administered by the gastrointestinal tract and supplemental calories, protein, and electrolytes are administered by vein. However, if enteral feedings are impossible, all essential nutrients should be provided in the parenteral diet and frequent monitoring of blood and urine levels of electrolytes and other major minerals is performed to determine the precise requirements of these dietary constituents.

The importance of the catheter to the success of long-term parenteral nutrition has been repeatedly emphasized, yet certain features of catheter insertion and care should be outlined for use of this technique in the thermally injured patient. Central venous catheters are placed in the superior caval system through unburned skin if at all possible. On occasion, catheters have been inserted into the inferior vena cava by way of the venopuncture at the groin, but this is associated with greater hazard of infection and thrombosis (16). The techniques of catheter placement are the same as in any patient. In the burn patient, the intravenous administration tubing, filter, and the dressing over the catheter site are changed daily. Withdrawal of blood or measurement of central venous pressure through the infusion ctaheter is discouraged, for these practices may allow the introduction of micro-organisms into the administration system. Standard parenteral fluid bottles or bags and infusion tubing are used to deliver the nutrient solution by gravity drip. The volume of fluid per unit time is marked on a strip of adhesive tape and attached to the bottle, so that the time of day corresponds with the level of fluid in the flask to ensure constant continuous administration rate of the hypertonic nutrient solution. Alternatively, infusion pumps may be used to insure delivery of a fixed predetermined volume per liter time.

Because of the increased fluid requirements of the burn patient*, more dilute solutions may be used to deliver adequate volumes of water and yet supply predicted caloric and protein requirements to preserve body mass following thermal injury. Solutions of 12-20% dextrose and 4-6% crystalline amino acids, or protein hydrolysates, are prepared daily for each patient in the hospital's manufacturing pharmacy in a laminar air flow hood. Peptides may not be fully utilized following injury and, therefore, we have preferred the crystalline amino acid solutions for preparation of the nutritional solution. Minerals and vitamins are added when indicated by laboratory determination or the clinical condition of the patient. The traumatized individual requires a higher quantity of nitrogen to maintain equilibrium than the patient in resting starvation. Therefore, solutions with a nitrogen-calorie ratio of 1:130 to 150 are considered optimum to provide adequate protein intake in proper proportion to total calorie intake. In addition, supplemental potassium is necessary to achieve equilibrium but rarely should concentrations exceed 40 mEq potassium per liter of solution.

The basic nutrient solution, composed of hypertonic glucose and crystalline amino acid or protein hydrolysate, is infused at a constant continuous rate through the venous catheter placed in the superior vena cava. Frequent determinations of blood and urine sugar are essential for this therapy to be safe and effective. It is usually best to begin administration of these hypertonic glucose solutions with one to two liters given over 24 hours and increase the dose in stepwise increments, allowing 2-3 days between each increment to permit adaptation to the large glucose load in order to minimize glucose intolerance. Regular insulin is administered if necessary by continuous intravenous infusion utilizing a syringe pump with the rate of administration based on blood glucose concentrations and adjusted for glucosuria that is measured every one to four hours. The amount of insulin administered may range between 50-300 units/day in seriously ill, thermally injured patients.

* Evaporative water loss can be predicted in burn patients by the formula: [(25 + % body surface burn) × body surface area in m^2 = ml H_2O lost/hr].

The overall nutritional goal is to provide adequate caloric requirements while maintaining blood glucose between 100-200 mg/100 ml. Increased potassium and phosphorus administration may be necessary as noted above. Phosphate requirements range from 15-25 mEq potassium dihydrophosphate per 1,000 calories administered.

In the critically ill patient, daily measurement of serum sodium, potassium, chloride and bicarbonate levels, CO_2, blood urea nitrogen, glucose, calcium, and phosphate is essential, and at times one or more of these determinations may be necessary two or three times a day in individual patients. Adjustments in the electrolyte and mineral concentrations are determined by their plasma levels and total output as measured in 24-hour collections. Because of the complications of septic thrombophlebitis and central venous thrombosis which have been associated with long-term indwelling catheters in the burn patient, catheters are changed every two to four days, rotated to the contralateral side if placement sites are available.

Use of fat emulsions

Fat emulsions are isotonic and contain 1-2 calories per ml, and may be administered by peripheral vein in order to avoid many of the hazards associated with central venous infusion of hypertonic glucose solutions. The emulsion, administered through a Y-connector with the connection below an in-line filter (the emulsion will not pass through a filter), is infused simultaneously with a solution containing 5-15% dextrose, 4-5% amino acids, electrolytes, vitamins, and minerals. Central venous cannulae may be necessary for the administration of more hypertonic solutions, but peripheral venous routes are frequently employed in the burn patient because of the increased fluid requirements allowing the infusion of dextrose and amino acid solutions containing less than 14% solute concentration. We have not observed alteration in coagulation or liver function with the use of soybean emulsion (9).

It should be remembered that carbohydrate, not fat, appears to be the critical energy-providing nutrient which stimulates insulin release, a key hormonal signal for storage of body fuels. Thus, carbohydrate remains an essential component of the diet of the critically ill patient. However, it appears that a certain portion of the caloric needs may be administered as fat with minimal effects on protein metabolism.

In most patients, up to 20% of the energy requirements can be provided by fat emulsions with no major deleterious effects on nitrogen balance, and with the safety of infusion of all nutrients via peripheral vein (12). Additional fat may be administered if a positive energy balance and significant weight gain are desired. As metabolic rate returns toward normal, the total carbohydrate load may be reduced in proportion to the decrease in metabolic activity.

ANCILLARY MEASUREMENTS

Hormonal administration

Our recent studies of the post-traumatic metabolic response indicate that increased adrenergic activity (increased catecholamine elaboration) alters organ blood flow, dampens the release of insulin, stimulates glucagon secretion, and has direct effects on the hormonal environment favoring proteolysis, gluconeogenesis, and ureagenesis. The effects of relative insulinopenia (relative to glucagon and catecholamines) may be modulated by administering insulin, glucose, and amino acids, a technique used by some for patients with varying degrees of stress, including burns, myocardial infarction, and infection. Coexisting sepsis may accentuate postinjury glucose intolerance, necessitating large doses of insulin. Since the need for such may quickly lessen if sepsis is brought under control, careful and frequent monitoring of the blood and urine glucose is essential in these patients.

Human growth hormone, the most potent anabolic agent known, has the unique physiologic role of promoting growth, improving storage of nitrogen, potassium, and phosphorus, and facilitating transport of amino acids. Administration of growth hormone to nine patients with large thermal injuries, in addition to the calories and nitrogen required to meet or exceed predicted energy requirements, resulted in marked augmentation of nitrogen retention, which appeared to be a dose related response (18). BUN decreased, blood glucose increased slightly, but, more important, serum basal insulin approximately doubled. A close relationship existed between nitrogen balance and basal insulin secretion, and increased insulin augmentation appeared to be the controlling mechanism for the improved nitrogen retention.

Physical therapy

Disposition and incorporation of amino acids into skeletal protein is facilitated by activity of the muscle cell. The mobility and physical activity of burn patients may be severely limited and a planned exercise program must be instituted to maintain an active and functional skeletal mass. With the help of the physical therapist, simple isometric exercises can be accomplished, while the patient remains in bed or an extremity is immobilized, to improve the vitality of muscles and encourage the movement of nitrogen to skeletal muscle cells once caloric and nitrogen equilibrium are achieved. Technological advances, such as air-fluidized and water beds, may improve patient care and minimize formation of decubiti but they discourage active use of muscle groups. These devices which provide unique suspension systems for patients, approximating the weightless state, may actually increase the breakdown of lean body mass if regular and specialized exercises are not instituted.

Timely closure of the burn wound

The initiator of the metabolic response to thermal injury is a large skin defect, thus every effort should be made to optimize its healing and reestablish a properly functioning surface barrier and interface between the individual and surrounding environment. The use of topical antimicrobial agents, biologic dressings, and early excision are aimed at minimizing infection in the burn wound and achieving early healing or grafting. However, it is not until satisfactory closure of the burn wound with cutaneous autografts is accomplished that a reversal of many of the metabolic sequelae occur. Following coverage of a large wound, the patient's appetite seems to improve, spirits rise, with increased exercise and improved morale. With wound closure and adequate nutritional support, convalescence is associated with a rebuilding of body mass, gain in weight, and the patient's return to an active productive life.

REFERENCES

1. Soroff, H. S., Pearson, E., Arney, G. K. and Artz, C. P., An analysis of alterations in body composition in burned patients. *Surg. Gynec. Obstet. 112*: 425 (1961).
2. Moore, F. D., Metabolic Care of the Surgical Patient. Philadelphia, W. B. Saunders Co., 1959, pp. 409-456.
3. Kinney, J. M., Long, C. L., Gump, F. E. and Duke, J. H., Jr., Tissue composition of weight loss in surgical patients. I .Elective operation. *Ann. Surg. 168*: 459 (1968).
4. Daws, T. A., et al., Evaluation of cardiopulmonary function and work performance in man during caloric restriction. *J. Appl. Physiol. 33*: 211 (1972).
5. Sutherland, A. B. and Batchelor, A. D. R., Nitrogen balance in burned children. In: Wallace, A. B. and Wilkinson, A. W. (editors): *Research in Burns*, Edinburgh, Livingstone, 1966.
6. Liljedahl, S. O. and Birke, G., The nutrition of patients with extensive burns. *Nutr. Metab. 14*: (supplement) 110 (1972).
7. Hinton, P., Allison, S. P., Littlejohn, S., and Lloyd J., Electrolyte changes after burn injury and effects of treatment. *Lancet 2*: 218 (1973).
8. Wilmore, D. W., Curreri, P. W., Spitzer, K. W., Spitzer, M. E. and Pruitt, B. A., Jr., Supranormal dietary intake in thermally injured hypermetabolic patients. *Surg. Gynec. Obstet. 132*: 881 (1971).
9. Wilmore, D. W., Moylan, J. A., Helmkamp, G. M. and Pruitt, B. A., Jr., Clinical

evaluation of a 10% fat emulsion for parenteral nutrition in thermally injured patients. *Ann. Surg. 178*: 503 (1973).

10. Curreri, P. W., Wilmore, D. W., Mason, A. D., Jr., Newsome, T. W., Asch, M. J. and Pruitt, B. A., Jr., Intracellular cation alterations following major trauma: effect of supranormal caloric intake. *J. Trauma 11*: 3890, (1971).
11. Wilmore, D. W., Long, J. M., Mason, A. D., Jr., Skreen, R. W. and Pruitt, B. A., Jr., Catecholamines: mediator of the hypermetabolic response to thermal injury. *Ann. Surg. 180*: 653-669 (1974).
12. Long, J. M., Wilmore, D. W., Mason, A. D., Jr. and Pruitt, B. A., Jr., Fat carbohydrate interaction: nitrogen sparing effect of varying caloric sources for total intravenous feeding. *Surg. Forum 25*: 61-63 (1974).
13. Soroff, H. S., Pearson, E. and Artz, C. P., An estimation of the nitrogen requirements for equilibrium in burned patients. *Surg. Gynec. Obstet. 112*: 159 (1961).
14. Levenson, S. M., et al., Ascorbic acid, riboflavin, thiamine, and nicotinic acid in relation to severe injury, hemorrhage, and infection in the human. *Ann. Surg. 124*: 840 (1946).
15. Brodribb, A. J. M. and Ricketts, C. R., The effect of zinc in the healing of burns. *Injury 3*: 25 (1971).
16. Warden, G. D., Wilmore, D. W. and Pruitt, B. A., Jr., Central venous thrombosis: a hazard of medical progress. *J. Trauma 13*: 620 (1973).
17. Hinton, P., Littlejohn, S., Allison, S. P. and Lloyd, J., Insulin and glucose catabolic response to injury in burn patients. *Lancet 1*: 767(1971).
18. Wilmore, D. W., Moylan, J. A., Bristow, B., Mason, A. D., Jr. and Pruitt, B. A., Jr., Human growth hormone and high caloric feeding: modification of the metabolic response following thermal injury. *Surg. Gynec. Obstet. 183*: 875 (1974).

3

Supplement techniques to central parenteral nutrition

The use of elemental diets

K. D. Bury, M.D., ScM., F.R.C.S. (C), F.A.C.S.

INTRODUCTION

Throughout the 1950's and 1960's, investigators at the National Institutes of Health developed a totally synthetic mixture of simple sugars, pure amino acids, and micro and macro nutrients which, when mixed with water, formed a clear, stable solution (1). Given orally, ad lib, as the sole nutritional source, this solution maintained small animals in good health throughout several generations (2). In 1965, healthy human volunteers received from 2100 to 3700 calories per day of a chemically formulated bulk free liquid diet and remained clinically and biochemically stable for up to 19 weeks (3). The development of total parenteral nutrition (TPN) significantly improved the survival of critically ill patients and re-emphasized the vital role of positive nutritional support in the treatment of many disease states (4). However, use of the gastro-intestinal tract as the route of alimentation whenever possible, remains attractive to many physicians, since the possibility of sepsis is excluded and the clinical management of such a support system is less complicated than TPN.

The digestive-absorptive function of the normal gut in the breakdown and transport of the components of a normal diet are still being explored and elucidated. The role of the intestinal epithelial cell in brush border enzymatic digestion of luminal disaccharides and small peptides followed by transmembrane, transcellular transport of the end products has been clarified and the characteristics and inter-relationships of many of the transport systems defined (5, 6, 7). In volunteers with a normally functioning gastro-intestinal tract, absorption of fat, carbohydrate and protein is most complete after ingestion of the complex nutrient source.

Starvation leads to a disproportionate atrophy of the small bowel with decreased mucosal cell production and migration, and depression of brush border and some intracellular enzymes (8). Knowledge of the combined effect of malnutrition and either a specific gastrointestinal disease state, immunosuppressive drugs, some antibiotics and antifungal agents, or therapeutic abdominal irradiation on gut morphology and function is sporadic and incomplete (9, 10).

The development of predigested, bulk free, liquid, chemically formulated diets which meet total nutritional requirements if over 16,000 calories per day are ingested was initially regarded as a major advance in clinical nutrition and expected to either substitute for the necessity of TPN in selected patients, or provide continuing nutritional support during the transition from intravenous to normal oral alimentation. The initial diet formulation was indeed made up of the end products of carbohydrate and protein digestion – glucose and pure L amino-acids with only enough fat to prevent fatty acid deficiency. Clinical trials with this diet at suggested dilution, providing 1 cal/ml, however, caused gastrointestinal side effects, particularly if infused intra-jejunally, mainly associated with the high osmolality of the product at normal dilution (11). Subsequent products require minimal digestion as the nutrient and/or nitrogen sources are larger sub-units of whole carbohy-

Table 1. Composition per 1,000 K Cal of four elemental diets

	Vivonex	Flexical	Enteropac-6	Precision isotonic
Nitrogen (GM)	3.37	3.5	6	4.8
Source	Synthetic L-amino acids	Casein hydrolysate	Casein hydrolysate	Egg albumin
Carbohydrate (GM)	212	155	Z195	150
Carbohydrate (GM)	212	155	195	150
Source	Glucose oligo-saccharides	Starch, oligo-saccharides, sucrose	Maltose	Glucose oligosaccharides
Fat (GM)	1.45	34.0	1.2	31.0
	Lineoleic acid	Soy oil 80% MCT 20%	Linoleic acid	Vegetable oil
Sodium (mEq)	37.4	15.2	32.7	34
Potassium (mEq)	29.9	38.2	28	25
Magnesium (mEq)	16	14.4	16	15.1
Calcium (mEq)	22.2	35	24	33
Chloride (mEq)	50.8	35.8	26	30

All diets contain trace elements, and vitamins in amounts usually exceeding daily maintenance requirements per 1800 calories.

Vivonex – Eaton Laboratories, Norwich, N.Y. 13815
Flexical – Mead Johnson and Company, Evansville, Indiana 47721
Precision - Doyle Pharmaceuticals Coi. Minneapolis, Minnesota 55416.
Enteropac-6 – Pharmacia (Canada), 2044 boul St. Regis Blvd., Dorval, Quebec H9P 1H6.

drate or protein sources. A comparison of the composition of some currently available products is listed in Table 1.

The following list of characteristics applies to most chemically defined or "elemental" diets.

1. When reconstituted with water, they form a solution or stable suspension.
2. They are free of bulk.
3. The protein source varies from pure amino acid, casein hydrolysate, or egg albumen.
4. The main caloric source is carbohydrate – either as oligosaccharide or disaccharide.
5. Fat content varies up to 30% of the total calories, but most are nearly fat free.
6. Essential fatty acid requirements are *probably* met by all diets.
7. If at least 1800 calories per day are ingested or infused daily, vitamin requirements are met.
8. Mineral content – particularly Sodium – varies with the diet source.
9. All are acidic – varying with the flavoring agents added.
10. All are hypertonic at normal dilution.
11. Unflavored and high nitrogen products are available.

Most of the studies performed to date utilizing the available diets confirm their ability to provide adequate nutritional support with positive caloric and nitrogen balance in those patients in whom a minimum of 1600 cal. was fed daily by mouth, through a naso-gastric feeding tube, or via a jejunostomy (12). Few animal or clinical studies have been performed to elucidate the physiologic effects of elemental diet administration. Unflavored products are not tolerated orally but reduce osmolality at normal dilution and are thus preferred for tube feeding. Flavoring agents decrease the pH and increase the osmolality of the final solution. However, the diets still are relatively unpalatable with an unpleasant sweetness and a prolonged aftertaste, making long-term complete oral feeding difficult. Delay in gastric emptying with bolus feeding (13) and inhibition of gastric acid secretion have been documented in animals and man (14). Prolonged intestinal transit time with a significant decrease in stool bulk is clinically obvious and has been documented (15) and a significant decrease in myoelectric activity of the small intestine has been shown (16). In spite of an initial report of a decrease in the types and numbers of stool microflora (17), no significant alteration could be found by several investigators (18, 19). The effects of elemental diets on upper gastrointestinal secretions remain controversial.

Table 2. Effects of elemental diets on pancreatic function

Investigator	Enzyme content	Volume of secretion	Bicarbonate content	Route of administration
Neviackas	Decreased lipase Decreased amylase Decreased trypsin	?	Unchanged	Oral
Wolfe	Increased protein	Increased	Unchanged	Duodenal perfusion
Ragins	Unchanged	Increased	Unchanged	Intraduodenal
	Unchanged	Unchanged	Increased	Intrajejunal

Oral and duodenal administration of an elemental diet containing only pure L amino-acids as the nitrogen source increases the volume of pancreatic secretion – probably via cholecystokinin release since the increase was similar to perfusion of a mixture of pure amino acids alone, or IV administration of cholecystokin. Ragins' work substantiates the clinical impression of many physicians that intrajejunal administration of the same diet either has no effect or decreases the volume of pancreatic secretion. One explanation for the lack of bicarbonate increase in the pancreatic effluent has been a relatively non-stimulatory effect of elemental diets on secretin – possibly because of inhibition of gastric acid secretion.

Originally, a clinical impression of decreased pancreatico-biliary secretion was documented and several investigators reported patients whose pancreatic fistulas closed while they were receiving complete nutritional support from elemental diets (20, 21). A review of the findings of various investigators interested in the effects of elemental diets on exocrine pancreatic function is summarized in Table 2 (22, 23, 24). Bounous has reported a protective prophylactic effect in both mice and men following several days of elemental diet ingestion on the intestinal lesions following 5-FU and radiation therapy (25, 26).

CLINICAL USES OF ELEMENTAL DIETS

These diets have been available for a long enough period of time that some assessment can be given of their usefulness in various clinical situations.

A. Pre-operatively

1. In chronically ill patients with low serum proteins, elemental diets probably should replace clear fluids as a mechanical bowel preparation for laparotomy, colonoscopy, and in some cases, radiography. Evidence of the effectiveness of such diets for bowel preparations is plentiful (27).

2. Malnourished patients requiring elective surgery may be metabolically improved by a 14 day period of nutritional replenishment with elemental diets.

GASTRO-INTESTINAL FISTULAS

Statistics accumulated from various reports on the nutritional management of gastro-intestinal fistulas with elemental diet suggest that such therapy in conjunction with improved local care of the fistula has dramatically reduced the previously high morbidity and mortality rates. An overall spontaneous closure rate of 70% has been achieved with a mortality of about 18% (28). Duodenal fistulas may be managed by jejunostomy feedings and low small bowel fistulas by intragastric alimentation. In most cases, the bowel perfused with the diet is healthy and one only has to be concerned about the presence of a sufficiently long segment to totally absorb the diet. The presence of gastrointestinal disease such as regional enteritis reduces the spontaneous closure rate and recurrences may occur (29, 30).

INFLAMMATORY BOWEL DISEASE

In critically ill patients, TPN is indicated. However, in patients with a moderate exacerbation of their disease, elemental diet vs. regular diet does "put the lower bowel at rest" and encourage early remission (31).

SHORT BOWEL SYNDROME

One of the earliest clinical applications of an elemental diet was in a patient with 6 inches of jejunum. Neither fluid, caloric or nitrogen requirements could be met without concomitant intravenous therapy (32). It is now generally recognized that patients with massive bowel resection should have an initial course of TPN. After several weeks, oral elemental diets may be well tolerated and provide the intraluminal nutrients some investigators feel are necessary for maximum intestinal adaptation to occur.

ACUTE DIVERTICULITIS

Since elemental diets are the ultimate in low residue diets, in selected cases, they may provide adequate nutritional support for the patient while his inflammatory process subsides.

PANCREATITIS AND PANCREATIC FISTULAS

Although the literature presents evidence of successful nutritional management of both acute pancreatitis (33) and pancreatic fistulas with elemental diets, experimental work and a review of the physiology of pancreatic secretion suggest that intragastric and intraduodenal feeding with elemental diets tends to increase the fistula drainage by stimulating the exocrine pancreas via release of cholecystokinin. Intrajejunal feeding may bypass this control system, provide adequate nutritional support, and lead to spontaneous fistula closure. In patients with severe pancreatitis, a gastrointestinal ileus usually precludes oral feeding. There is evidence that pancreatic storage enzymes are decreased after chronic administration of elemental diet (34).

PAEDIATRICS

Elemental diets have successfully been used in young children and infants to treat chronic and acute diarrhoeas of unknown aetiology (35). Diets in which the nitrogen source is entirely composed of pure L amino-acids are non-allergenic and have proven useful in both infant and adult malabsorptive states which may involve an allergenic component.

LACTASE DEFICIENCY

All available elemental diets are lactose free and thus well absorbed in patients with both congenital and acquired lactase deficiency.

POST-OPERATIVE NUTRITION

It has been shown that the small bowel regains normal motility and absorptive capacity within 24 hours after abdominal surgery. A small jejunostomy tube inserted at surgery may be used for infusion of elemental diet almost immediately post-operatively, providing nutritional support and in some cases, avoiding the necessity for TPN (36). These diets have also been found useful after head and neck surgery because they can be infused through a very small catheter.

SUPPLEMENTAL NUTRITIONAL SUPPORT

Patients with excessive protein and caloric requirements due to severe burns, multiple trauma, etc., may require over 5,000 k cal/day, for positive nitrogen and caloric balance. This may be achieved by a combination of TPN and enteral elemental diet therapy. I have listed some specific disease entities and clinical situations in which elemental diets have been successfully used to provide complete nutritional support. Naturally there is some overlap in both directions. Many patients who tolerate gastrointestinal elemental diet feeding would also digest and absorb a blended liquid diet – such as Isocal. These diets are composed of whole protein and carbohydrate – such as corn syrup, and soy protein – but *not* natural foods such as beef, carrots, peas, etc. Such tube feeding liquid diets may be nearly isotonic, contain no lactose, and are balanced nutritionally. The main advantage elemental diets have here is that they can more readily through a very small nasogastric or jejunostomy feeding tube, while whole protein may clog the system. There is also less residue and thus fewer and smaller bowel motions with elemental diet therapy. Thus it occasionally is a matter of hygiene and nursing convenience in comatose and severely debilitated patients which dictates the type of gastrointestinal feeding ordered by the physician.

I have emphasized the properites and clinical uses of products which are marketed as chemically defined or elemental. The preparation of these diets is always "clearly stated on the package". The method of administration may be either oral, via nasogastric tube, or via jejunostomy catheter. It is important to begin administration of the diet at near isotonic concentration, particularly if feeding is via jejunostomy. Continuous 24 hour infusion results in fewer gastrointestinal side effects than bolus oral feeding. A pump is seldom necessary but may be helpful for jejunostomy infusion when a very slow rate per hour is desirable to initiate the alimentation. More specific information on proper clinical administration of these diets is present in several review articles (38).

In summary, elemental diets have been shown to provide complete and adequate nutritional support in a wide variety of clinical situations. If the gastrointestinal tract is available for feeding purposes, and at least 100 cm is available for perfusion by the diet, then feeding via the gut should probably be tried. More and more use is being made of jejunostomy feedings, especially for post-operative nutrition. It is the low residue feature of these diets that makes them so attractive – since they run well through either a number 5 or number 8 paediatric feeding tube, or a number 16 polyethylene catheter.

Although no crossover studies have been reported, it is my clinical impression that diets containing only pure L amino acids as their nitrogen source are absorbed equally as well as diets containing a casein hydrolysate. More work needs to be done to elucidate the site of absorption of such diets, the advantage of varying carbohydrate and protein sources, and the comparison of elemental versus blended liquid diets in similar situations.

REFERENCES

1. Greenstein, J. P., Otey, M. C., Birnbaum, S. M. and Winitz, M., Formulation of a Nutritionally Complete liquid diet. *J. Nat. Can. Inst. 24*: 211 (1960).
2. Greenstein, J. P., Birnbaum, S. M., Winitz, M. and Otey, M. C., Quantitative Nutritional Studies with Water Soluble, Chemically Defined Diets. I. Growth, Reproduction and Lactation in Rats. *Arch. Biochem. Biophys. 72*: 396 (1957).
3. Winitz, M., Seedman, D. A. and Graff, J., Studies in Metabolic Nutrition Employing Chemically Defined Diets. Extended Feeding of Normal Human Adult Males. *Am. J. Clin. Nutrition 23*: 525 (1965).
4. Steiger, E., Daly, J. M., Allen, T. R., Dudrick, S. J. and Vars, H. M., Post-operative Intravenous Nutrition: Effects on Body Weight, Protein, Regeneration, Wound Healing and Liver Morphology. *Surgery 73*: 686 (1973).
5. Gray, G. M., Carbohydrate Digestion and Absorption. *Gastroenterology 58*: 96 (1970).
6. Gray, G. M., Protein Digestion and Absorption. *Gastroenterology 61*: 535 (1971).
7. Nivon, S. E. and Mawer, G. E., Th3 Digestion and Absorption of Protein in Man. *Br. J. Nutr. 24*: 227 (1970).
8. Achord, J. L., Acute Effects of Fasting on Gastro-intestinal Structure and Function. *Med. Times 95*: 441 (1967).
9. Binder, H., Jejunal Absorption of Water and Electrolytes in Inflammatory Bowel Disease. *J. Lab. Clin. Med. 76*: 915 (1970).
10. Sodikali, F., Depeptidase Activity and Malabsorption of Glycylglycine in Disease States. *Gut 12*: 276 (1971).
11. Stephens, R. V. and Randall, H. T., Use of a Concentrated, Balanced-Liquid Elemental Diet for Nutritional Management of Catabolic States. *Ann. Surg. 170*: 642 (1969).
12. Miller, J. M. and Taboada, J. C., Clinical Experience with an Elemental Diet. *Am. J. Clin. Nutr. 28*: 46 (1975).
13. Bury, K. D. and Jambunathan, G., Effects of Elemental Diets on Gastric Emptying and Gastric Secretion in Man. *Am. J. Surg. 127*: 59 (1974).
14. Rivilis, J., McArdle, H., Wlodek, G. and Gurd, F. N., Effects of an Elemental Diet on Gastric Secretion. *Ann. Surg. 179*: 226 (1974).
15. Perrault, J., DeVroede, G. and Bounous, G., Effects of an Elemental Diet in Healthy Volunteers. *Gastroenterology 64*: 569 (1973).
16. Moore, E. P., Copeland, E. M., Dudrick, S. J. and Weisbradt, N. W., Effect of an Elemental Diet on the Electrical Activity of the Small Intestine in Dogs. Abstract. Presented at annual meeting of Association of Academic Surgery, 1975.
17. Winitz, M., Adams, R. F. and Seedman, D. A., Studies in Metabolic Nutrition Employing Chemically Defined Diets: II. Effects on Gut Microflora Population. *Am. J. Clin. Nutrition 23*: 546 (1970).

18. Bornside, G. H. and Cohn, I., Stability of Normal Human Fecal Flora During a Chemically Defined, Low Residue Liquid Diet. *Ann. of Surgery 181*: 58 (1975).
19. Bounous, G. and DeVroede, G., Effects of an Elemental Diet on Human Fecal Flora. *Gastroenterology 66*: 210 (1974).
20. Voitk, A. J., Echanve, E., Brown, R. A., McArdle, A. H. and Gurd, I. N., Elemental Diet in the Treatment of Fistulas of the Alimentary Tract. *S.G. and O. 137*: 68 (1973).
21. Stephens, R. V. and Randal, H. T., Use of a Concentrated, Balanced-Liquid Elemental Diet for Nutritional Management of Catabolic States. *Ann. Surg. 170*: 642 (1969).
22. Ragins, H., Levenson, S. M., Signer, R., Stamford, W. and Seifter, E., Intrajejunal Administration of an Elemental Diet at Neutral pH Avoids Pancreatic Stimulation. *Am. J. Surg. 126*: 606 (1973).
23. Neviackas, J. A. and Kerstein, M. D., Pancreatic Enzyme Response with an Elemental Diet. *S.G. and O. 142*: 71 (1976).
24. Wolfe, B. M., Keltner, R. M. and Kaminski, D. L., The Effect of an Intraduodenal Elemental Diet on Pancreatic Secretion. *S.G. and O. 140*: 241 (1975).
25. Bounous, G., Gentile, J. M. and Hugon, J., Elemental Diet in the Management of the Intestinal Lesion Produced by 5-Fluorouracil in Man. *Can. J. Surg. 14*: 312 (1971).
26. Hugon, J. S. and Bounous, G., Elemental Diet in the Management of the Intestinal Lesions Produced by Radiation in the Mouse. *Can. J. Surg. 15*: 18 (1972).
27. Johnston, W. C., Oral Elemental Diet: A New Bowel Preparation. *Arch. Surg. 108*: 32 (1974).
28. Bury, K. D., Elemental Diets. Chapter 20. Fischer, J. E., *Total Parenteral Nutrition*, Little, Brown and Co., Boston, 1976.
29. Bury, K. D., Stephens, R. V. and Randall, H. T., Use of a Chemically Defined, Liquid, Elemental Diet for Nutritional Management of Fistulas of the Alimentary Tract. *Am. J. Surg. 121*: 174 (1971).
30. Voitk, A. J., Schave, U., Brown, R. A., McArdle, A. H. and Gurd, F. N., Elemental Diet in the Treatment of Fistulas of the Alimentary Tract. *S.G. and O. 137*: 68 (1973).
31. Rocchio, M. A., Chung-Ja, C., Haas, K. and Randall, H. T., Use of a Chemically Defined Diet in the Management of Patients with Inflammatory Bowel Disease. *Am. J. Surg. 127*: 469 (9174).
32. Thompson, W. R., Stephens, R. U., Randall, H. T. and Bowen, J. R., Use of the "Space Diet" in the Management of a patient with Extreme Short Bowel Syndrome. *Am. J. Surg. 117*: 449 (1969).
33. Voitk. A., Brown, R. A., Echave, U., McArdle, A. H., Gurd, F. N. and Thompson, A. G., Use of an Elemental Diet in the Treatment of Complicated Pancreatitis. *Am. J. Surg. 125*: 223 (1973).
34. Brown, R. A., Thompson, A., McArdle, A. and Gurd, F. N., Alteration of Exocrine Pancreatic Storage Enzymes by Feeding an Elemental Diet: A Biochemical and Ultrastructural Study. *Surgical Forum 21*: 391 (1970).
35. Sherman, J. O., Hamly, D. and Khachadurian, A. K., Use of an oral Elemental Diet in Infants with Severe Intractable Diarrhea. *The J. of Paediatrics 86*: 518 (1975).
36. Page, C. P., Ryan, J. A. and Haff, R. C., Continual Catheter Administration of an Elemental Diet. *S.G. and O. 142*: 184 (1976).
37. Bury, K. D., Stephens, R. V., Chung-Ja, C. and Randall, H. T., Chemically Defined Diets. *Can. J. Surgery 17*: 1 (1974).
38. Russell, R. I., Progress Report Elemental Diets. *Gut 16*: 68 (1975).

Research on peripheral administration of parenteral nutrition in the postoperative period

F. W. Ahnefeld and R. Dölp

In "hyperalimentation" as described by Dudrick (1968) the infusion fluids must be administered via a central venous catheter due to their high osmolality. It is, however, well-known that the caval catheter is accompanied by numerous complications (Burri, 1971) which prohibit routine application in the postoperative period. To make it possible for amino acid and energy substitutes to be administered via peripheral veins, even in routine therapy, the osmolarity of infusion fluids must not be higher than 1,000 to 1,200 mosm/l, i.e. the amount of amino acids and carbohydrates which can be administered is limited. We have, therefore, been engaged for the past several years (Ahnefeld, 1973) in an intensive study of a medium-term "minimal diet" within our concept of postoperative infusion therapy. It includes the intake of nitrogen and energy as a basic supply, i.e. at least the endogenous nitrogen balance minimum and the BMR are covered by parenteral substitution in the postoperative period. The first results of the administration of such an infusion fluid via the peripheral veins were published in 1974 (Dölp).

Other authors (Blackburn, 1973; Greenberg, 1976) have also reported on their studies involving other nutritive mixtures that can be infused into the peripheral veins.

In this respect, Blackburn (1973) inspired discussions about whether in the so-called post-aggression syndrome amino acid substitution alone will produce a sufficient endogenous gain in energy because of lipolysis, to achieve a more favorable nitrogen balance than would result from a combination of amino acids and carbohydrates or sugar alcohols. We have decided in favour of the second combination, because we believe that the positive effect of amino acid substitution on the nitrogen balance described by Blackburn (1973) is attributable to the amino acids infused rather than endogenous fat mobilization. Greenberg (1976) confirmed this in recent studies.

During the research work in our Institute, the question arose whether a significant difference is found in a basic electrolyte solution when the nitrogen and energy supply is reduced (A).

In a further step, we increased the nitrogen content of the infusion mixture and subsequently recorded a number of parameters in a screening procedure to find out which of them changes significantly with respect to the control group, i.e. which require further testing in the future (B).

METHODS

A) Three groups of postoperative patients were picked at random (pyelolithotomy). Group I received a basic electrolyte solution (control group), group II received a 1% amino acid solution, and group III a 1.5% amino acid solution,[1] each at a dosage of 40 ml/kg body weight per day over a postoperative period of 4 days.

Statistical evaluation was carried out with the Student-t test.

B) In a further test series we compared two groups: one group received a mixture of 5% glucose and lactated Ringer's solution in a ratio of 2:1 (control), the other group received a 2.5% amino acid solution with 12.5% sorbitol (TPE 1800)[2] over a postoperative period of 6 days at a dosage of 40 ml/kg body weight per day.

35 blood and 8 urine parameters were recorded daily to determine in a screening procedure which metabolic effects are influenced by infusion solution II in the postoperative period in comparison with the control group.

The statistical evaluation of the data obtained was performed according to a method (computer program) suggested by Koch (1969) whereby the total series of the individual groups are compared (in contrast to the Student-t test which only compares single days), thus obtaining strong evidence with a small number of cases.

RESULTS

A) 1. While the serum *urea* concentration in the control group decreases

[1] The infusion fluids were kindly supplied by J. Pfrimmer and Co. Erlangen. Solution I: Tutofusin OPS, solutions II and III: amino acid pattern corresponding to Aminofusin L 600.

[2] The solutions were kindly supplied by J. Pfrimmer and Co. Erlangen. Solution II: TPE 1800, the amino acid pattern corresponds to that of Aminofusin L 600.

Content / Liter		Control	AA 1%	AA 1,5%
Na^+	(mVal)	100	90	90
K^+	(mVal)	18	25	25
Mg^{++}	(mVal)	6	6	6
Ca^{++}	(mVal)	4	-	-
Cl^-	(mVal)	90	125	126
Acetate	(mVal)	38	-	-
Zinc	(mg)	-	2,5	2,5
Tot. Amino Acids	(g)	-	10,0	15,0
Tot. Nitrogen	(g)	-	1,6	2,4
Sorbitol	(g)	50,0	50,0	50,0
Xylitol	(g)	-	25,0	25,0
Aethanol	(g)	-	-	21,3
Tot. Calories	(kcal)	200	340	500
N-free Calories	(kcal)	200	300	450
Cal / N	(kcal/g)	-	188	188
Osmolality	(mOsmol/kg)	500	800	1400
Vitamins		-	+	+

Table 1. Composition of the infusion fluids Test A

Content / Liter		2/3 Glucose 5% 1/3 Ringers Lactate	AA 2,5%
Na^+	(mVal)	43,6	51,5
K^+	(mVal)	1,3	30,0
Ca^{++}	(mVal)	1,0	5,0
Mg^{++}	(mVal)	0,7	6,0
Cl^-	(mVal)	37,0	34,0
Lactate	(mVal)	9,0	-
Acetate	(mVal)	-	25,0
Phosphate	(mMol)	-	10,0
Tot. Amino Acids	(g)	-	25,0
Tot. Nitrogen	(g)	-	3,8
Glucose	(g)	33	-
Sorbitol	(g)	-	125
Tot. Calories	(kcal)	130	600
N-free Calories	(kcal)	130	500
Cal / N	(kcal/g)	-	132
Osmolality	(mOsmol/kg)	+	1167
Vitamins		-	+

Table 2. Composition of the infusion fluids Test B

<u>Blood Parameters</u>

pH
pCO_2
pO_2
Base Excess
Osmolality
Electrophoresis
  Tot. Protein
  Albumin
  α_1, α_2, β, γ-Glob
Na^+
K^+
Cl^-
Ca^{++}
Creatinine
SGOT
SGPT
Alkal. Phos.
Total Bili.
Uric Acid
Urea
Cholesterol
Phosphate
Lactate
Glucose
PTT
Prothrombin Time
Fibrinogen
Thrombo.
Hematocrit
Ery.
Leuko.
  Stab.
  Segs.

<u>Urine Parameters</u>

Volume
pH
Osmolality
Total Nitrogen
N-Balance
Glucose
Urea
α-Amino-N

Table 3. Blood and urine parameters

significantly until the third postoperative day, it increases in the two other groups while still remaining within the normal range.

Urea excretion – an indicator of the degree of catabolism – is therefore significantly higher in these groups than in the control group.

2. As was expected, the postoperative *nitrogen balance* constantly remained negative. It was computed as the difference between the nitrogen substitution – an average of 16.8 g/96 h in group II and 24 g/96 h in group III – and the nitrogen loss through urine, drainage (Redon) and intestine during the same period of time. For the latter a fixed value of 1 g N/day was assumed (Jürgens, 1968).

Group I revealed a nitrogen deficit of 33.7 $\pm$ 11.7 g during 4 days, an order of magnitude which we already reported 2 years ago for a similar group of patients (Dölp, 1974). Group II had a negative nitrogen balance of 29 $\pm$ 9.9 g and did therefore differ significantly from the control group. Only in group III was a positive effect of nitrogen substitution found. In this group, the negative nitrogen balance was reduced to 18.6 $\pm$ 12.7 g, i.e. approximately 65% of the administered amino acids were utilized anabolically when compared to the control group.

3. Evidence for *local tolerance* was indicated by the frequency of the need to change the indwelling cannula (Braunüle), which occurred in the event of reddening, swelling and/or pressure pain in the area of the puncture wound. During the observation period, a change of the Braunüle was necessary 1.3 times per patient in group I, 1.5 times in group II and 1.6 times in group III. The general tolerance was good, i.e. no apparent side-effects.

B) The evidence of the statistically determined differences between the groups (control group, TPE group) suggests the necessity for further parameter observation. The indication of standard deviations or confidence intervals would be useless for this small number of cases as they would represent pseudovalues which might induce wrong conclusions. The following metabolic parameters differed significantly ($P < 0.05$) with respect to the control group: uric acid, glucose, total N in the urine and nitrogen balance.

1. From almost identical initial values, the serum *uric acid* concentration of the TPE was markedly higher than that of the control group, although it remained within the normal range. The investigation of blood *glucose* concentration shows a higher postoperative increase in the control group than in the group having received the amino acid mixture although an increase was evident here also.

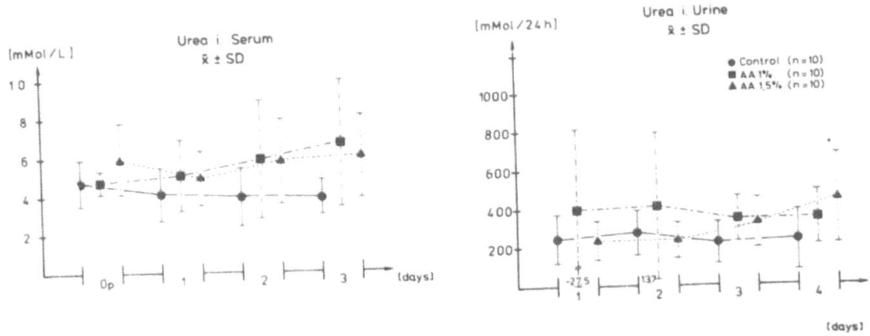

Figure 1. Serum and urinary urea

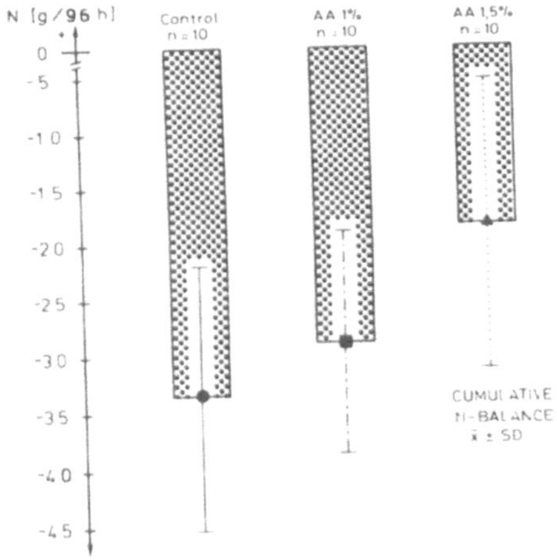

Figure 2. Cumulative nitrogen balance

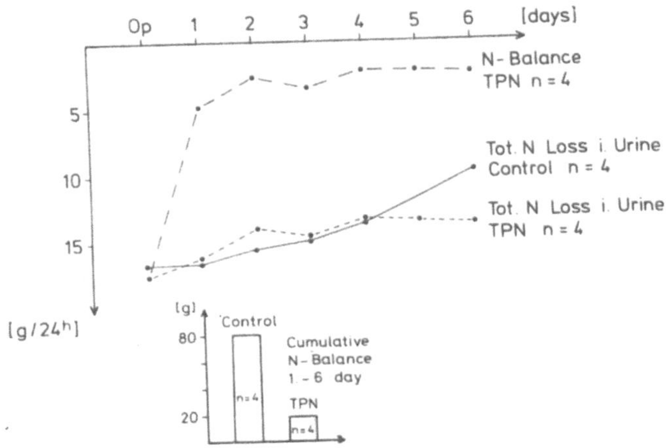

Figure 3. Nitrogen balance

2. The daily mean nitrogen excretion in urine was 13.7 g for the control group, and 14.3 g for the other group.

Thus, a favorable *nitrogen balance* was obtained in the TPE group which improved to approximately −2 g/day. The calculation of the cumulative nitrogen balance also reveals that the test group with a nitrogen loss of 17.4 g during 6 days was considerably better off than the control group with 82.7 g.

3. A change of the Braunüle was necessary twice in the control group during the test period in comparison to 3 times in the TPE group, which signifies an adequate *local tolerance* of the test solution. General intolerance reactions were not observed.

DISCUSSION

The evaluation of our results clearly indicates that the nitrogen balance when compared with that of a control group does not change anymore when the nitrogen supply falls below a certain level. This was shown by the nitrogen balance of the group of patients who received a 1% amino acid solution. These amino acids were utilized catabolically and appeared as increased urea excretion in the urine. An additional catabolic effect was evident in the group receiving a 1.5% amino acid solution which produced, when evaluated with respect to the control group, an anabolic utilization of the substituted amino acids in the approximate order of magnitude of only 65%; the nitrogen balance, however, was distinctly more favorable. Thus, by increasing the supply, the utilization of the substituted amino acids for the synthesis of protein structures is not only improved relatively but also absolutely up to a definite limit. A similar finding was reported by VAN WAY (1975). He showed that the nitrogen loss was higher when the nitrogen and calorie supplies were low than when the nitrogen supply was increased. He concluded from his studies that a nitrogen balance which is in equilibrium or positive may be achieved with a nitrogen substitution of 8 to 11 g as well as an energy supply of 1,800 to 2.300 kcal per day in adult patients after moderate surgical trauma (e.g. cholecystectomy). Decisive is, of course, that the amino acid mixtures used are always in equilibrium as far as their amino acid pattern is concerned, i.e. that they are adapted to the requirements of the patient.

The results of our study with the 2.5% amino acid solution (TPE 1800) indicate, when evaluated with respect to the control group, an anabolic amino acid utilization of 94% during the test period as well as a nitrogen balance which is almost in equilibrium. This is an ideal value and corresponds with the data made available by VAN WAY. Due to the low number of cases involved, however, this study cannot be regarded as conclusive but may instead be considered as a trend analysis that at least shows the order of magnitudes correctly.

For our study B we chose such a small group of patients in order to record a large number of parameters during an observation period of 6 days and still be able to obtain quick results to allow further pertinent research work. We selected the parameters (see table 3) according to the requirements of the FDA in the USA where much stricture regulations are enforced for the clinical testing of infusion fluids than in the Federal Republic of Germany. We therefore investigated a total of 43 parameters in the blood and urine and evaluated their statistical significance in comparison to a control group according to a method of KOCH (1967) which applies for a small number of cases.

Four parameters of the metabolism were found to be significantly different, whereby nitrogen metabolism was the most obvious. As previously mentioned, the nitrogen balance showed an improvement almost as high as the entire intake. This is especially remarkable since in 1974 DÖLP in another test series with a 1.5% amino acid solution, we found an anabolic utilization of approximately only 50%. It has to be pointed out, however, that in this particular group of tested patients the infusion solutions were administered by infusion pumps, i.e. at a constant rate within 24 hours providing optimal conditions for the desired utilization. We are in agreement with DUKE (1970) and KINNEY (1972) that during a post-aggression period, the amount of protein calories in the total calorie consumption increases above normal, while the energy requirements as a whole remain within the normal range after selective interventions. In other words, the postoperative nitrogen requirements increase much more than the energy requirements.

In test A no peculiarities could be detected in the blood glucose that warrant discussion. In test B, at a relatively low glucose substitution of 100 g per day in the control group, we found on the first postoperative day an average blood glucose concentration of 176 mg% due to the well-known disturbance of glucose utilization. This value corresponds closely with the results of a study published by us (DÖLP 1975) in which another problem was considered. The TPE group showed a significantly lower blood glucose concentration.

In all solutions tested, the electrolytes (sodium, potassium, magnesium, calcium, chloride) were balanced so that no differences in the groups nor within the series were obtained.

Since the peripheral vein tolerance was also satisfactory, the infusion solution TPE 1800 introduced here will certainly become part of our routine clinical infusion therapy.

We are presently investigating a large number of cases to support the described findings, but are nevertheless already able to recommend a regimen (Dick, 1976) whereby the nutrients may be supplied parenterally according to a progressive plan.

In the *primary stage*, a nutritive solution should be available which on the one hand supplies nitrogen (in the form of amino acids) and energy (in the form of sorbitol and xylitol) in sufficient amounts (25 g/l amino acids and 150 kcal/g N) and on the other hand can be administered into peripheral veins. Most of the routine parenteral nutrition in a hospital may be performed with this *basic nutrition*.

When it appears that this basic parenteral nutrition is no longer adequate with regard to time, quantity or quality, either the composition or the concentration of the solution must be changed, i.e. a shift from a basic nutrition to a *requirement-adapted* nutrition must be made. This includes an initial stage for – apart from the central venous supply – adaptations of dose and composition to the metabolic situation of the patient (post-aggression syndrome, micro-circulatory disturbances, etc.). A discussion of the recommended quantities and qualities according to a specific scheme is not possible here.

SUMMARY

In two comparative studies, we tested a 1% and a 1.5% amino acid solution as well as a 2.5% amino acid solution – all solutions containing a supplementary amount of energy – to determine their clinical value for routine postoperative infusion therapy.

The purpose was to achieve an evident improvement in the nitrogen balance and – through peripheral intravenous administration – an acceptable local tolerance. Moreover, metabolic parameters which are known to change under the influence of parenteral nutrition should deviate from the initial (zero) value as little as possible.

We found that no significant improvement in the nitrogen balance could be achieved with the 1% amino acid solution in comparison to that of the control group. In contrast, the 2.5% amino acid solution yielded a nitrogen balance on the approximate order of magnitude of the nitrogen intake which was more favorable than that of the control group – the number of cases, however, was small. Important changes in metabolic parameters were not encountered with this solution. The local tolerance was also satisfactory so that the clinical value is established.

Since the nitrogen balance improves greatly with increasing nitrogen supply – up to an order of magnitude not yet defined – it is recommended that the nitrogen supply in the postoperative period should be as high as possible. Thus, we have exceeded the "minimal diet" which we defined (AHNEFELD, 1973) and have entered the range which may be defined as "basic nutrition". Central venous administration of complete parenteral nutrition would be the last step in the postoperative infusion therapy program.

REFERENCES

Ahnefeld, F. W., Dölp, R. und Fodor, L., Differenzierte postoperative Substitution: Bedingungen und Konzeption. *Infusionstherapie Sonderheft 2*: 79-84 (1973).

Blackburn, G. L. and Flatt, J. P., et al., Protein sparing therapy during periods of starvation with sepsis or trauma. *Ann. Surg. 177*: 588-593 (1973).

Burri, C., Komplikationen beim Cava-Katheter in: Lang, K. (ed.), Bilanzierte Ernährung in der Therapie. Thieme-Verlag, Stuttgart, 1971.

Dölp, R., Grab, E., Knoche, E. und Ahnefeld, F. W., Stoffwechselverhalten und Verwertung parenteral zugeführter Kohlenhydrate in der postoperativen Phase. *Infusionstherapie 2*: 103-110 (1975).

Dölp, R., Bauer, H., Ahnefeld, F. W. und Seeling, W., Klinische Untersuchungen über die routinemäßige Infusionstherapie mit 1,5%-igen Aminosäurenlösungen der operativen Medizin. *Infusionstherapie 1*: 615-622 (1973/74).

Dudrick, S. J., et al., Long-term total parenteral nutrition with growth, development and positiven nitrogen balance. *Surgery 64*: 134-142 (1968).

Duke, J. H. and Jørgensen, S. B., et al., Contribution of protein to calorie expenditure following injury. *Surgery 68*: 168-174 (1970).

Greenberg, G. R. and Marliss, E. B., et al., Protein-sparing therapy in postoperative patients. *N. Engl. J. Med. 294*: 1411-1416 (1976).

Jürgens, P. und Dolif, D., Die Bedeutung nichtessentieller Aminosäuren für den Stickstoffhaushalt des Menschen unter parenteraler Ernährung. *Klinische Wochenschrift 46*: 131-137 (1968).

Kinney, J. M., Calories/Nitrogen: Disease and injury relationships Symposium on Total Parenteral Nutrition, Tennessee, 1972.

Koch, G. G., Some aspects of statistical analysis of "split plot" experiments in completely randomized layouts. *Journ. Am. Statist. Ass. 64*: 485-505 (1969).

The rationale for using a fat emulsion ('intralipid') as part energy substrate during intravenous nutrition

H. A. Lee, B.Sc., M.B., B.S., F.R.C.P.

Any consideration of intravenous substrates used for total parenteral nutrition in the post traumatic phase must take into consideration the normal metabolic processes that occur during this time. A distinction should also be made between so-called protein sparing therapy (1, 2) effective over the first 3-4 days of inanition due either to gastrointestinal failure or other causes and total parenteral nutrition (3, 4, 5) supplying full energy and nitrogen substrates.

It is accepted that in most western civilisations a normal dietary intake includes 40% of the calories from a fat source, approximately 40% from carbohydrates and 20% from protein. It is also acknowledged that the greatest store of reserve energy in the body is in the fat depots mainly as triglyceride (Table 1). In the immediate post-traumatic phase there is a

Table 1. Fuel reserves and requirements

Estimated energy reserves of 70 kg man			
Substrate	Quantity kg	Duration	Kcal
Carbohydrate (Mainly liver glycogen)	0.2	6-12 h	800
Fat (Adipose triglyceride)	12–15	20–25 days	108–135,000
Protein (Mainly muscle)	4– 6	10–12 days	16– 24,000

Estimated daily needs	Protein g	Energy Kcals
Medical patient (Uncomplicated)	45– 75	1500–2000
Surgical patient (Uncomplicated)	75–125	2000–3500
Hypercatabolic state e.g. Major burn	125–300	3500–5000

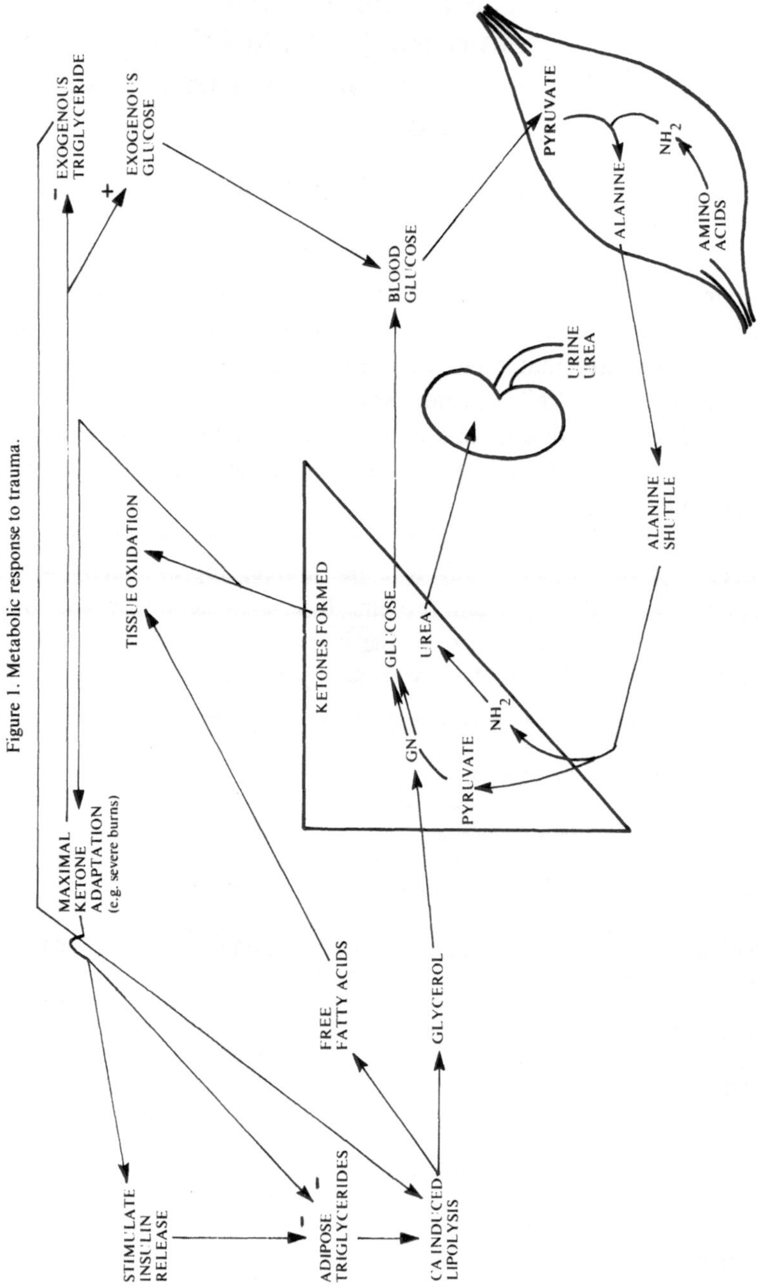

Figure 1. Metabolic response to trauma.

metabolic response that strives to maintain normal energy levels for the vital processes of cell function, which includes the breakdown of cell protein for this purpose (gluconeogenesis) (Fig. 1). Thus the immediate post-traumatic phase is characterised by an increase in the catabolic hormones, adrenaline, cortisol and glucagon and a suppression of the principal anabolic one, insulin. The reserve stores of carbohydrate as glycogen, are rapidly mobilised and used (within 12 hours) and the triglyceride depots release free fatty acids which are then converted by the liver into ketones, (6) betahydroxybutyrate and aceto-acetate, energy substrates that can be utilised by other organs including the brain. The liver is the only organ that contributes significantly to blood ketone levels. The tissue concentrations of free fatty acids dependent upon lipolysis of adipose triglycerides, the principal ketogenic precursors, are the main regulators of hepatic ketogenesis. Whereas the liver has enzymes allowing utilisation of free fatty acids and ketones, other tissues such as heart and kidney can utilise triglycerides in addition to these substrates. The rate of ketogenesis may also be affected by the availability of non-fat substrates. Muscle protein is broken down, with the release of aminogroups which are carried to the liver via the alanine shuttle, whereby the NH_2 groups are detached to form urea and the

Table 2. Energy substrate changes in post-operative period

1. Gluconeogenesis principally from muscle protein precursors
2. Lipolysis of adipose triglycerides provides 70-80% of energy requirements
3. Ketone bodies
   (i) Adaptive brain metabolism
   (ii) Improved nitrogen conservation of ketosis
   (iii) Limit oxidation of muscle tissue amino acids
   (iv) Maintain muscle protein synthesis
4. Carbohydrate feeding induced insulin resistance
5. Carbohydrate inhibition of lipolysis and ketogenesis
6. In maximal ketone adaptation further energy must be provided as glucose

Figure 1. Metabolic response to trauma.

GN = Cortisol induced gluconeogenesis.

CA = Catecholamines; alanine shuttle carries carbon moieties and amino groups from muscle to liver. Alanine is formed by transamination of pyruvate in muscle. Note liver virtually unable to utilize ketones (23). Provision of additional exogenous triglyceride in a maximally keto-adapted subject cannot be expected to further improve nitrogen conservation. Increased ureagenesis in the unfed patient represents dissolution of muscle mass.

carbon moieties resynthesised to pyruvate and lactate and the formation of glucose.

Thus it is seen that it is normal in the post-traumatic phase for the metabolic fuel substrate to alter so that there is increased utilisation of fat (7). It has been variously estimated that fat may provide up to 70-80% of the total energy requirements during this phase. (8) Other adaptive metabolic facets are shown in Table 2. Equally it should be stressed that usually during the post 24-36 hours after trauma from a therapeutic standpoint one is not so much concerned with nutrition as such but with the restitution of physiological homeostasis by correction of blood and plasma deficits, maintenance of normal gaseous exchange, correction of early electrolyte deficits and subsequently nutrition. Thus the appropriateness of fat versus carbohydrate calories in so-called stress is a moot point. Furthermore, if one considers anaesthesia as one of the most stressful situations then there is evidence to show that carbohydrate metabolism is specifically inhibited whilst fat metabolism is left unimpaired. (9)

There has been a long debate as to whether a fat calorie is equal to a carbohydrate calorie during intravenous nutrition. This has arisen because nitrogen balance studies have shown a deterioration when carbohydrate has partially or wholly replaced fat but this has been a transitory phenomenon until adaptation to fat metabolism has occurred. (10, 11) Likewise, as might be expected, infusions of "Intralipid" into normal volunteers has not shown any beneficial effect upon nitrogen balance other than could be anticipated from the glycerol content (12). It cannot be over-emphasised that it is not valid to extrapolate results obtained in normal subjects to acutely ill catabolic patients, who have an entirely different internal metabolic environment. It is not disputed that there are many good reports that show where energy has been solely derived from carbohydrate, that nitrogen balance has been achieved with clinical benefit to the patient and restitution of nutritional status. Equally, in those regimes where the provision of energy from fat has contributed up to 60% of the total equally good results have been obtained. Over the past year interesting studies on energy substrate hormone interactions have shown that the metabolic profile adapts according to the energy provided. (13) Thus during intravenous carbohydrate administration, the plasma profile alters towards increases of pyruvate, lactate, alanine and immunoreactive insulin with suppression of free fatty acids and ketone bodies, whereas during fat infusion free fatty acids and ketone bodies are elevated and lactate, pyruvate, alanine and immunoreactive insulin are suppressed.

Table 3. Comparative composition of human breast milk and soybean oil ("intralipid")

Fatty acids		Breast milk %	Intralipid	
			Soybean oil	Phospholipids
Butyric	C4:0	0.5	–	–
Caproic	C6:0	Trace	–	–
Caprylic	C8:0	Trace	–	–
Capric	C10:0	2	–	–
Lauric	C12:0	6	–	–
Myristic	C14:0	9	0.035	0.09
Palmitic	C16:0	23	9.18	32.51
Stearic	C18:0	7	2.87	15.69
Arachidic	C20:0	1	0.12	0.132
Behenic	C22:0	–	0.059	3.41
Others		Trace		
Caproleic	C10:1	Trace	–	–
Lauroleic	C12:1	Trace	–	–
Myristoleic	C14:1	0.5	–	–
Palmitoleic	C16:1	3	0.026	0.37
Oleic	C18:1	37	26.41	32.05
Linoleic	C18:2	8	54.27	11.33
Linelenic	C18:3	0.5	7.18	0.297
Arachidonic	C20:4	1.0	–	0.15
Others		1.5		0.222

Table 4. I.V. Energy regime. Carbohydrate (50% cals) and fat (50% cals) to supply 3,000 kcals per day for 70 kg man

Glucose	– 50% solution + potassium ± insulin
	– 750 ml* – 375 g glucose (1500 kcals) per 24 hr
	– 5.36 g/kg body weight/day
	– 0.223 g/kg/hr
Fat	– 20% soybean emulsion ("intralipid")
	– 750 ml – 150 g fat (1500 kcals) per 24 hr
	– 2.14 g/kg body weight/day
	– 0.089 g/kg/hr
Total caloric volume	– 1500 ml
Caloric osmolar load	– 129 mOsm/hr
% Lost of daily caloric load	– less than 5%

* Either as 32 ml hourly boluses or continuous infusion via central venous catheter.

These findings are of fundamental importance since they illustrate quite clearly that energy provision should not be given so as to match the anticipated hormonal profile but be given to ensure adequate utilisation in the sure knowledge that in the vast majority of patients the hormonal profile will adapt. It is equally important to be safe in the knowledge that both carbohydrate calories or fat calories can maintain nitrogen balance and produce suitable a:v amino acid differences, suggesting utilisation of intravenous amino acid nitrogen. Some patients have been shown to be slow in becoming keto adapted (14) whereas others may be totally ketone adapted e.g. severe burn patients so that provision of more fat can only result in triglyceride accumulation in the blood stream and not improve metabolic homeostasis. It has been shown that infusion of ketones in normal fasting man can cause a reduction in plasma free fatty acids. This is thought to result because ketones above a certain level inhibit lipolysis and they may stimulate insulin release which also inhibits lipolysis. Differences in degree of ketone adaptation may also explain why the liver of well fed rats does not increase ketogenesis upon addition of free fatty acids to the same degree as in starved rats. In such groups of patients, therefore, provision of carbohydrate seems ideal. In some patients who may be unable to secrete adequate amounts of insulin or who become insulin resistant, it may be important to rely more on intravenous fat. It is for many of the foregoing reasons that the author routinely uses an intravenous energy substrate regime that derives 50% energy from carbohydrate and 50% from fat (See Table 3).

The intravenous fat substrate used is "Intralipid" soybean oil emulsion (15) of the composition shown in Table 4. It is seen that 50% of this fat emulsion is derived from the unsaturated fatty acid linoleic acid. The osmolalities of the 10 and 20% "Intralipid" emulsions have the advantage that they are near isotonic i.e. 280-350 mOsm/1, whilst 50% glucose contains 3,800 mOsm/1. The physico-chemical characteristics of "Intralipid" are very similar to those of naturally occurring chylomicrons. Many investigations have shown that intravenously infused soybean oil emulsion is not only cleared from the bloodstream like normal chylomicrons but actually utilised for energy processes (Table 5). The most important studies have shown that the effects of "Intralipid" on respiratory quotient are to reduce it toward 0.7 indicative of fat combustion for energy processes. Studies on the elimination of C14 labelled carbon dioxide after the infusion of C14 labelled fatty acids and the appearance of ketone bodies after "Intralipid" infusion have confirmed metabolic utilization. Furthermore, studies which have depended either on carbohydrate or fat only or carbohydrate and fat in 50% propor-

Table 5. Methods of investigating utilization of soybean oil emulsion ("intralipid")

1. Similarity to chylomicron kinetics
2. Increased fractional elimination rate (K_2) in post-operative period
3. Nitrogen balance studies
4. Effects on respiratory quotient i.e. approaches 0.7
5. ^{14}C-labelled CO_2 expired air elimination studies
6. Formation of ketones after infusion of intralipid

Table 6. Intravenous non-protein energy substrates: some complications

Disturbance	Substrate
Metabolic acidosis: lactic acidosis	Fructose: sorbitol: ethanol-carbohydrate combinations
Hyperosmolar dehydration syndrome	Hypertonic: glucose 40%, 50% sorbitol 30%
Hyperuricaemia	Sorbitol: fructose: xylitol
Oxalaemia and oxaluria	Xylitol
Hyperbilirubinaemia	Xylitol, sorbitol
Triglyceridaemia	Xylitol, fructose, sorbitol
Hyperlipidaemia	Fat emulsion
Essential fatty acid deficiency	Fat free I.V. regime
Hypophosphataemia	Fat free I.V. regime with phosphorus poor amino acid solution
Folate metabolism abnormalities	Ethanol
Complications of vein access sites	Hypertonic carbohydrate solutions

Table 7. Optimal observations and precautions during I.V. feeding regime

1. Strict aseptic measures
2. Full instruction to nursing staff
3. Maintain constancy of infusion rate
4. Check fat clearing capacity by centrifuging blood after 6 hr fat free period
5. Measurements of fluid balance
6. Daily weight
7. Measurement of serum electrolytes
8. Check liver function tests
9. Serum and urine osmolality
10. Serum phosphate
11. Blood sugar (urinary glucose not sufficient) – Keep below 10 mmol/l i.e. renal threshold
12. Any specific tests dictated by underlying condition

tions have shown that the energy requirement for maintaining nitrogen equilibrium is very similar i.e. 45 kcals/kg body weight. (16) It is interesting to note that many of the most serious metabolic complications of parenteral nutrition are related to the intravenous non-protein energy substrates (see Table 6). By using a regime which derives in equal proportion energy from fat and glucose the majority of these complications can be avoided. The use of such regimes demands limited but mandatory daily observations as outlined in the accompanying Table 7. No matter what regime is used for parenteral nutrition it must be conceded this can never be considered as a short cut to metabolic success.

There are few contraindications to the use of fat emulsions in parenteral nutrition. Thus patients with known disorders of lipid metabolism e.g. hyperlipoproteinaemias or who are maximally keto adapted e.g. early treatment of severe burns patients, are best provided with glucose energy. Other patients may sometimes show a delay in becoming keto adapted, so that a gradual transition from total glucose calories to a glucose-fat ("Intralipid") combination may be indicated. In those patients where insulin resistance may be very high, a greater proportion of the energy can be derived from fat. I do not recommend exceeding 50% of total energy derived from fat. "Intralipid" fat tolerance for adults is 3-5 g per kg body weight. The advantages of using a combined glucose and fat emulsion regime are shown in the accompanying Table 8.

If the general philosophy is accepted that certain deficiency states will arise when a given nutrient is absent from the intravenous nutritional

Table 8. Some advantages of using combined glucose-intralipid in intravenous feeding regime

1. Large amounts of energy in small volume
2. Large amounts of energy in *near isotonic* preparation
3. Source of essential fatty acids
4. Minimal vein irritation – may be given peripherally
5. Good long-term tolerance
6. Metabolised like naturally occurring substrate (i.e. chylomicrons)
7. No urinary or faecal losses
8. No interference with immune response mechanisms
9. No effect on coagulation mechanisms
10. Very good tolerance in paediatrics
11. Smaller requirements of exogenous insulin
12. Diminishes risk of hyperlipidaemia problems
13. Relies on sources similar to normally metabolised substrates
14. Minimizes known potential metabolic problems

regime then it seems reasonable to provide this ab initio. Such reasoning can apply to essential fatty acid deficiency. It seems totally inappropriate to recommend that this may be provided by the infusion of plasma or by the occasional infusion of a fat emulsion. Essential fatty acid deficiency may occur much more rapidly than previously thought in acutely ill patients with profound disturbances (17) (see Table 9). This can be avoided by giving the fat emulsion "Intralipid". Although at one stage it was considered that "Intralipid" phospholipid content might be a useful source of phosphorus, some doubts have arisen as a result of some recent observations. Thus it is recommended that even in intravenous nutritional regimes using fat emulsions as part energy substrate, the phosphorus requirement should be met by a separate provision of inorganic phosphate (18).

The indications for "Intralipid" are those where parenteral nutrition is generally indicated. Recent studies have shown that this includes its use in pancreatitis. Though the question is often posed as to whether this is advisable, it should be recorded that the integrity of the pancreas so far as its exogenous enzymes are concerned, has no bearing upon the metabolism of intravenously administered lipid. A number of studies have shown the value of lipid emulsions in this setting. Even with hepatic disorders a tolerance level of 1.5 g/kg body weight with a variety of liver pathologies has been clearly demonstrated. The importance, perhaps, of the provision of an energy intravenous substrate regime derived on a 50% basis each from carbohydrate and fat is illustrated by recent findings during home parenteral

Table 9. Essential fatty acid deficiency

1. Biochemistry (Changes may appear after only 10 days)
Serum linoleic acid falls
5, 8, 11-Eicosatrienoic acid (20:3 N-9) appears
Later arachidonic acid (20:4 N-6) falls
$\frac{\text{Triene (20:3)}}{\text{Tetrene (20:4)}}$ rises above 0.4
2. Clinical
Skin changes – scaling, desquamation, exudation
Hepatomegaly
Gastro-intestinal mucosal damage
Defective immune responses
Prostaglandin deficiencies
Cell membrane phospholipid changes

nutrition. (19) In those patients receiving the major portion of their energy from carbohydrate a tendency towards hypertriglyceridaemia (Type IV hyperlipoproteinaemia) has been noted. Whereas, in patients receiving mainly a fat emulsion "Intralipid" a tendency towards hypercholesterolaemia (Type II hyperlipoproteinaemia) has been the case.

Some doubts have been cast as to whether infusion of fat emulsions might compromise pulmonary ventilation-diffusion-perfusion functions. This arose from some studies in rabbits that suggested the red cell might be coated by the fat emulsion and interfere with the transport of oxygen. Furthermore, it had also been noted that a proportion of fat was cleared through the lungs and histological studies in animals had shown deposition of fat in this location. However, some studies in the most catabolic of patients i.e. burns, have shown increased elimination of fat and no interference with xenon ventilation-perfusion evaluations. (17) Similarly, recently in normal control subjects in Sweden (20) and in the United States (21) the degree of change shown on arterial oxygen carrying capacity, lung compliance and diffusion gradients has been shown not to be significant. As has clearly been indicated beforehand, it is important that with all intravenous nutritional regimes a certain number of mandatory observations are carried out otherwise iatrogenic lipoidosis may occur. (22) Dependent on these results it is clearly indicated whether a change from one substrate to another is necessary.

In view of the foregoing there clearly should not be any argument as to whether a fat calorie is better or less good than a carbohydrate calorie. There is no need to look beyond fat or glucose calories to provide intravenous energy substrates. Either, with the appropriate nitrogen provision, can maintain nitrogen homeostasis and prevent the consequences of negative nitrogen balance. Flexibility in the design of intravenous regimes is allowed for by use of either greater or lesser amounts of the two energy substrates dependent upon the individual's metabolic environment.

Table 10. Clinical applications of intralipid

1. I.V. Feeding in post-operative period
2. Renal disease – e.g. ARF, CRF
3. Gastro-intestinal disorders e.g. fistulae, ulc. colitis
4. Severe trauma
5. Paediatric practice
6. Home parenteral nutrition
7. Hepatic and pancreatic disorders
8. Intensive care patients

REFERENCES

1. Hoover, H. C., Grant, J. P., Gorschboth, C. and Ketcham, A. S., *New Engl. J. Med. 293*: 172 (1975).
2. Blackburn, G. L., Flatt, J. P. and Hensle, T. W., In: Total Parenteral Nutrition, pp. 363-394. Ed. Fischer, J. E., *Publ.* Little, Brown and Company (Inc.) (1976).
3. Lee, H. A. (ed.), Parenteral Nutrition in Acute Metabolic Illness, *Academic Press*, London and New York (1974).
4. Ghadimi, H. (ed.), Total Parenteral Nutrition: Premises and Promises. John Wiley and Sons, Inc. (1975).
5. Fischer, J. E. (ed.), Total Parenteral Nutrition. Little, Brown and Company (Inc.) (1976).
6. Biebuyck, J. F. In: Parenteral Nutrition in Infancy and Childhood. pp. 54-70. Ed. Bode, H. H. and Warshaw, J. B., Publ. Plenum Publishing Corp. New York (1973).
7. *Lancet 2*: 263 (1975).
8. Cahill, G. F., *New Engl. J. Med. 282*: 668 (1970).
9. Biebuyck, J. F., *Anesthetiology 39*: 188 (1973).
10. Munro, H. N., *Physiol. Rev. 31*: 449 (1951).
11. Munro, H. N. and Naismith, D. J., *Biochem. J. 54*: 191 (1953).
12. Brennan, M. F., Fitzpatrick, G. F., Cohen, K. H. and Moore, F. D., *Ann. Surg. 182*: 386 (1975).
13. Jeejeebhoy, K. N., Anderson, G. H., Nakhooda, A. F., Greenberg, G. R., Sanderson, I. and Marliss, E. B., *J. Clin. Invest. 57*: 125 (1976).
14. Smith, R., Fuller, D. J., Wedge, J. H., Williamson, D. H. and Alberti, K. G. M. M., *Lancet 1*: 1 (1975).
15. Wretlind, A. In: Parenteral Nutrition in Acute Metabolic Illness, pp. 77-96. Ed. Lee, H. A. Publ. Academic Press Ltd., London and New York (1974).
16. Hartley, T. F. and Lee, H. A., *Nutrit. Metabol. 19*: 201 (1976).
17. Wilmore, D. W., Moylan, J. A., Helkamp, G. M. and Pruitt, B. A., *Ann. Surg. 178*: 503 (1973).
18. Tovey, S., Benton, K. G. F. and Lee, H. A., *Postgrad. Med. J. 53*: 289 (1977).
19. Broviac, J. W., Riella, M. C. and Scribner, B. H., *Am. J. Clin. Nutr. 29*: 255 (1976).
20. Sundstrom, G., Zaunder, C. W. and Arborelius, M., *J. Appl. Physiol. 34*: 816 (1973).
21. Greene, H. L., Hazlett, D. and Demaree, R., *Am. J. Clin. Nutr. 29*: 127 (1976).
22. Freund, U., Krauz, Y., Levij, I. S. and Eliakim, M., *Am. J. Clin. Nutr. 28*: 1156 (1975)
23. Williamson, D. H. and Hems, R. In: Essays in cell metabolism. p. 257. Ed. Bartley, W., Kornberg, H. L. and Quayle, J. R., Wiley-Interscience, London (1970).

Lipid emulsions and technique of peripheral administration in parenteral nutrition

Arvid Wretlind

After the introduction of a safe fat emulsion around 1960, the supply of sufficient amounts of energy in parenteral nutrition was no longer a problem (1). This was the last link in a long series of investigations pertaining to complete intravenous nutrition starting with the studies on intravenous amino acid supply by Elman (2) 40 years ago.

With intravenous fat emulsions - in combination with not less than 20 cal percent of carbohydrates - the required amount of energy can readily be supplied. The advantages of a fat emulsion in parenteral nutrition are summarized in Table 1. By using a fat emulsion, large amounts of energy can be given in small volumes of isotonic fluid. Fat produces 9 kcal per g which is more than twice the energy obtained from either carbohydrates or protein. Because of their isotonicity, the fat emulsions may be given through peripheral veins in contrast to the concentrated glucose solutions, which have to be administered via catheters into a central vein. Thrombophlebitis is seldom encountered with an isotonic fat emulsion. The infusions do not cause diuresis and, furthermore, no losses are observed either in the urine or feces. Fat emulsions also supply the body with essential fatty acids and triglycerides, which are a part of our ordinary food. In this way the normal lipid composition of the cell membrane and other parts of the body may be maintained or restored. During starvation after operations, trauma, etc., the main source of energy is the body fat. The metabolic pathways of fat

Table 1. Advantages of using fat emulsions in parenteral nutrition

1. Large amount of energy in small volume
2. Supply of essential fatty acids
3. Maintenance of normal lipid composition of the body
4. Metabolic pathways of fat not impaired
5. No loss in urine or feces
6. Isotonic solution. No thrombophlebitis
7. Complete intravenous feeding via peripheral veins

oxidation do not seem to be impaired in the postoperative period and in other conditions with increased energy requirements.

I. COMPOSITION OF FAT EMULSIONS

Two of the commercial fat emulsions now available – Intralipid and Lipofundin S – contain soybean oil as fat (Table 2). Egg yolk phospholipids are

Table 2. Composition of fat emulsions

	Intralipid[1] g	Lipiphysan[2] g	Lipofundin S[3] g
Soybean	100 or 200		100 or 200
Cottonseed oil		150	
Egg yolk phospholipids	12		
Soybean lecithine	20		
Soybean phospholipids			7.5 or 15
Glycerol	25		
Sorbitol		50	
Xylitol			50
DL-*-tocopherol		0.5	
Distilled water to a volume (ml) of:	1,000	1,000	1,000

[1] Vitrum, Stockholm, Sweden.
[2] Egic, Loiret, France.
[3] Braun, Melsungen, Germany.

Table 3. Fatty acids in soybean oil and egg yolk phospholipids in Intralipid

		Soybean oil %	Egg yolk phospholipids %
Myristic acid	C14	0.04	0.09
Palmitic acid	C16	9	33
Palmitoleic acid	C16:1	0.03	0.4
Stearic acid	C18	3	16
Oleic acid	C18:1	26	32
Linoleic acid	C18:2	54	11
Linolenic acid	C18:3	8	0.3
Arachidic acid	C20	0.1	0.1
Arachidonic acid	C20:4	–	0.2
Behenic acid	C22	0.06	3
Unidentified acids		–	0.2

used as emulsifiers in Intralipid, soybean phospholipids in the other emulsion. Lipiphysan contains cottonseed oil emulsified with soybean phospholipids. The fatty acid contents of the soybean oil and egg yolk phospholipids are shown in Table 3.

There are two preparations – Nutrifundin and Trivemil – containing fat as an emulsion mixed with amino acids and sorbitol or xylitol. The composition of these products is shown in Table 4.

Schoefl (3) and *Fraser* and *Håkansson* (4) carried out electron microscope studies on Intralipid and chylomicrons. These investigations showed that the size of the fat particles in Intralipid 10% (mean diameter 0.13 μm) was about the same as that of chylomicrons (the mean diameter varied between 0.096 and 0.21 μm). The particles in Intralipid 20% were somewhat larger (mean diameter 0.16 μm). These, and a number of other investigations, have shown many physical and biochemical similarities between chylomicrons and the fat emulsion Intralipid.

A fat emulsion like Intralipid is quite stable. It can be stored for at least 18 months at a temperature between 0 and 4°C. There are no significant changes in any of the physical and chemical properties. Intralipid has also been stored for 2½ years at + 4°C and at 20°C without any changes. Tests in both dogs and man did not show any decreased tolerance. The margin for the recommended storage conditions seems to be great.

Heparin and emulsions containing fat-soluble vitamins can be added to Intralipid. No other solutions are recommended for mixing with Intralipid. However, Intralipid may be given simultaneously with any infusion solutions via the same cannula or catheter by using a Y-shaped tube. Again, with

Table 4. Fat-polyol-amino acid preparations

Constituents	Nutrifundin[1] g	Trivemil[2] g
Soybean oil fract.	38	38
Soybean lecithine		7
Soybean phospholipids fract.	3.8	
Sorbitol		100
Xylitol	100	
Amino acid mixture	60	60
Distilled water to	1000	1000

[1] Braun, Melsungen, Germany.
[2] Egic, Loiret, France.

regard to the mixing of Intralipid with other infusion solutions, the margin is great. *Solassol* and *Joyeux* (5) mix Intralipid with amino acids, glucose and all other nutrients in a container holding two liters for daily use. The mixture may be stored 3 months at + 4°C according to the authors. This method of mixing should only be used by experts, who are also able to check every container bacteriologically.

II. EXPERIMENTAL STUDIES WITH FAT EMULSIONS

Experimental studies show that there are marked biological differences between the various fat emulsions. *Because of these pronounced differences it is not correct to speak of fat emulsions in general. The name of the fat emulsion should always be given and its exact composition stated.*

A. Tolerance

Comparative investigations of different fat emulsions in dogs were performed by *Håkansson* (6). He infused 9 g of fat per kg/day. The tests were made with two cottonseed oil emulsions as well as the emulsion with soybean oil, Intralipid. Each investigation period was four weeks and the amount of fat supplied corresponded to the total energy requirement. The dogs which received the soybean oil emulsion were alert and well with normal weight gain. They showed only slight anemia. All the dogs given the cottonseed oil emulsion died and had severe anemia. These dogs had blood in the feces and in the urine. They were dull, vomited, had leukocytosis and diarrhea. The symptoms after Lipiphysan were worse than those after Lipofundin. Lipiphysan also caused a large reduction in the serum albumin content. The cottonseed oil emulsion produced fatty infiltration in the liver and centrolobular necrosis. Jaundice was a constant finding and a pronounced leukocytosis was recorded after the cottonseed oil emulsions.

The results of *Håkansson* (l.c.) were confirmed by *Jacobson* and *Wretlind* (7), who extended the experiments to include Lipofundin S. Surprisingly, the Lipofundin S which contains soybean oil in the same concentrations as Intralipid was as toxic as the previously investigated cottonseed oil preparations. The toxic factor is thus likely to be found in the soybean phospholipids.

Berg et al. (8) have also partly confirmed Håkansson's results. They infused Lipofundin S into the superior vena cava of dwarf pigs in various doses. Five received less than 5 g of fat/kg/day and survived; the other five were given more than 5 g/kg/day and all succumbed. They showed no lipemia but general fatty infiltrations in different organs. One pig had fatal enteral hemorrhages. The others died from "idiopathic and metabolic" heart insufficiency.

B. Fat emulsions and lipoprotein lipase

The effect of induced serum lipoprotein lipase on different fat emulsions has been investigated by *Boberg* and *Carlson* (9). They found that the artificial fat emulsion Intralipid and chylomicrons had similar effects, whereas other substrates or fat emulsions had quite different properties in that respect.

C. Elimination of fat emulsion from the bloodstream

It is desirable that the fat particles in an artificial fat emulsion have the same biological properties as those of the natural chylomicrons, including among other things transport in the blood, and distribution and utilization in the body.

Temporary hyperlipemia occurs after every fat infusion. According to investigations by *Hallberg* (10, 11), the kinetic principle for the elimination of fat particles after an Intralipid infusion in dog and man is practically identical with that for the elimination of natural chylomicrons. The kinetic principle is characterized by the fact that above a certain "critical particle concentration", elimination is maximal. Below this critical concentration, elimination is exponential. The maximum elimination for a person who has fasted overnight corresponds to 3.8 g of fat per kg per 24 hours (35 kcal/kg/24 hours). After starving for 38 hours the elimination capacity is increased to 52 kcal/kg/24 hours. During the postoperative period, while starving for 48 hours, the elimination capacity rises to 100 kcal/kg/24 hours. *Wilmore et al.* (12) have also confirmed this increased fat elimination capacity in the catabolic state in patients suffering from burns. *Forget et al.* (13) found an increase in the fat elimination rate when the intravenous supply of Intralipid during an infusion period of 28 days was successively increased from 3 to 8 g of fat/kg/day in a child. At the same time an increase in the postheparin lipoprotein lipase activity was observed.

Infusion of Intralipid results in maximum serum triglyceride levels at the end of the infusion, but the serum free fatty acid level gradually reaches a maximum within 4 hours after the infusion and falls to preinfusion levels after 6-8 hours (14). Serum triglyceride clearance seems to be independent of the total amount of energy given. However, the disappearance rate of serum free fatty acid is increased by a larger energy supply.

Coran and *Nesbakken* (15) studied the effect of the fat emulsion Intralipid on plasma triglycerides and free fatty acids in neonates. They found that neonates were able to eliminate fat as rapidly as adults. Moreover, it was observed that heparin increased the elimination rate of triglycerides and raised the level of free fatty acids.

Gustafsson et al. (16) reported that prematures, with normal birthweight for length of pregnancy, had a maximum fat elimination capacity from the bloodstream of approximately 6 grams of fat/kg/24 hours, i.e. as high as that for healthy, adult subjects. For neonates with a birthweight that was low-for-date, the maximum fat elimination capacity was lower. These infants showed a distinct tendency with each dose of fat to accumulate lipids in the plasma, mostly in the chylomicron fraction. In some cases, an intravenous heparin dose of 50 IU/kg appreciably improved the infant's capacity to eliminate fat. This finding supports the assumption that in neonates who were undernourished during their intrauterine life, the functions of the lipoprotein lipases are in some way not fully developed. However, it should be possible to improve the elimination capacity by combining the supply of Intralipid with heparin.

On the basis of observations regarding the elimination of Intralipid from the bloodstream, an Intra-Venous Fat Tolerance Test (IVFTT) has been developed by *Carlson* and *Hallberg* (17), *Boberg et al.* (18) and *Carlson* and *Rössner* (19).

The effect of an intravenous supply of fat on the triglyceride concentration in blood has been studied. One group of patients with burns was given 100 g of fat intravenously daily in the form of 500 ml of Intralipid 20% for five weeks (20, 21). There were no significant differences in the mean concentration of plasma triglycerides between the group given fat and a group with no fat infusions. The studies on the fasting free fatty acid level in blood showed a decrease in the group with fat. These investigations indicated that burn patients tolerated the fat emulsion very well.

The elimination of fat from the bloodstream after infusion of Lipiphysan and Lipofundin S is much faster than after Intralipid (22, 23). It is likely that this is caused by the uptake of the fat particles by the reticulo-endothelial system (24). The elimination rate of Nutrifundin from the bloodstream seems to be about the same as that of Lipofundin S.

D. *Influence of fat emulsion on the reticuloendothelial system and the immunological factors*

Gigon et al. (25) have shown by studies in man that, after infusion of Intralipid, some of the fat particles are absorbed by the endothelial cells in the pulmonary vessels. They did not observe any signs of aggregation of the fat particles.

Scholler (26) reported that fat from some fat emulsions is accumulated in the reticuloendothelial cells. This accumulation was found to depend on the composition of the emulsions and the size of the fat particles. The investigations were performed by electron microscope studies of liver biopsies from man and rats. After intravenous infusions of Lipofundin S the fat particles were taken up by the reticuloendothelial cells by phagocytosis in both man and experimental animals. The reticuloendothelial system was partly blocked, and antibody formation was significantly reduced. After infusion of Intralipid no accumulation of fat particles in the Kupffer's cells was observed.

No significant reduction in the formation of antibodies was found in guinea pigs after Intralipid. Because of the impairment of the resistance of the body by the accumulations of particles in the reticuloendothelial system, it has been stated that only those fat emulsions - such as Intralipid - which are not taken up by the reticuloendothelial cells should be used clinically (26).

Huth et al. (27) have shown interesting differences between the cottonseed oil emulsions and the egg yolk phospholipids-soybean oil emulsion Intralipid in studies on tolerance for endotoxin from *Escherichia coli*. Infusions of cottonseed oil in rabbits caused a decreased tolerance against the endotoxin. After Intralipid infusions only insignificant effects were found.

Carpentier et al. (28) found that the fat emulsion Intralipid did not reduce the formation of immunoglobulins.

E. Fat emulsion and the coagulation system

The influence on the coagulation mechanism has been thoroughly studied by several researchers. *Duckert* and *Hartmann* (29), *Hartmann* (30), *Cronberg* and *Nilsson* (31) and *Kapp et al.* (32) found, after very extensive experimental and clinical investigations, that Intralipid did not have any effect on coagulation nor on the fibrinolytic system. There is no reason to anticipate a greater disposition toward thrombosis after fat infusions. Consequently, it did not seem necessary to administer heparin together with the fat infusions.

Huth et al. (27) showed that Lipofundin S had pronounced effects on the coagulation mechanism resulting in disseminated intravascular coagulation in rabbits. This effect was not observed after intravenous administration of Intralipid.

F. Fat emulsion and the pulmonary function

Steinbereithner and *Wagner* (33) investigated the effect of intravenous infusions of Intralipid on the oxygen arterial tension in patients with serious cranial trauma and chronic hypoxic syndrome. The results of these studies showed no reduction of the oxygen tension and no interference with oxygen supply to the tissues.

Measurement of the steady state pulmonary diffusing capacity and membrane diffusing capacity in normal human volunteers, before and after administration of 500 ml of 10% Intralipid intravenously, has shown a decrease in these functions for at least 4 hours following the infusion in 6 out of 10 subjects (34). These changes returned to control levels within 24 hours in all 6 subjects. Simultaneous infusion of heparin with Intralipid prevented the decrease in both the steady state pulmonary diffusing capacity and membrane diffusing capacity. This finding might support the concept of adding heparin to Intralipid when the pulmonary function is impaired.

The pulmonary diffusing capacity, determined by ^{133}Xenon perfusion-diffusion and carbon monoxide rebreathing techniques, was found to be normal following the infusion of Intralipid (12). Blood gas levels did not change after infusion of single or multiple units of the fat emulsion.

Sundström et al. (35) investigated pulmonary function parameters in healthy human males before, during and after infusion of fat emulsion. The pulmonary diffusing capacity for carbon monoxide decreased in this study by about 15 percent. Alveolar oxygen tension did not change and the alveolar-arterial difference for oxygen tension decreased.

Table 5. Osmolality of solutions for intravenous nutrition and of plasma

Solution	mOsm per kg water
Plasma	290
0.9% NaCl	308
10% Intralipid	280
20% Intralipid	330
5% Glucose	278
10% Glucose	523
20% Glucose	1,250
30% Glucose	2,100
50% Glucose	3,800
3.3% Aminosol	555
10% Aminosol	925
Vamin*	1,275

* 7% crystalline amino acids and 10% carbohydrates.

G. Fat emulsion and osmolality

It is important that the osmotic pressure of the blood does not change. Consequently, isotonic solutions should be used. Table 5 shows the osmolality of different infusion solutions used for intravenous nutrition. It is evident that large amounts of energy can be administered by means of fat emulsions without changing the osmotic pressure of the blood. If hypertonic solutions are used they must be given slowly during the whole 24 hours, according to the technique described by *Dudrick et al.* (36). *Bernhoff* (37) showed that the contractile strength of the myocardium in dogs was reduced when hypertonic infusion solutions were used. On the other hand, iso-osmotic solutions such as 5.5% glucose and 10% and 20% Intralipid had no negative effect on the myocardium.

H. Nutritional aspects of fat emulsions

(a) Energy source

Investigations have shown that intravenously supplied fat emulsions are utilized, in principle, in the same way as alimentary fat. This is evident from studies which have demonstrated that fat emulsions can be used as a source of energy to improve the nitrogen balance (38, 39, 40, 41, 42, 43).

In many studies the effects of the nonprotein energy sources, glucose and fat, on the nitrogen balance have been compared. *Jeejeebhoy et al.* (44) gave patients on total parenteral nutrition nonprotein energy in the form of either glucose alone (glucose system) or 83% fat (Intralipid) and 17% glucose (lipid system). This nonprotein energy was administered with a constant supplement of 1 g amino acids per kg body weight per day. The results of 27 studies in 24 patients using either system for 7 days showed that the nitrogen balances were positive with both systems. However, during the first four days of each test period the nitrogen balance was significantly higher with the glucose than with the lipid system. During the last three days no differences were recorded. This indicates that the gain in nitrogen was a temporary phenomenon.

Eighteen preoperative and postoperative patients, divided into two groups, underwent total parenteral nutrition with either fat or glucose as the main nonprotein energy source for an average period of 15 and 16 days, respectively (45). Estimation of nitrogen balance showed no differences between the two groups. Both groups demonstrated weight gain, but it was more marked with the glucose system.

The ability of a fat emulsion to produce nitrogen sparing in the absence of nitrogen intake was examined by *Brennan et al.* (46) in healthy man. It was found that the nitrogen sparing seen when an intravenous fat emulsion was given as sole source could be reproduced completely by the infusion of the same amount of glycerol as is found in the fat emulsion.

Using fat and glucose in varying proportions, *Long et al.* (47) have shown that nitrogen sparing was proportional to the glucose intake with no effect related to the amount of infused fat.

Bark et al. (48) investigated the question of whether there is any difference in the nitrogen balance when the main energy source is a hypertonic carbohydrate solution or a fat emulsion. The nitrogen balance of nine patients was examined during the first six postoperative days after gastric resection. All of them were given crystalline amino acids corresponding to 0.3 g N/kg body weight per day together with fructose, electrolytes and vitamins. Five of the patients were also given 50 kcal/kg body weight per day mainly as fat emulsion (Intralipid). The other four patients received the same amount of energy mainly in the form of a 54% glucose solution. The investigation showed that it was possible to obtain nitrogen equilibrium during the immediate postoperative course, whether the main nonprotein supply consisted of a hypertonic carbohydrate solution or a fat emulsion. There was no significant difference between the two energy sources in this respect.

All investigations in this field indicate that under adequate nitrogen intake, the nitrogen balance is influenced by changes in energy supply whether they come from glucose or fat with glucose. It appears that glucose will spare more nitrogen than fat. These differences seem to be small in most patients. However, in catabolic phases, the differences might be significant. Hypocaloric amounts of glucose or fat (< 11 kcal/kg) do not affect the nitrogen balance in patients receiving 1 g of amino acids per kg body weight (49).

It has been found that intravenously administered fat emulsions are oxidized in the body as calculated (50, 51, 52). An intravenous infusion technique in rats has been used to determine the oxidation rate of the fatty acids in a fat emulsion (53, 54). A soybean oil emulsion (Intralipid) labelled with ^{14}C palmitic, oleic or linoleic acid has been used. The peak of $^{14}CO_2$ in the expired air, indicating complete oxidation of the fat, occurred two hours after the injection. The total amount of fat oxidized during the first 12 hours after the injection was 40 to 70 percent depending on – among many different factors – the nutritional state of the rat. *Reid* (43) found a decrease in the respiratory quotient when fat emulsions were administered, which showed a combustion of the fat supplied.

When a positive energy balance was attained by intravenous nutrition with Intralipid, the weight increase expected in relation to energy storage was obtained; this also indicates that the fat is utilized in the same way as the fat in our usual diet (7).

In a number of studies most of the energy supply was given in the form of fat. Thus, *Peaston* (55, 56) and *Stell* (57) gave 200 g of fat (about 3 g/kg) per day, corresponding to 60-80 percent of the total energy supply. *Bergström et al.* (58) supplied about 40 percent of the energy in the form of fat, corresponding to about 2 g of fat/kg. This quantity was previously recommended by *Hallberg et al.* (42), *Steinbereithner* (59) and *Allen* and *Lee* (60). *Deitel* and *Kaminsky* (61) used for infusion through a peripheral vein a 'lipid system' consisting of 3 g of fat/kg, 1.5 g of glucose/kg and all other nutrients.

Rickham (62) gave neonates on intravenous nutrition 2.5-3 g fat/kg/day (Intralipid). *Børresen* and *Knutrud* (63), *Børresen et al.* (64, 65), *Grotte* (66) and *Grotte et al.* (67) administered 3-4 g of fat (Intralipid)/kg/day to neonates and infants as a part of a complete intravenous feeding resulting in normal growth.

(b) Source of essential fatty acids

The essential fatty acid deficiency in dogs on intravenous feeding was described by *Meng* and *Early* (68). In 1970 *Pensler et al.* (69) demonstrated essential fatty acid deficiency in three children on prolonged total parenteral alimentation. There were changes in the plasma fatty acid patterns, consisting of a reduction in the levels of linoleic and arachidonic acid, and an increase in oleic, palmitoleic and 5, 8, 11-eicosatrienoic acid. Scaly lesions on the skin were the main clinical symptom observed.

Caldwell et al. (70) reported that infants on low-fat intravenous nutrition developed eczema, and that this condition was readily cured by an infusion of fat emulsion. A 25-week-old baby on parenteral nutrition who had received no fat emulsions since its eighteenth day of life suffered from scaly skin lesions, sparse hair growth and thrombocytopenia. Analysis of the fatty acids in the plasma phospholipids showed low levels of linoleic and arachidonic acid and a high content of 5, 8, 11-eicosatrienoic acid indicating an essential fatty acid deficiency. On administration of sufficient fat emulsion (Intralipid) to provide 4 percent of the daily energy requirement in the form of linoleic acid, the levels of linoleic and arachidonic acid rose and the level of 5, 8, 11-eicosatrienoic acid decreased, the skin lesions healed, and the thrombocytopenia was corrected.

Infants less than six months old on intravenous nutrition with glucose, protein hydrolysate and no fat were found to have a low content of essential fatty acids in the serum and dermatitis (71).

For a long time there was no definite evidence that the essential fatty acids were required by adults. An adult male patient, however, maintained on intravenous nutrition without fat for 100 days developed a skin rash. The fatty acids in the serum phospholipids were found to have a high content of 5, 8, 11-eicosatrienoic acid and a low content of arachidonic acid (72). Intralipid administered intravenously (22.8 grams of linoleic acid per day) caused the serum phospholipid content of eicosatrienoic acid to drop and the level of arachidonic acid to rise. Simultaneously, the rash disappeared.

Table 6. Some reports on the use of intralipid in adults

g of fat/kg/day	Infusion period	Authors	Year
1-3	Single infusions. Up to 28 days	Schuberth and Wretlind (1); Buchner and Cesnik (74)	1961-1962
1-2	Single infusions.	Ôstergaard (75); Schuberth (76); Freuchen (77); Jones et al. (78); Schärli (79)	1963-1964
1-3	Single infusions. Up to 150 days	Lawson (80); Lee and Shortle (81); Hadfield (82); Steinbereithner (59); Peaston (55); Hallberg et al. (42); Freuchen and Østergaard (83); Hartmann (30); Vlaardingerbroek (84)	1965-1967
2-5	Up to 7 months	Hartmann (85); Feischl and Hiotakis (86); Stell (57); Liljedahl (87); Bergström et al. (58); Jacobson (88); Zumtobel and Zehle (89); Geremy et al. (90)	1968-1972
2-5	Up to more than 5 years	Jeejeebhoy et al. (44, 73); Wilmore et al. (12); Solassol and Joyeux (5); Deitel and Kaminsky (61); Lamke et al. (21); Kessler (91)	1973-1976

In five out of thirteen patients with severe burns it was found that the essential polyunsaturated fatty acids, as well as phosphatidylserine and phosphatidylethanolamine, were much reduced in the erythrocyte membranes (12). The deficiency was not correlated with the degree of the burns. Stress or alcoholism was mentioned as a possible additional etiological factor. Fat emulsion (Intralipid) given parenterally restored the fat composition of the erythrocyte membrane.

When a patient was given intravenous nutrition without fat for a period of 9 months, fatty degeneration of the hepatic tissues occurred (73). When

50-100 g of fat (Intralipid) were administered daily for one month, followed by 50-100 g of fat per week, the fatty degeneration of the liver diminished successively during the next period of 5 months. It seems that the essential fatty acids are required to prevent fatty degeneration of the liver.

III. CLINICAL STUDIES WITH THE SOYBEAN OIL-EGG YOLK PHOSPHOLIPID EMULSION INTRALIPID

The broadest clinical experience with fat emulsions has been obtained with Intralipid (Table 6).

A. Adults

A large number of investigations has demonstrated that it is possible to administer complete intravenous nutrition with Intralipid as the source of fat for a long period in adult man.

In a series of investigations dealing with complete intravenous nutrition *Lawson* (80) gave about 3 g of fat/kg for a period varying between 8 and 36 days. Liver biopsies after 30 and 36 days showed as the only change a pigmentation of Kupffer's cells. No appreciable changes were observed in the bromsulphalein retention, bilirubin content in serum or serum transaminases.

Hadfield (82) gave intravenous nutrition using Intralipid in amounts up to 12 g of fat/kg/day for 15 days to a patient with ulcerative colitis, and for 4 weeks to a patient with severe malabsorption.

Hallberg et al. (92) reported complete intravenous nutrition administered to a patient with Crohn's disease. The patient received daily 2-2.5 g of fat/kg (Intralipid), 0.4-6.2 g of glucose/kg and up to 1.2 g of amino acids/kg (Aminosol) regularly during a period of more than 5 months. The total amount of fat was 15 kg.

In one case, complete intravenous nutrition was administered for 7 months and 13 days (7, 58). The patient was a woman, 43 years of age, who lost consciousness as a result of severe cerebral injury caused by carbon monoxide poisoning. The amino acids were given in the form of Vamin, and fat in the form of Intralipid 20%. Fructose and glucose were used as carbohydrates. The average daily energy supply was about 2,000 kcal. For 6 months, 408 ml of Intralipid 20% were given daily, corresponding to 816 kcal. The increase in weight during the period of intravenous nutrition was 10 kg, from 40 to 50 kg, without any appreciable change in the body fluid volume. Histopathological studies were conducted by means of repeated needle biopsies of the liver (93). The parenchymal cells did not show any significant light or electron microscopic changes during the period of intravenous nutrition. The Kupffer's cells, however, showed focal proliferations, enlargement, accumulation of fat droplets and occurrence of a lipofuscin-like pigment. The evidence suggested that droplets of neutral fat in the Kupffer's cells were segregated in lysosome-like bodies, which subsequently underwent structural reorganization and transformation into lipofuscin-like granules. After cessation of the intravenous therapy there was a slow decrease in the number of lipofuscin-like bodies in the Kupffer's cells during the following 1.5 years. The observed changes did not signify any liver cell damage.

Jacobson (88) administered intravenous nutrition to a 70-year-old patient during a period of 69 days after a massive resection of the small intestine and 25 cm of the ascending colon because of acute occlusion of the superior mesenteric artery. The mean daily supply was 3.58 l of water, 2,850 kcal, 70 g of amino acids, 405 g of carbohydrates, 100 g of fat (Intralipid) and all other essential nutrients. After the period of intravenous nutrition the patient was able to resume oral nutrition.

Jeejeebhoy et al. (73) have a patient who has been nourished intravenously exclusively since 6 October 1970. The patient, who is a housewife (born 1934), stayed for the first 9 months in the hospital. After that, she remained in her own home, attending to the intravenous nutrition herself. The infusions are given during the night through a catheter of silicon rubber inserted in the superior vena cava. For this purpose an amino acid mixture is used (Amigen) together with glucose, fat (500 ml of Intralipid 10%), electrolytes and vitamins. The total energy supply is 2,000 kcal or 34 kcal/kg. Two liver biopsies were performed after fat had been supplied for 3 and 5 months, respectively. They showed that the hepatic tissue was entirely normal. This case, where intravenous nutrition has been continued for about 6 years, shows that a nutritional condition can be maintained which enables the patient to perform daily work in a satisfactory manner. The studies mentioned and a number of other studies on adult patients show that by means of complete intravenous nutrition, including fat emulsions, patients can be kept in a good nutritional condition for a comparatively long time.

Yeo et al. (94) treated 12 patients for 7 to 28 days during the postoperative period with 3 g of fat/kg/day (Intralipid) as part of a total intravenous feeding administered through a peripheral vein. Ten patients recovered and were discharged. Two patients died of causes unrelated to the parenteral nutrition.

B. Neonates and infants

Complete intravenous nutrition with fat, i.e. Intralipid, has been thoroughly studied in neonates and infants (Table 7). *Børresen* and *Knutrud* (63) and *Børresen et al.* (65) administered such intravenous nutrition via a peripheral vein. By giving 3-4 g of fat per kg it was possible to avoid hypertonic carbohydrate solutions (hyperalimentation). The infusions via a peripheral vein were given for periods of 1 to 3 weeks. One report dealt with 32 neonates, who had been operated on for gastrointestinal malformations and subsequently required complete intravenous nutrition. Of these, 26 survived. In another series complete parenteral nutrition was administered to 14 infants suffering from severe surgical complications. All of these patients survived. Similar results were obtained by *Grotte et al.* (66, 67) using a program for *total* parenteral nutrition based on fat (Intralipid) and amino acids (Vamin) with the addition of standardized doses of electrolytes, trace minerals and vitamins.

There are many reports on infants who have received complete

Table 7. Some reports on the use of intralipid in neonates and infants

g of fat/kg/day	Infusion period	Authors	Year
2.5-4	3-50 days	Rickham (62); Bôrresen et al. (65)	1967-1970
1-4	3-84 days	Coran (95); Caldwell et al. (96); Heird et al. (97); Wei et al.(9 8); Børresen (99)	1971-1973
3-8	3-205 days	Grotte et al. (67); Forget et al. (13); Coran (100); Pendray (101); Puri et al. (102); Schärli and Rumlova (103)	1974-1976

intravenous nutrition with Intralipid after operations for severe congenital malformations. Despite the major surgical intervention, a positive nitrogen balance could be achieved on the same order of magnitude as that of normal bottle-fed infants.

Children treated with intravenous nutrition in different USA hospitals have received 28-69 percent of the amount of energy supplied in the form of fat (Intralipid). The daily supply of fat varied between 1.1 and 6 g per kg.

The total infusion time per child varied between 8 and 122 days. All the infusions were given via a peripheral vein. The majority of these severely ill children showed satisfactory growth.

IV. CLINICAL STUDIES USING THE EMULSIONS LIPIPHYSAN, LIPOFUNDIN S, NUTRIFUNDIN AND TRIVEMIL

The cottonseed oil emulsion Lipiphysan should, according to the manufacturers, be given in limited amounts. The recommended average daily dose for adults is 0.8 to 1.2 g of fat per kg body weight. The total dose should not exceed 1000 to 1500 g of fat corresponding to about 15 to 20 units of 500 ml 15% emulsion. For children, the recommended average dose is 2 g of fat.

According to *Eckart et al.* (52) there were no adverse reactions to Lipofundin S when given in the dose of 1 g of fat/kg/day. *Schmidtsdorf* (104) used it for surgical patients after large operations for periods of up to 3 weeks.

Lipofundin S is readily taken up by the reticuloendothelial cells. *Lemperle* and *Reichelt* (105) have thus used Lipofundin S to assess the phagocytic activity in patients.

The preparation Nutrifundin, which contains amino acids, xylitol and soybean oil, is according to *Voss* and *Schnell* (106) galenically stable and causes no adverse reactions in dogs. *Witzel et al.* (107) have reported single infusions of Nutrifundin in 15 volunteer test subjects. The infusion of 500 ml caused no side effects. Twenty-three patients were treated with 1003 infusions. The daily dose was 1000 ml containing 42 g of lipids. Six patients were on parenteral nutrition exclusively for an average of 27 days. Leukocytes, transaminases, alkaline phosphatase and other tests remained unchanged. Histological examinations of liver biopsies after 23 days of infusions showed no pathological findings. The amount of fat given in the form of Nutrifundin by others varied between 0.5 and 1 g/kg/day (108).

A preparation similar to Nutrifundin – Trivemil (EB 51) – has been used in France. *Cailar et al.* (109) found the product to be well-tolerated in a daily dosage of 1000-1500 ml. Many investigators have reported that Trivemil appears to be nontoxic, efficient and valuable. The infusions were given to patients after surgery or with medical diseases. The amount of fat given daily was 38 to 57 g.

V. INFUSION TECHNIQUE

The infusion technique varies considerably. The tendency has been, and still is, to find simple infusion methods without serious side effects. Infusion via a peripheral vein is preferable to infusion via a catheter in a central vein because complications are then minor and easy to diagnose.
via a peripheral vein is preferable to infusion via a catheter in a central vein because complications are then minor and easy to diagnose.

In adults on intravenous nutrition including fat for shorter periods (7-14 days), infusion through a cannula in a peripheral vein is recommended. Preferably, the cannula should not be left in the same place in the vein longer than 8-12 hours a day to avoid the risk of mechanical irritation leading to thrombophlebitis. *Weiss* and *Nissan* (110) have demonstrated a markedly reduced incidence of thrombophlebitis when the infusion via a peripheral vein is limited to a daily period of 12 hours instead of maintaining a continuous infusion. By using a so-called lipid system of 3 g of fat, 1.5 g of glucose and 1 g of amino acids per kg body weight per day, it was possible for *Deitel* and *Kaminsky* (61) to administer complete intravenous nutrition via peripheral veins for periods of up to 78 days. If total parenteral nutrition in adults is indicated for several weeks or months a central vein catheter in the superior vena cava might be necessary.

In many reports on infants and children receiving intravenous nutrition including a fat emulsion (Intralipid), the infusions have been given via peripheral veins (64, 67, 100). Scalp vein needles have been used in most cases. In older children, the veins of the dorsum of the hand have been used (67, 100, 101). The fat emulsion may be mixed with amino acid and glucose solutions before it is infused into the vein with the aid of a 3-way connector and a constant infusion pump. Half the calculated requirement of each solution is given on the first day, and this is gradually increased to the full requirement by the 3rd day.

VI. INDICATIONS

In principle, complete intravenous nutrition including a fat emulsion is indicated in all cases when nutrients cannot be adequately supplied either orally or enterally (1).

VII. ADVERSE REACTIONS AND CONTRA-INDICATIONS

Acute adverse reactions have been observed only in a small percentage of the patients receiving the soybean oil-egg yolk phospholipid emulsion, Intralipid. The few adverse reactions noted were febrile responses (30), chills, sensation of warmth, shivering, vomiting and pain in the chest and back. Thrombophlebitis has only occasionally been observed (42, 92). Adverse reactions during long-term administration of Intralipid to adults as well as infants have been rare. In all, there are only reports of one hundred cases of mild or moderate reactions, and seven cases of severe complications – two in adults (111, 112) and five in infants (113, 114, 115).

Krediet and *De Gens* (116) also described a 29-year-old woman on parenteral nutrition for ten weeks because of cachexia and a large defect in the abdominal wall after a colectomy. After forty-seven days, in which she received 4.2 kg of fat in the form of Intralipid, high fever, jaundice and thrombocytopenia occurred. These symptoms disappeared when the infusion of fat emulsion was discontinued.

Liver damage was discussed earlier as a contraindication for the use of fat emulsion. Careful studies have been performed with 41 patients with moderate and severe liver damage on parenteral nutrition including Intralipid (100 g of fat/day) for 10 to 30 days postoperatively (89). Liver function tests, platelet counts, coagulation time and plasma clearing capacity were not affected. Histological examination of liver biopsy specimens showed no fat accumulation. *Michel et al.* (117) investigated 16 patients with alcohol cirrhosis who were given intravenous nutrition including Intralipid for 15 days. No effects on liver function tests could be related to the fat infusions.

The administration of Intralipid is contraindicated in patients with a disturbed fat metabolism and in patients with severe disturbances of fat metabolism such as pathological hyperlipemia and lipoid nephrosis (118). In order to avoid administering fat to a patient unable to eliminate the fat from the bloodstream, the following simple test should be performed. In the morning after the first infusion of fat emulsion, a citrated blood sample is centrifuged at 1200–1500 r.p.m. If the plasma is then highly opalescent or milky, further infusions should be postponed or smaller daily amounts of fat emulsion should be given. In the great majority of cases, the plasma is completely clear 12 hours after the conclusion of an infusion of fat. This test should be repeated at weekly intervals. It is extremely rare to find a patient who cannot eliminate the fat particles from the circulation.

VIII. DOSAGE

The basal amounts of fat, amino acids and carbohydrates stated in Table 8 should be supplied to avoid loss of weight in adults and to ensure growth in infants. The patient should also receive all other essential nutrients. In some cases after severe trauma, operations, etc., it may of course be necessary to increase the supply of for example energy, water, amino acids, carbohydrates and fat.

Table 8. Tentatively recommended daily allowance of energy, water, amino acids, carbohydrates and fat for complete intravenous nutrition

Energy and nutrients	Adult Amount per kg per day to cover		Newborns and infants Amount per kg per day
	basal or normal need	high need	
Energy	25-30 kcal	50-60 kcal	90-120 kcal
Water	25-30 ml	50-60 ml	120-150 ml
Amino acids	1 g	2 g	2.5 g
Glucose, fructose	2 g	5 g	12-18 g
Fat	2 g	3 g	4 g

SUMMARY

Fat metabolism is of vital importance for the energy supply required under both normal and starving conditions. Fat can be given in large amounts with glucose as a source of nonprotein energy and as part of a well-balanced complete nutrition.

Great differences in tolerance for the various fat emulsions have been reported. The fat emulsion of choice seems to contain soybean oil and egg yolk phospholipids. It has been shown to be well-tolerated in both animals and man. Investigations have indicated that this fat emulsion has about the same biochemical properties and is metabolized in about the same way as orally supplied fat entering the bloodstream as chylomicrons.

In a large number of experimental and clinical investigations it has been shown that an adequate complete intravenous nutrition can be achieved by using chemically well-defined nutrients including fat.

The complete intravenous nutrition including a fat emulsion could be given via a peripheral vein. This always seems to be the safest and easiest access for parenteral feeding.

Our present knowledge of complete intravenous nutrition, including fat emulsions, is such that it could and should be used to prevent and treat malnutrition with its complications in patients who do not receive proper enteral nutrition.

REFERENCES

1. Schuberth, O. and Wretlind, A., Intravenous infusion of fat emulsions, phosphatides and emulsifying agents. Clinical and experimental studies. *Acta Chir. Scand.*, Suppl. 278, 3 (1961).
2. Elman, R., Amino-acid content of the blood following intravenous injection of hydrolysed casein. *Proc. Soc. exp. Biol. Med.37*: 437 (1937).
3. Schoefl, G. I., The ultrastructure of chylomicra and of the particles in an artificial fat emulsion. *Proc. Roy. Soc. B. 169*: 147 (1968).
4. Fraser, R. and Häkansson, I., Personal communication (1976).
5. Solassol, C. et Joyeux, H., Nouvelles techniques pour nutrition parentérale chronique. *Ann. Anësth. Franc. Spécial II*: 75 (1974).
6. Häkansson, I., Experience in long-term studies on nine intravenous fat emulsions in dogs. *Nutr. Dieta 10*: 54 (1968).
7. Jacobson, S. and Wretlind, A., The use of fat emulsions for complete intravenous nutrition. In: Fox, Jr., C. L. and Nahas, G. G. (eds.), Body Fluid Replacement in the Surgical Patient. Grune and Stratton, New York, p. 334 (1970).
8. Berg, G., Teichmann, K. D., Wörrle, G., Bergner, D. und Hahn, H., Langfristige parenterale Applikation von Fettemulsionen beim Zwergschwein. *Zschr. für Ernährungswiss. 10*: 1 (1970).
9. Boberg, J. and Carlson, L., Determination of heparin-induced lipoprotein lipase activity in human plasma. *Clin. Chim. Acta 10*: 420 (1964).
10. Hallberg, D., Studies on the elimination of exogenous lipids from the blood stream. The kinetics for the elimination of a fat emulsion studied by single injection technique in man. *Acta Physiol. Scand 664*: 306 (1965).
11. Hallberg, D., Elimination of exogenous lipids from the blood stream. An experimental, methodological and clinical study in dog and man. *Acta Physiol. Scand.*, Suppl. 65: 254 (1965).
12. Wilmore, D. W., Moylan, J. A., Helmkamp, G. M. and Pruitt, B. A., Jr., Clinical evaluation of a 10% intravenous fat emulsion for parenteral nutrition in thermally injured patients. *Ann. Surg. 78*: 503 (1973).
13. Forget, P. P., Fernandes, J. and Haverkamp-Begemann, P., Enhancement of fat elimination during intravenous feeding. *Acta Paediatr. Scand. 63*: 750 (1974).
14. MacFadyen, B., Maynard, A. and Dudrick, S. J., Triglyceride and free fatty acid clearances and linoleic acid repletion using 10% soybean oil emulsion in patients receiving standard parenteral hyperalimentation. Abstracts of short communication presented at the IXth International Congress of Nutrition in Mexico City, p. 198, Sept. 3-9 (1972).
15. Coran, A. G. and Nesbakken, R., The metabolism of intravenously administered fat in adult and newborn dogs. *Surgery 66*: 922 (1969).
16. Gustafsson, A., Kjellmer, I., Olegärd, R. and Victorin, L., Nutrition in low-birthweight infants. *Acta Paediatr. Scand. 61*: 149 (1972).
17. Carlson, L. A. and Hallberg, D., Studies on the elimination of exogenous lipids from the blood stream. The kinetics of the elimination of a fat emulsion and of chylomicrons in the dog after single injection. *Acta Physiol. Scand. 59*: 52 (1963).
18. Boberg, J., Carlson, L. A. and Hallberg, D., Application of a new intravenous fat tolerance test in the study of hypertriglyceridaemia in man. *J. Atheroscl. Res. 9*: 159 (1969).
19. Carlson, L. A. and Rössner, S., A methodological study of an intravenous fat tolerance test with Intralipid emulsion. *Scand. J. Clin. Lab. Invest. 29*: 243 (1972).
20. Carlson, L. A. and Liljedahl, S.-O., Lipid metabolism and trauma. IV. Effect of treat-

ment with intravenous fat emulsion on plasma lipids, protein and clinical condition of burned patients. *Acta Chir. Scand. 137*: 123 (1971).
21. Lamke, L.-O., Liljedahl, S.-O. et Wretlind, A., Aspects nutritionnels et cliniques de la nutrition intra-veineuse chez les brulés. *Ann. Anësth. Franc. Spécial II, 15*: 27 (1974).
22. Warembourg, H., Biserte, G., Jaillard, J., Bertrand, M. et Sezille, G., Etude comparée des cinétiques d'épuration plasmatique de deux émulsions lipidiques injectables chez l'homme et chez l'animal. *C.R. Soc. Biol. 160*: 1234 (1966).
23. Lemperle, G., Reichelt, M. and Denk, S., The evaluation of phagocytic activity in men by means of a lipid-clearing-test. Abstract from 6th International Meeting of the Reticuloendothelial Society, p. 83 (1970).
24. Dewailly, P., Trupin, N., Nouvelot, A., Fruchart, J. C., Jaillard, J. et Sezille, G., Etude métabolique de trois émulsions lipidiques utilisées dans l'alimentation parentérale. II. Etude par perfusion de foie de rat isolé. *Nutr. Metabol. 19*: 318 (1975).
25. Gigon, J. P., Enderlein, F. und Scheidegger, S., Über das Schicksal infundierter Fettemulsionen in der menschlichen Lunge. *Schweiz. Med. Wschr. 96*: 71 (1966).
26. Scholler, K. L., Transport und Speicherung von Fettemulsionteilchen. *Z. prakt. Anästh. Wiederbel. 3*: 193 (1968).
27. Huth, K. W., Schoenborn, W. und Börner, J., Zur Pathogenese der Unverträglichkeitserscheinungen bei parenteraler Fettzufuhr. *Med. Ernähr. 8*: 146 (1967).
28. Carpentier, Y., Delespesse, G. et Collett, H., Evolution des capacités immunologiques des patients sous nutrition parentérale. A propos de 20 cas. Abstract de Congrès International de Nutrition Parentérale, Montpellier, p. 48, Sept. 12-14 (1974).
29. Duckert, F. und Hartmann, G., Intravenöse Fettinfusion und Blutgerinnung. *Schweiz. Med. Wschr. 96*: 1205 (1966).
30. Hartmann, G., Fettemulsionen (Intralipid) in der inneren Medizin. *Wien. Med. Wschr. 117*: 51 (1967).
31. Cronberg, S. and Nilsson, I.-M., Coagulation studies after administration of a fat emulsion intralipid. *Thromb. Diath. Haemorrh. 18*: 364 (1967).
32. Kapp, J. P., Duckert, F. and Hartmann, G., Platelet adhesiveness and serum lipids during and after Intralipid (R) infusions. *Nutr. Metabol. 13*: 92 (1971).
33. Steinbereithner, K. und Wagner, O., Das Verhalten des arteriellen Sauerstoffdrucks nach intravenöser Fett- und Laevulosebelastung bei schweren Schädelverletzten. *Agressologie 8*: 389 (1967).
34. Greene, H., Hazlett, D., Demarre, R. and Dramesi, J., Effect of Intralipid on pulmonary function in normal humans and on electron microscopy of rabbit lung and liver. Abstracts of short communications presented at the IXth International Congress of Nutrition in Mexico City, p. 197, Sept. 3-9 (1972).
35. Sundström, G., Zauner, C. W. and Arborelius, M., Decrease in pulmonary diffusing capacity during lipid infusion in healthy men. *J. Appl. Phys. 34*: 816 (1973).
36. Dudrick, S. J., Wilmore, D. W., Vars, H. M. and Rhoads, J. E., Can intravenous feeding as the sole means of nutrition support growth in the child and restore weight loss in adult *Ann. Surg. 169*: 974 (1969).
37. Bernhoff, A., Negative inotropic effect of hyperosmotic infusion fluids. *Opusc. Med. 15*: 162 (1970).
38. Schärli, A., Praktische Gesichtspunkte bei der vollen parenteralen Ernährung. *Int. Z. Vitaminforsch. 35*: 52 (1965).
39. Abbott, W. E., Davies, J. H., Benson, J. W., Krieger, H. and Levey, S., Metabolic alterations in surgical patients. VI. The effect on weight and nitrogen balance of providing varying caloric intakes by intravenous carbohydrate, fat and amino acids in gastrectomized patients. *Surg. Forum 5*: 501 (1955).

40. Wadström, L. R. and Wiklund, P. E., Effect of fat emulsions on nitrogen balance in the postoperative period. *Acta Chir. Scand.* Suppl. *325*: 50 (1964).
41. Larsen, V. and Brôckner, J., Nitrogen balance and operative stress. Effect of early postoperative nutrition on nitrogen balance following major surgery. *Acta Chir. Scand.* Suppl. *343*: 191 (1965).
42. Hallberg, D., Schuberth, O. and Wretlind, A., Experimental and clinical studies with fat emulsion for intravenous nutrition. *Nutr. Dieta 8*: 254 (1966).
43. Reid, D. J., Intravenous fat therapy. II. Changes in oxygen consumption and respiratory quotient. *Brit. J. Surg. 54*: 204 (1967).
44. Jeejeebhoy, K. N., Andersson, G. H., Nakhooda, A. F., Greenberg, G. R., Sanderson, I. and Marliss, E. B., Metabolic studies in total parenteral nutrition with lipid in man. Comparison with glucose. *J. Clin. Invest. 57*: 125 (1976).
45. Gazzaniga, A. B., Bartlett, R. H. and Shobe, J. B., Nitrogen balance in patients receiving either fat or carbohydrate for total intravenous nutrition. *Ann. Surg. 182*: 163 (1975).
46. Brennan, M. F., Fitzpatrick, G. F., Cohen, K. H. and Moore, F. D., Glycerol: Major contributor to the short-term protein sparing effect of fat emulsions in normal man. *Ann. Surg. 182*: 386 (1975).
47. Long, J. M., Wilmore, D. W., Mason, A. D. and Pruitt, B. A., Fat carbohydrate interaction: Effects on nitrogen sparing in total intravenous feeding. *Surg. Forum 25*: 61 (1974).
48. Bark, S., Holm, I., Häkansson, I. and Wretlind, A., Nitrogen sparing effect of fat emulsion compared to glucose in the postoperative period. *Acta Chir. Scand.* To be published (1977).
49. Greenberg, G. R., Marliss, E. B., Anderson, G. H., Langer, B., Spence, W., Tovee, E. B. and Jeejeebhoy, K. N., Protein-sparing therapy in postoperative patients. Effects of added hypocaloric glucose or lipid. *New Engl. J. Med. 294*: 1411 (1976).
50. Geyer, R. P., Chipman, J. and Stare, F. J., Oxidation *in vivo* of emulsified radioactive trilaurin administered intravenously. *J. Biol. Chem. 176*: 1469 (1948).
51. Lerner, S. R., Chaikoff, I. L., Enteman, C. and Dauben, W. G., The fate of C^{14}-labelled palmatic acid administered intravenously as a tripalmitin emulsion. *Proc. Soc. exp. Biol. Med. 70*: 384 (1949).
52. Eckart, J., Tempel, G., Kaul, A. und Shürbrand, P., Untersuchungen zur Utilization parenteral verabfolgter Triglyceride nach Operationen und Traumen. *Infusionstherapie 2*: 138 (1973/74).
53. Lindmark, L. and Wretlind, A., Personal communication (1975).
54. Yokoyama, K., Okamoto, H., Tsuda, Y and Suyama, T., Metabolism of intravenously injected fat emulsion. Abstracts of Xth International Congress of nutrition in Kyoto, Japan, p. 226, August 3-9 (1975).
55. Peaston, M. J. T., Design of an intravenous diet of amino acids and fat suitable for intensive patient-care. *Brit. Med. J. 2*: 388 (1966).
56. Peaston, M. J. T., Maintenance of metabolism during intensive patient-care. *Postgrad. Med. J. 43*: 41 (1967).
57. Stell, P. M., Esophageal replacement by transposed stomach. *Arch. Otolaryng. 91*: 166 (1970).
58. Bergström, K., Blomstrand, R. and Jacobson, S., Long-term complete intravenous nutrition in man. *Nutr. Metabol.* Suppl. *14*: 118 (1972).
59. Steinbereithner, K., Problems of artificial alimentation in an intensive therapy unit. (Possibilities and limitations). In: Evans, F. T. and Gray, T. (eds.), Chapter 11, Modern Trends in Anaesthesia. Butterworths, London (1966).
60. Allen, P. C. and Lee, H. A., A clinical guide to intravenous nutrition. Blackwell, Oxford (1969).

61. Deitel, M. and Kaminsky, V., Total nutrition by peripheral vein – the lipid system. *CMA Journal III*: 152 (1974).
62. Rickham, P. P., Massive small intestinal resection in newborn infants. Hungarian lecture delivered at the Royal College of Surgeons of England. *Ann. Roy. Coll. Surg. Engl. 41*: 480 (1967).
63. Børresen, H. C. and Knutrud, O., Parenteral feeding of neonates undergoing major surgery. *Acta Paediatr. Scand. 59*: 420 (1969).
64. Børresen, H. C., Coran, A. G. and Knutrud, O., Postoperative parenteral ernaering av nyfôdte. *Nord. Med. 85*: 1089 (1970).
65. Børresen, H. C., Coran, A. G. and Knutrud, O., parenteral feeding of newborns undergoing major surgery. In: Berg, G. (ed.), Advances in Parenteral Nutrition. Symposium of the International Society of Parenteral Nutrition, Prague, Sept 3-4, 1969. G. Thieme Verlag, Stuttgart, p. 93 (1970).
66. Grotte, G., Nutrition parentérale du nourrisson. In: Nahas, G.-G. et Viars, P. (eds.), Les Solutés de Substitution et Rééquilibration Métabolique. Librairie Arnette, Paris, p. 509 (1971).
67. Grotte, G., Esscher, T., Hambraeus, L. and Meurling, S., Total Parenteral Nutrition in pediatric surgery. In: Proceedings Meeting, Vancouver, published by Pharmacia (Canada) Ltd., 2044 St.Regis Blvd., Dorval, Quebec, p. 140 (1974).
68. Meng, H. C. and Early, F., Study of complete parenteral alimentation on dogs. *J. Lab. Clin. Med. 34*: 1121 (1949).
69. Pensler, L., Whitten, C., Paulsrud, J. and Holman, R. T., A study of fat metabolism during fat-free IV therapy. American Pediatric Society and Society for Pediatric Research. Abstracts, p. 1677 (1970).
70. Caldwell, M. D., Meng, H. C. and Jonsson, H. T., Essential fatty acids deficiency (EFAD) – Now a human disease. *Fed. Am. Soc. exptl. Bipl.* 57th Annual Meeting, N.J., No. 3913, April 15-20 (1973).
71. Paulsrud, J. R., Pensler, L., Whitten, C. F., Stewart, S. and Holman, R. T., Essential fatty acid deficiency in infants induced by fat free intravenous feeding. *Amer. J. Clin. Nutr. 25*: 897 (1972).
72. Collins, F. D., Sinclair, A. J., Boyle, J. P., Coats, D. A., Maynard, A. Y. and Leonard, R. F., Plasma lipids in human linoleic acid deficiency. *Nutr. Metabol. 13*: 150 (1971).
73. Jeejeebhoy, K. N., Zohrab, W. J., Langer, B., Phillips, M. J., Kuksis, A. and Andersson, G. H., Total parenteral nutrition at home for 23 months without complication and with good rehabilitation. *Gastroenterology 65*: 811 (1973).
74. Buchner, H. und Cesnik, H., Erfahrungen über parenterale Fettzufuhr bei schwer Verletzten. *Med. Klin. 57*: 1482 (1962).
75. Østergaard, J., Parenteral nutrition of operated patients. *Nutr. Dieta 5*: 408 (1963).
76. Schuberth, O., Klinische Erfahrungen mit Fettemulsionen für intravenöse Anwendung. *Berliner Med. 14*: 235 (1963).
77. Freuchen, I., Intravenous fat emulsion. *Nutr. Dieta 5*: 403 (1963).
78. Jones, E., Robinson, J. S. and McConn, R., Maintenance of metabolism during intensive patient care. Parenteral Nutrition Colloquium. Lowe and Brydone Printers, Ltd., London, p. 32 (1964).
79. Schärli, A., Beitrag zur parenteralen Ernährung bei chirurgisch Kranken. *Praxis 53*: 1215 (1964).
80. Lawson, L. J., Parenteral nutrition in surgery. *Brit. J. Surg. 52*: 795 (1965).
81. Lee, H. A. and Shortle, W. P. J., Parenteral nutrition. *King's Coll. Hosp. Gaz. 44*: 192 (1965).
82. Hadfield, J. I. H., High calorie intravenous feeding in surgical patients. *Clin. Med. 73*: 25 (1966).

83. Freuchen, I. und Østergaard, J., Die parenterale Ernährung von Operationspatienten. *Wien. Med. Wschr. 117*: 49 (1967).
84. Vlaardingerbroek, V. M., Experiences with intravenous nourishment. *Nederlands Tijdschr. Geneeskd. 111*: 415 (1967).
85. Hartmann, G., Fettemulsionen (Intralipid) in der inneren Medizin. *Wien. Med. Wschr. 117*: 51 (1967).
86. Feischl, P. und Hiotakis, K., Vollständige parenterale Ernährung bei schwerem Tetanus. *Med. Klin. 64*: 2296 (1969).
87. Liljedahl, S.-O., Burn treatment at Karolinska hospital in Stockholm. *Opusc. Med. 15*: 179 (1970).
88. Jacobson, S., Long-term parenteral nutrition following massive intestinal resection. *Nutr. Metabol. 14*: 150 (1972).
89. Zumtobel, V. und Zehle, A., Postoperative parenterale Ernährung mit Fettemulsionen bei Patienten mit Leberschäden. *Langenbeck's Arch. klin. Chir.* Suppl. *Chir. Forum*, p. 179 (1972).
90. Geremy, F., Nguyen-Huy-Dung et Deligné, P., Etude par bilans azotés en periode catabolique post-operatoire d'une nouvelle solution de l-amino-acids (V 15 001 ou Vamin). *Ann. Anésth. Franc. 12*: 583 (1972).
91. Kessler, E., Hyperalimentation in the management of gastrointestinal cutaneous fistulae. *South Afr. J. Surg. 12*: 101 (1974).
92. Hallberg, D., Holm, I., Obel, A.-L., Schuberth, O. and Wretlind, A., Fat emulsion for complete intravenous nutrition. *Postgrad. Med.42*: A71, A87, A99, A149 (1967).
93. Jacobson, S., Ericsson, J. and Obel, A.-L., Histopathological and ultrastructural changes in the human liver during complete intravenous nutrition for seven months. *Acta Chir. Scand. 137*: 335 (1971).
94. Yeo, M. T., Gazzaniga, A. B., Bartlett, R. H., Shobe, J. B. and Irvine, R. N., Total intravenous nutrition. Experience with fat emulsions and hypertonic glucose. *Arch. Surg. 106*: 792 (1973).
95. Coran, A. G., The intravenous use of fat for the total parenteral nutrition of the infant. *Lipids 7*: 455 (1972).
96. Caldwell, M. D., Jonsson, H. T. and Othersen, H. B., Essential fatty acid deficiency in an infant receiving prolonged parenteral alimentation. *J. Ped. 81*: 894 (1972).
97. Heird, W. C., Driscoll, J. M., Jr., Schullinger, J. N., Grebin, B. and Winters, R. W., Intravenous alimentation in pediatric patients. *J. Ped. 80*: 351 (1972).
98. Wei, P., Hamilton, J. R. and LeBlanc, A. E., A clinical and metabolic study of an intravenous feeding technique using peripheral veins as the initial infusion site. *CMA Journal, 106*: 969 (1972).
99. Børresen, H. C., Balanced intravenous nutrition in pediatric surgery. *Nutr. Metabol.* Suppl. *14*: 114 (1972).
100. Coran, A. G., Total intravenous feeding of infants and children without the use of a central venous catheter. *Ann. Surg. 179*: 445 (1974).
101. Pendray, M. R., Peripheral vein feeding in infants: Technique, results and problems. Proceeding Meeting Vancouver, published by Pharmacia (Canada) Ltd., 2044 St. Regis Blvd., Dorval, Quebec, p. 158 (1974).
102. Puri, P., Guiney, E. J. and O'Donnell, B., Total parenteral feeding in infants using peripheral veins. *Arch. Dis. Childh. 50*: 133 (1975).
103. Schärli, A. und Rumlova, E., Parenterale Ernährung in der Kinderchirurgie. Ergebnisse von Bilanzuntersuchungen. *Infusionstherapie 2*: 51 (1975).
104. Schmidtsdorf, G., Aspekte der parenteralen Ernährung. *Zbl. Chir. 97*: 11 (1972).
105. Lemperle, G. und Reichelt, M., Der Lipofundin-Clearance-Test. *Med. Klin. 68*: 48 (1973).
106. Voss, U. und Schnell, J., Parenterale Ernährung mit einer aminosäurehaltigen Fett-

emulsion im Tierversuch. In: Berg, G. (ed.), Advances in Parenteral Nutrition. G. Thieme Verlag, Stuttgart, p. 117 (1970).
107. Witzel, L., Berg, G., Grabner, W. und Bergner, D., Parenterale Ernährung mit eine kombinierten Fett-Kohlenhydrat-Aminosäurelösung. *Med. Ernähr. 11*: 177 (1970).
108. Rudolph, P., Brackwede, M., Bartoscheck, H. D. und Weis, K.-H., Die kombinierte Anwendung verschieden zusammengesetzter Nährlösungen in der Intensivmedizin. *Infusionsthérapie 4*: 287 (1973/74).
109. Cailar, J., Crastes de Paulet, A.. Bornier, B. M., Crastes de Paulet, Mme, Kieulen, J. et Becker, H., L'EB 51 (Trivemil) nutriment complet pour l'alimentation parentérale. *Ann. Anésth. Franç. Spécial II*: 103 (1974).
110. Weiss, Y. and Nissan, S., A method for reducing the incidence of infusion phlebitis. *Surg. Gynecol. Obstet. 141*: 73 (1975).
111. Horisberger, B., Severe pulmonary and cerebral circulation disturbances after high doses of parenterally supplied fat emulsions. A case of extraordinary therapeutic complication. *Schweiz. Med. Wschr. 96*: 1065 (1966).
112. Depisch, D., Bedrohliche Hyperlipämie im Rahmen eines allergischen Schocks bei parenteraler Ernährung einer Tetanuspatientin. *Anaesthesist 20*: 437 (1971).
113. Chaptal, J., Jean, R., Crastes de Paulet, A., Guillaumont, R., Morel, G. et Maurin, A., Apports énergétiques et azotés au cours du traitement des états de déshydration aiguë du nourrisson. *Rev. Pract. 14*: 199 (1964).
114. Chaptal, J., Jean, R., Crastes de Paulet, A., Guillaumont, R., Crastes de Paulet, P., Maurin-Belay, B. et Morel, G., Etude sur l'alimentation parentérale lipiqidue et azotée chez l'enfant et chez le nourrisson déshydraté. *Ann. Péd. 11*: 441 (1964).
115. Hanc, I., Klezkowska, H. and Rodkiewicz, B., On intravenous infusions of fat emulsions in pediatric surgery. *Ped. Polska 43*: 1355 (1968).
116. Krediet, R. T. en De Gens, A., Parenchymateuze icterus en thrombocytopenie na langdurige behandeling met een intraveneuze vetemulsie (Intralipid). *Ned. T. Geneeskd. 119*: 1766 (1975).
117. Michel, H., Raynaud, A., Crastes de Paulet, Mme, Nalet, B., Orsetti, A. et Bertrand, L., Tolérance du cirrhotique aux lipides intra-veineux. Congrès International de Nutrition Parentérale. Montpellier, Sept. 12-14 (1974).
118. Freund, U., Krausz, Y., Levy, I. S. and Eliakim, M., Iatrogenic lipidosis following prolonged intravenous hyperalimentation. *Am. J. Clin. Nutr. 28*: 1156 (1975).

Amino acid infusion after surgical injury

George L. Blackburn, M.D., Ph.D./ Hugh Rienhoff, B.A./ John D. B. Miller, M.B., F.R.C.S., Ed./ Bruce R. Bistrian, M.D., Ph.D./ Jean Pierre Flatt, Ph.D./ Baltej S. Maini, M.D.

INTRODUCTION

After injury, the body concerns itself with regaining and preserving its integrity. There is an immediate immunologic response to meet entering pathogens; hemostasis is achieved and the healing process begins. Fundamental to the fight for integrity is the conservation of all of those tissues that contribute to this effort. The preservation of the body cell mass depends upon an adequate source of nutrition, primarily a source of amino acids and energy.

The body's response to any environmental stimulus or insult is conditional upon the nutritional state. It has been repeatedly demonstrated that any form of stress aggravates underlying protein deficiencies. In designing optimal nutritional therapy to deal with stress, the nutritional history is as important a consideration as the present anabolic needs. When protein reserves are depleted or allowed to be, the effects of stress and protein deficiencies are seen more readily and sooner.

FUNCTIONAL REDISTRIBUTION OF NITROGEN

The preservation of the body cell mass during injury related stress is difficult to accomplish. Dietary protein intake is usually diminished owing to anorexia. Also the uptake and utilization of dietary protein in the bowel is less efficient. The nitrogen necessary for synthesis is provided by tissues whose function is dispensable during periods of stress; muscle makes the greatest contribution. This is the basis for the concept of the functional redistribution of protein (Figure 1).

The amount of protein synthesized each day in a normal 70 kg man has been estimated at 385-425 gms using the N^{15} labelled amino acid isotope technique (1). This rate requires five to six times the recommended daily allowances (0.89 gms per kg per day) of a protein of high biologic value. This implies an extensive reutilization – approximately 80% – of amino acid released after cellular catabolism. In injury this reutilization is considerably diminished, causing dietary protein requirements to go up (2).

A mechanism has evolved by which intrinsic nitrogen is mobilized and used by those tissues that are directly involved in the healing and defense of the body. Muscle represents the largest reservoir of protein for such use. 39% of total body protein is contained in these tissues. The sarcoplasm, owing to its shorter half-life makes a greater contribution to the free amino acid pool than do the more stable structural proteins of muscle, myosin and actin. The digestive tract is another source of nitrogen. Containing 11% of the body protein, it synthesizes over 50 gms of protein each day. During diet-free periods, these tissues are in a state of net catabolism; thus making a significant contribution of amino acids during periods of stress. Integumental tissue is relatively inert except during injury. Increased hydroxyproline losses indicate net catabolism of this tissue which provides precur-

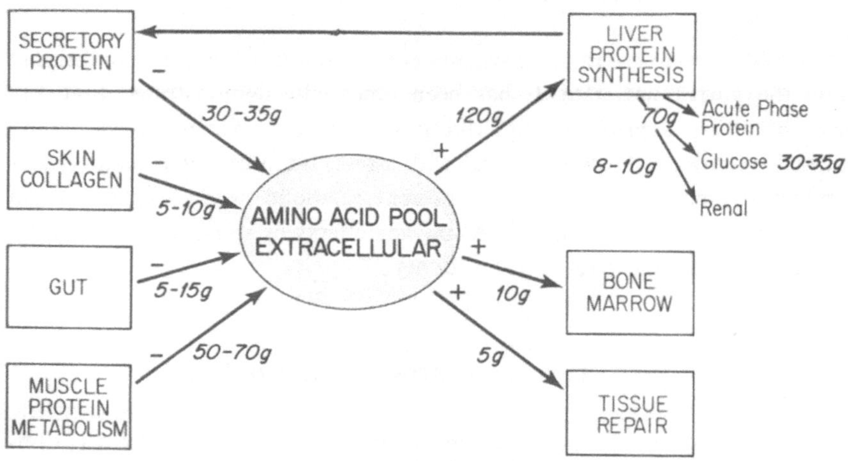

Figure 1. Functional redistribution of body cell mass. The manifold requirements for new proteins during injury require redistribution of body cell mass. This is accomplished by a decrease in circulatory amino acid concentrations creating net protein catabolism (protein synthesis protein catabolism) in muscle, skin, digestive tract, and certain secretory proteins (e.g. albumin). A concomitant 2-3 fold increase in protein synthesis of acute phase protein and visceral tissue enzymes occurs. Leukocytic activity, red cell production,wound healing and immune protein synthesis all require a larger share of amino acids than normal. Finally, increased rates of gluconeogenesis are observed, in part secondary to an increase in amino acid precursors (alanine and glutamine).

sors needed for wound healing. These aforementioned tissues provide the majority of endogenous nitrogen. Brain, kidney, heart, and lung remain in steady state; they neither contribute nor extract an unusual amount of amino acids from the free pool (1).

On the other hand, the liver which contains less than 5% of the total body protein synthesizes up to 20% of the total amount of protein made each day: over 30 gms of plasma proteins including albumin, fibrinogen, alpha and beta globulins, and transferrin. The tissue itself has a high rate of turnover – 7 to 8 days – and places greater demands for amino acids in stress. Bone marrow and leukocyte synthesis also require a constant supply of amino acids.

The metabolism of muscle is unique among protein tissues in the manner in which it reacts to injury. Muscle consumes only the branched-chain amino acids (BCAA) when alternative fuels are not available (3). Muscle protein catabolized *in situ* for energy results in the release of the remaining

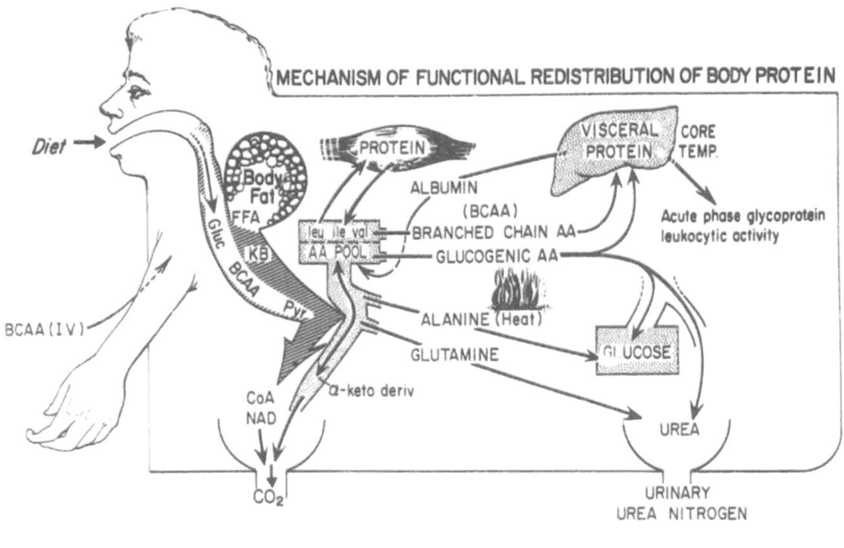

Figure 2. Mechanism of muscle proteolysis during illness. The rate of net amino acid release from muscle is controlled by oxidation of branched chain amino acid (BCAA) to ATP, CO_2, H_2O, (CO_ANAD). The consequence is redistribution of body cell mass and a substantial production of alanine and glutamine. The resulting work of gluconeogenesis produces heat to preserve core temperature as well as to produce hyperglycemia.

Effective nutritional support to reduce this proteolysis requires the provision of alternative keto-acids such as ketone body or dietary BCAA. This mechanism which is initiated by changes in muscle metabolism is key to the role protein metabolism plays in host survival. The capacity to produce adequate flux of muscle protein (i.e. nutritional status) significantly affects morbidity and mortality during infection.

amino acids that cannot be oxidized by muscle (4). The quantity and fate of these amino acids is largely dependent upon nutritional therapy. In injury there is an increase in the consumption of branched-chain amino acids as well as the release of them by muscle. By providing glucose exogenously, muscle is forced to rely on branched-chain amino acids and glucose; ketone bodies and free fatty acids are not available because of the antilypolytic, antiketogenic nature of insulin. Free amino acids including the branched-chain amino acids are either converted to C_3 fragments and then to glucose in the liver, or are used for visceral protein synthesis according to the local demands (5).

It is clear that the metabolic environment in the muscle compartment is the factor that determines how much amino acid is released from muscle and how and where it is used. Up to 120 gms of amino acids are liberated from muscle if the nutritional support provided takes advantage of this mechanism that adapts the body to the stresses of injury (Figure 2). A study was designed to test two therapies – 3.5% crystalline amino acids vs. 5% dextrose in water – to see which favored a more rapid recovery from injury (5).

CLINICAL STUDY

A combination of dextrose and amino acids is not feasible, primarily because the osmolality of such a solution is not tolerated by a peripheral vein. Even a well buffered solution, which dextrose is not, cannot be tolerated easily if the osmolality exceeds 600 mOsm. For a one liter peripheral solution, 100 mM are in the form of mineral and electrolytes including potassium, phosphate, sodium, chloride, calcium, and magnesium. To meet nitrogen requirements, 3.5% amino acid solution will provide enough nitrogen to minimize amino acid oxidation. This adds 350 mOsm. This would allow for the addition of 25 gms of glucose, an amount that has been shown to be ineffective in surgical patients and others for stress producing carbohydrate intolerance and insulin resistance (6).

A prospective randomized group of 20 patients were divided evenly into two groups, one receiving a 3.5% amino acid solution, the other receiving 5% dextrose solution. Each solution contained the electrolytes determined by the needs of individual patients. Only adult patients undergoing routine elective operations for pancreatic, biliary, inflammatory bowel, liver or colon conditions requiring intravenous fluid replacement for 6-10 days were considered for the study. No patients who were classified as severely depleted nutritionally according to the accepted parameters of nutritional status were considered, nor were any severely hypermetabolic patients as measured by urea nitrogen excretion in 24 hours accepted. Patients with diabetes mellitus, heart failure, renal failure, liver failure, shock, or any other disease causing gross alterations in metabolism and body chemistry were excluded (7).

Each patient received 3 liters of solution with electrolyte, vitamin, and mineral requirements as tolerated within fluid requirements (Figure 3). Additional fluid requirements were met with a balanced electrolyte solution. Routine laboratory tests were performed on the first day and every second day thereafter. These included serum electrolytes, liver function tests including albumin, and renal function tests. In addition, serum insulin, free fatty acids, ketone bodies, and glucose levels were measured every other day. The urine was collected every 24 hours and analyzed for creatinine, urea nitrogen, and electrolytes. The presence or absence of ketones and glucose was determined several times a day on the wards. Finally, those parameters of nutritional status – transferrin, delayed hypersensitivity skin tests, and anthropometrics – were determined and recorded before and at the end of the study.

The results of the study were conclusive: those patients receiving the solution of amino acids had a better nitrogen balance than those receiving the glucose solution (Figure 4). Initially, the average losses were similar (10.7 ± 4.3 vs. 8.5 ± 0.4 gms), the amino acid group being the latter and receiving only 1 liter of 3.5% solution that day. However, by the sixth day

---

Daily Additives
30-45 mEq/day potassium monophosphate
75-100 mEq/day sodium cloride
9.0 mEq/day calcium gluconate
8.0 mEq/day magnesium sulfate
1 ampoule B complex vitamins
40-60 potassium chloride
(as indicated) sodium acetate

Weekly Additives
1 amp multivitamins (including vitamin A and D)
1 mg folic acid
100 μg vitamin B_{12}
10 mg vitamin K

Figure 3.

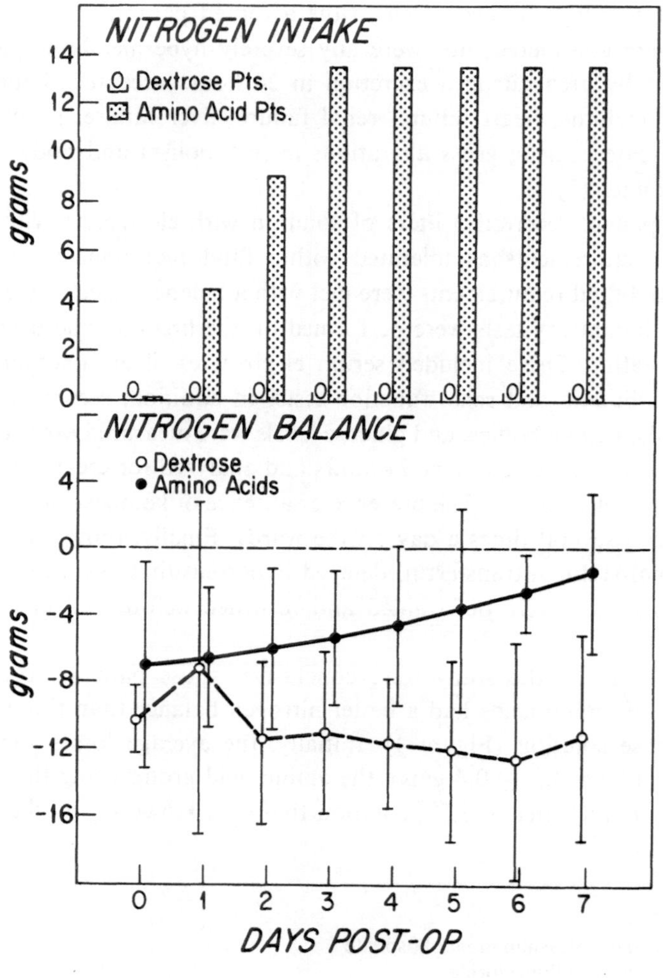

Figure 4. Nitrogen intake and nitrogen balance for study patients. Nitrogen balance in the amino acid group is significantly improved compared to patients receiving dextrose post-operatively. The amino acid group received less than 4.5 grams of nitrogen on day 1. This amount was increased approximately 5 gms per day until day 3.

the losses were significantly ($p < .001$) different (12.3 g $\pm$ 2.7 vs. 3.8 $\pm$ 1.0 g); again the amino acid group receiving 3 liters of solution on this day, represented by the latter figure. No patients in the dextrose group developed ketonuria. In the dextrose-free group, urinary ketones were manifested between days 1 and 3. In no case did these ketonuric patients revert to a negative test for urinary ketones. In the dextrose patients, plasma glucose levels diminished from an average high of 146 mg/day on the first day, to 129 mg/day where they remained for the course of therapy. In the dextrose-free patients, glucose levels steadily declined from 127 on the first day to 83 on the fourth day, where they remained. The FFA levels in the dextrose patients did not change significantly, remaining at 530 mM. The ketone bodies in the same patients were constantly depressed, ranging from .01 to .05 mM. The energy substrate profile for the amino acid group was quite different. The FFA levels on day 0 were comparable to the dextrose group but were significantly ($p < .001$) higher on the last day at 1133 $\pm$ 51 mM. This was also the situation for ketone bodies. On day 0, ketones were significantly highest ($p < .005$) at a level of .43 mM. The last day showed a greater difference ($p < .001$) with ketone levels at 1.74 mM. Insulin levels tended to parallel serum glucose concentrations. In the dextrose group, insulin values declined from 54 to 28. In the other group, the values progressed from 41 to 15. Only the day 0 values were not significantly different.

DISCUSSION OF RESULTS

The surgical patient is at considerable risk of developing visceral protein attrition and its attendant complications (2). Predisposing factors include the stress of operation, the need to rely on intravenous support in the early postoperative period, as well as the potential postoperative complications such as infection. All of these stresses compound protein deficiencies, a condition which is often pre-existent. It can be argued on the basis of this and other studies that while neither regimens affected the initial catabolic response associated with trauma, infused amino acids encouraged a greater rate of protein synthesis in the convalescent phase (8).

O'Keefe has shown that the rate of protein catabolism is roughly equivalent before and after trauma (9). The difference is in the rate of synthesis. The rate limiting factor in the production of protein is the availability of amino acids. If they are not supplied exogenously, there are simply fewer amino acids available for anabolism. Skillman (10) has conclusive evidence that the synthesis of albumin proceeds at a greater rate when amino acid solutions are administered rather than the usual dextrose. This study emphasized an important difference between glucose and amino acid therapy: the latter supports the viscera while the former supports some other tissue, mainly muscle.

Cellular Immunity

The major cause for the impairment of cellular immunity is inadequate nutrients to allow the anabolic blast transformation necessary for immune function. Thus when lymphocytes are exposed to an antigen challenge, such as during cutaneous delayed hypersensitivity tests using candida antigen, function appears depressed or absent. This condition is most frequently seen in marasmic patients, who at less than 85% of ideal weight, have recently experienced at least a 5 pound weight loss while on a diet with inadequate amounts of protein.

When these lymphocytes are evaluated by *in vitro* tests, which utilize nutrient-rich media, they appear to function normally. The exception is in advanced malnutrition (less than 60% of ideal body weight), particularly in patients demonstrating decreased synthesis of secretory proteins such as albumin. In any event, depressed or absent cell-mediated immunity represents an advanced stage of malnutrition making nutritional support mandatory.

AMINO ACIDS: THE METABOLIC RATIONALE

The infusion of dextrose postoperatively has been justified by the data originating with Gamble (11) who shows it to be nitrogen-sparing. The rationale was that dextrose stimulated the release of insulin which in turn enhanced amino acid uptake and protein synthesis while reducing protein degradation; protein loss, from muscle tissue especially, was less. When given in amounts ranging from 100 to 150 gms a day, dextrose appeared to have the extra advantage of preventing ketosis, the sign of starvation. Insulin resistance, catabolic hormones and gluconeogenesis were given as the cause for nitrogen loss in spite of carbohydrate administration.

The administration of carbohydrate counteracts the catabolic response to injury in muscle tissue, but at the expense of depleting the visceral compartment (12) (Figure 1, 2). Visceral attrition, a quasi-Kwashiorkor state, is frequently observed in patients receiving intravenous glucose. It is documented by hypoalbuminemia, impairment of cellular immunity, and depressed leukocyte counts. All of these conditions are a consequence of glucose administration in hypocaloric amounts. The optimal therapy would be one which harmonizes with the metabolic response to illness. Dextrose is proteinsparing but because of the profound effect it has on BCAA uptake in muscle, that tissue will be preserved. The resulting high insulin level reduces fat mobilization thus depriving the body of natural and efficient source of fuel. Ketone bodies, which can be used by the brain and other vital tissue in the absence of glucose, are produced in insignificant amounts when insulin and glucose levels are high. The hyperglycemia that normally occurs after injury further increases insulin concentration, promoting the storage of fat, an unnecessary process which increases the energy requirements of the body. Further carbohydrate administration increases blood glucose due to insulin resistance during infection.

Ketonemia indicates the successful adaptation to starvation. It is important that ketonemia occur, the manifestation of endogenous fat use, and hence an adequate supply of energy. In the event that ketonemia does not occur, carbohydrate calories are necessary if energy requirements are to be met.

The positive nitrogen balance indicates an overall prevalence of synthesis of protein because there is no storage of inactive nitrogen compounds. Nitrogen balance has its limitations in failing to reflect the exchange of nitrogen between tissues, particularly between muscle and visceral tissue, as

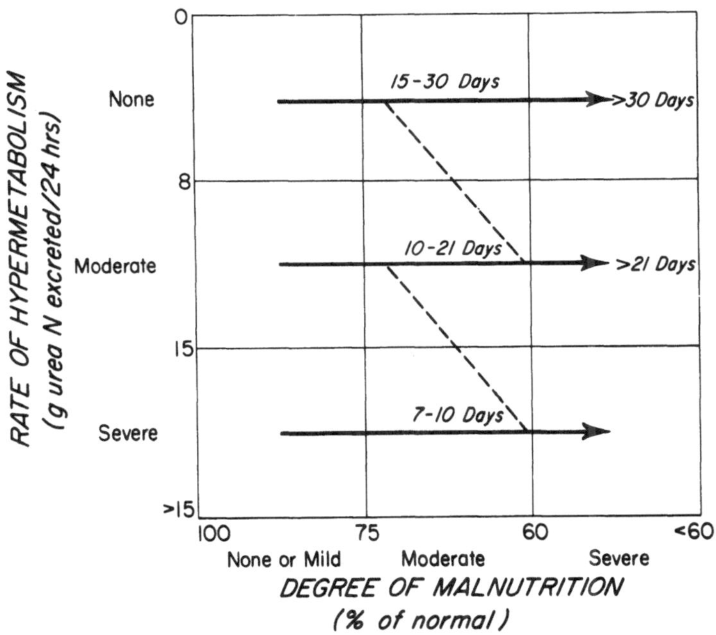

Figure 5. Dynamics of nutritional depletion. This shows schematically the dynamics of nutritional depletion in patients on regimes that induce a state of semi-starvation. The two variables, rate of hypermetabolism, and degree of malnutrition, determine the development of malnutrition and its attendant conditions.

well as in failing to reflect the rate of turnover in any given tissue (5); net protein synthesis can occur in one tissue while net catabolism occurs in another. Nitrogen balance does have its use in determining nitrogen requirements, the overall nitrogen economy, and the degree of catabolism.

NUTRITIONAL THERAPY

Figure 5 shows schematically* the dynamics of nutritional depletion in patients on regimes that induce a state of semi-starvation. Such regimes are invariably protein deficient, e.g. D_5W, fruit juice, gelatin, pudding. The two variables, rate of hypermetabolism, and degree of malnutrition, deter-

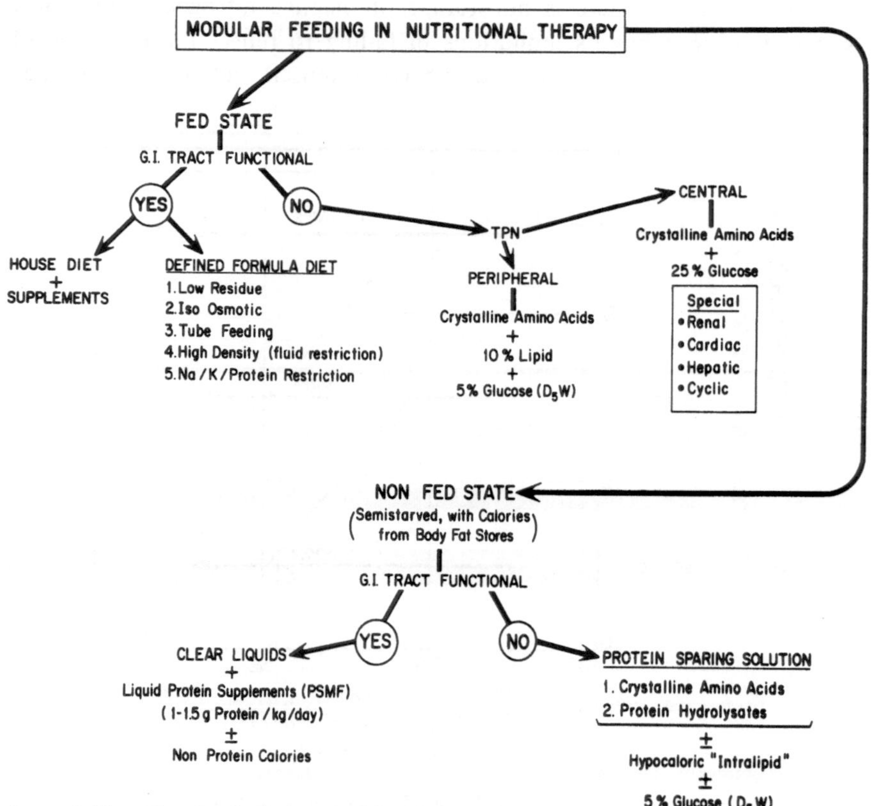

Figure 6. Algorithm for designing nutritional support.

* Model after S. S. Dudrick.

mine the development of malnutrition and its attendant conditions (2). Those patients not burdened by fever, sepsis, multiple trauma, or burns will lose body protein at a fairly constant rate. The presence of any combination of these clinical conditions considerably aggravates the loss of body protein which progresses exponentially. Weight loss may or may not confirm those changes; so other biochemical and immune function parameters such as nitrogen balance and skin testing are required.

The goal of nutritional support therapy for the injured patient is the maintenance of normal organ function which assures immune defense leukocytic activity and the synthesis of proteins. In designing such therapies, the first consideration is whether the patient should be in the semi-starved or fed state. The second consideration is whether the GI tract is functional. In postoperative patients who have adequate fat reserves but who don't

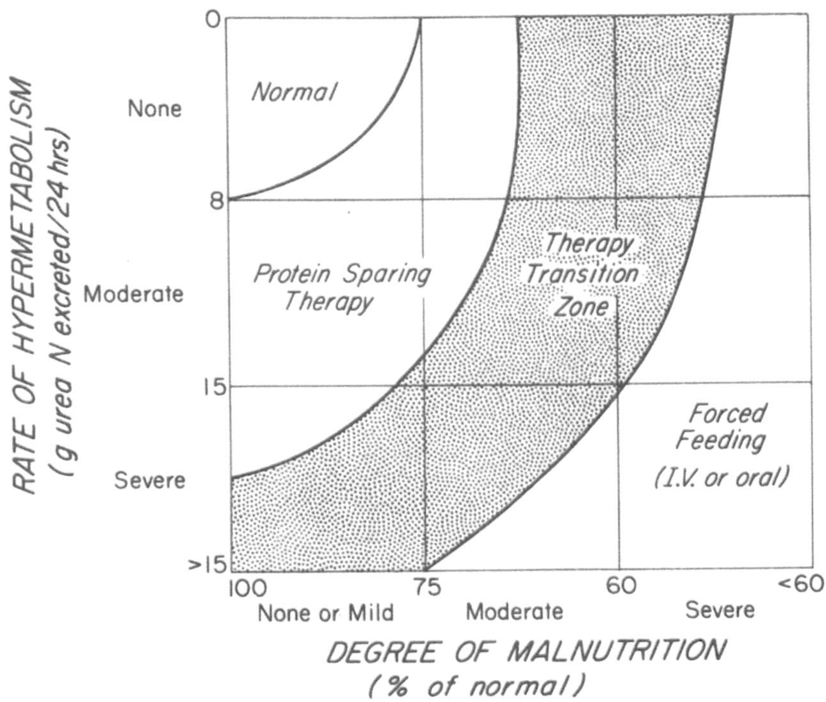

Figure 7. Indications for nutritional support. Protein-sparing therapy using amino acids alone is effective nutritional support when patients are moderately depleted and hypermetabolic. When patients begin to approach either severe categories, forced feeding becomes necessary to meet the energy and nitrogen needs.

have the use of their GI tract, crystalline amino acid solution is indicated. This algorithm for designing nutritional support therapy is diagrammatically illustrated in Figure 6. Figure 7 represents the superimposition of the two preceding figures, the algorithm and the matrix. Protein-sparing therapy using amino acids alone is effective nutritional support when patients are moderately depleted and hypermetabolic. When patients begin to approach either severe categories, forced feeding becomes necessary to meet the energy and nitrogen needs (13).

SUMMARY

The functional redistribution of body protein, primarily muscle, is a mechanism that has evolved for the purpose of meeting nitrogen needs crucial to survival in the face of diminished dietary intake. Muscle consumes branched-chain amino acids, ketone bodies and free fatty acids to meet the demands for energy. Those amino acids not oxidized by muscle are available for protein synthesis elsewhere particularly the viscera where the demand is the greatest and most crucial. This is the natural metabolic response to injury. The administration of glucose interferes with this response; insulin levels rise forcing amino acids to be used as fuel rather than for anabolism. Dextrose does spare protein tissue, but a distinction must be made as to which tissue: muscle in the case of glucose administration; viscera in the case of amino acid infusion. The use of glucose therapeutically should be limited to those patients who are unable to meet their energy needs with endogenous stores. Otherwise its use exaggerates the stress of injury and prolongs morbidity.

REFERENCES

1. Wannamacher, R. W., Jr., Protein metabolism. In: *Total Parenteral Nutrition: Premises and Promises*. H. Ghadimi (ed.). New York: John Wiley and Sons, p. 85 (1975).
2. Blackburn, G. L. and Bistrian, B. R., Nutritional care of the injured and/or septic patient. G. H. A. Clowes, Jr. (ed), *Surgical Clinics of North America 56*: 1195-1224 (1976).
3. Benotti, P. N., Balckburn, G. L., Miller, J. D. B., Bistrian, B. R., Flatt, J. P. and Trerice, M., Role of branched-chain amino acid (BCAA) intake in preventing muscle proteolysis. *Surgical Forum 27*: 7 (1976).
4. O'Donnell, T. F., Jr., Clowes, G. H. A., Jr. and Blackburn, G. L., et al., Proteolysis associated with a deficit of peripheral energy fuel substrates in septic man. *Surgery 80*: 192-199 (1976).
5. Blackburn, G. L., Nitrogen metabolism after surgical injury. In: Physiology in Medicine. *New England Journal of Medicine* (in press) (1977).
6. Blackburn, G. L., Flatt, J. P. and Heddle, T. E., Peripheral amino acid infusions. In: *Total Parenteral Nutrition*. J. Fischer (ed.), Ch. 19, pp. 363-394. Boston: Little, Brown and Company (1976).
7. Miller, J. D. B., Bistrian, B. R., Blackburn, G. L., Flatt, J. P.. Rienhoff, H. Y., Jr. and Trerice, M., Failure of postoperative infection to increase nitrogen excretion in patients maintained on peripheral amino acids. *Am. J. Clin. Nutrition* (in press) (1977).
8. Bristian, B. R., Winterer, J. C., Blackburn, G. L. and Scrimshaw, N. S., Failure of

yellow fever immunization to produce a catabolic response in individuals fully adapted to a protein-sparing modified fast. *Am. J. Clin. Nutr.* (in press) (1977).
9. O'Keefe, S. J. D., Sender, P. M., Clark, G. C. and James, W. P. T., The effect of varying the postoperative parenteral regime on the dynamics of protein metabolism following operative trauma. Proceedings of the International Congress of Parenteral Nutrition, Université de Montpellier, p. 333 (1976).
10. Skillman, J. J., Rosenoer, V. M., Smith, P. C. and Fang, M. S., Improved albumin synthesis in postoperative patients by amino acid infusion. *New. Engl. J. Med. 295*: 1037 (1976).
11. Gamble, J. L., Physiologic information gained from studies on the life raft ration. *Harvey Lectures 42*: 247 (1946).
12. Felig, P., Intravenous Nutrition: Fact and Fancy (Editorial). *New Engl. J. Med. 294*: 1455 (1976).
13. Blackburn, G. L. and Bistrian, B. R., Protein-calorie curative therapy. In: *Nutritional Support of Medical Practice.* H. Schneider (ed.), Ch. 6. New York: Harper and Row (1976).

Relationship of energy and protein input to nitrogen retention and substratehormone profile

K. N. Jeejeebhoy

INTRODUCTION

Total parenteral nutrition (TPN) has been invaluable in providing nutrients and aiding the restoration of body mass in patients with serious gastrointestinal diseases and malnutrition. A major metabolic objective in such patients is to conserve or augment the lean body mass. Since the basic structural constituent of lean tissue is protein, it is clear that the retention and efficient utilization of amino acids for protein synthesis is central to a successful programme of TPN.

In animal studies it is recognized that both non-protein calories and amino acids aid nitrogen retention (1) and by inference this suggests that these two factors are likely to promote protein synthesis.

In human subjects, it has been known for some time that giving hypocaloric glucose (i.e. calories insufficient to meet energy requirements) will reduce nitrogen loss from the body or spare nitrogen (2). Thus for many years post-operative patients were given daily 2 litres of 5% glucose in water (i.e. 100 gm glucose) in the belief that such an infusion would spare nitrogen – which it does, up to a point. More recently Blackburn et al (3). have suggested that when the total calories infused were insufficient to meet the needs of the patient, the infusion of amino acid was preferable to that of glucose. They also felt that in the hypocaloric state a substrate-hormone profile consistent with fat mobilization (high plasma free fatty acids and ketones) would aid nitrogen retention (3). In this context it was felt that under certain circumstances infusing glucose might reduce nitrogen retention by inhibiting mobilization of fat. Hence the questions raised during hypocaloric infusions were first whether amino acids were essential to nitrogen-sparing and secondly whether a specific substrate-hormone profile was especially important in promoting nitrogen retention in the hypocaloric state.

In contrast to the hypocaloric situation most systems of TPN provide calories in excess of the requirements. The technique used in the USA has

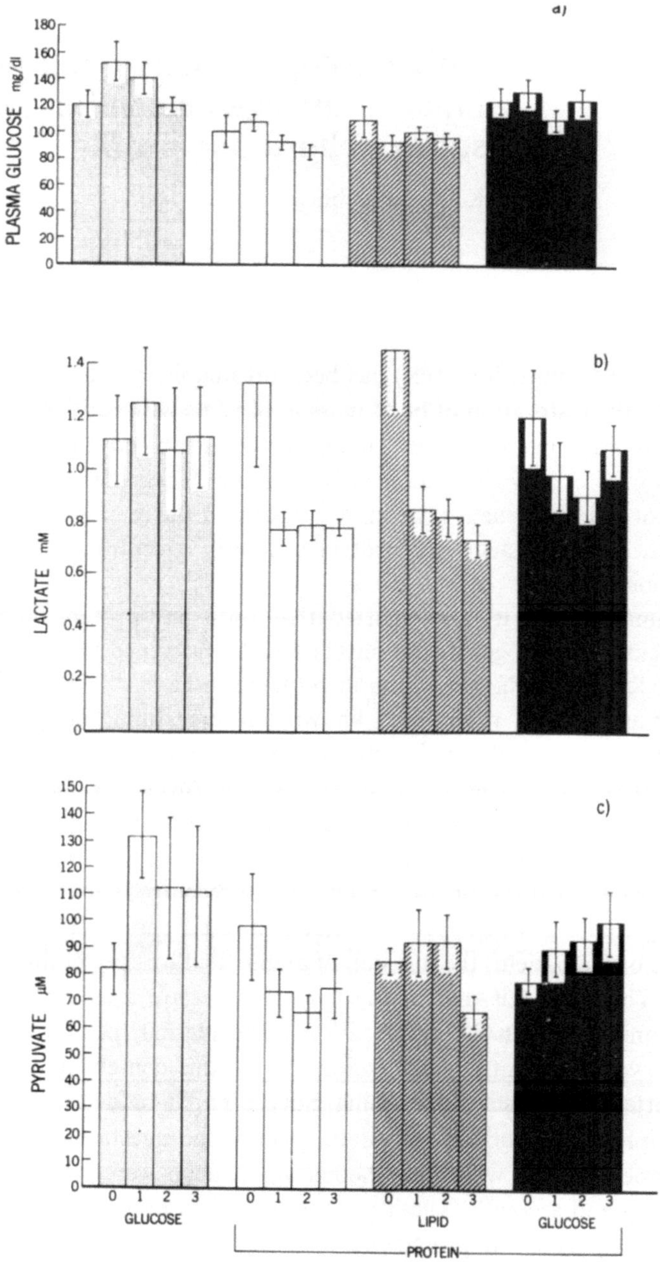

Figure 1. Plasma glucose (a), blood lactate (b) and blood pyruvate (c) levels during infusions of glucose, protein, protein plus lipid and protein plus glucose after operation (0) and on the first, second and third post-operative days. Values are mean ± S.E.M.

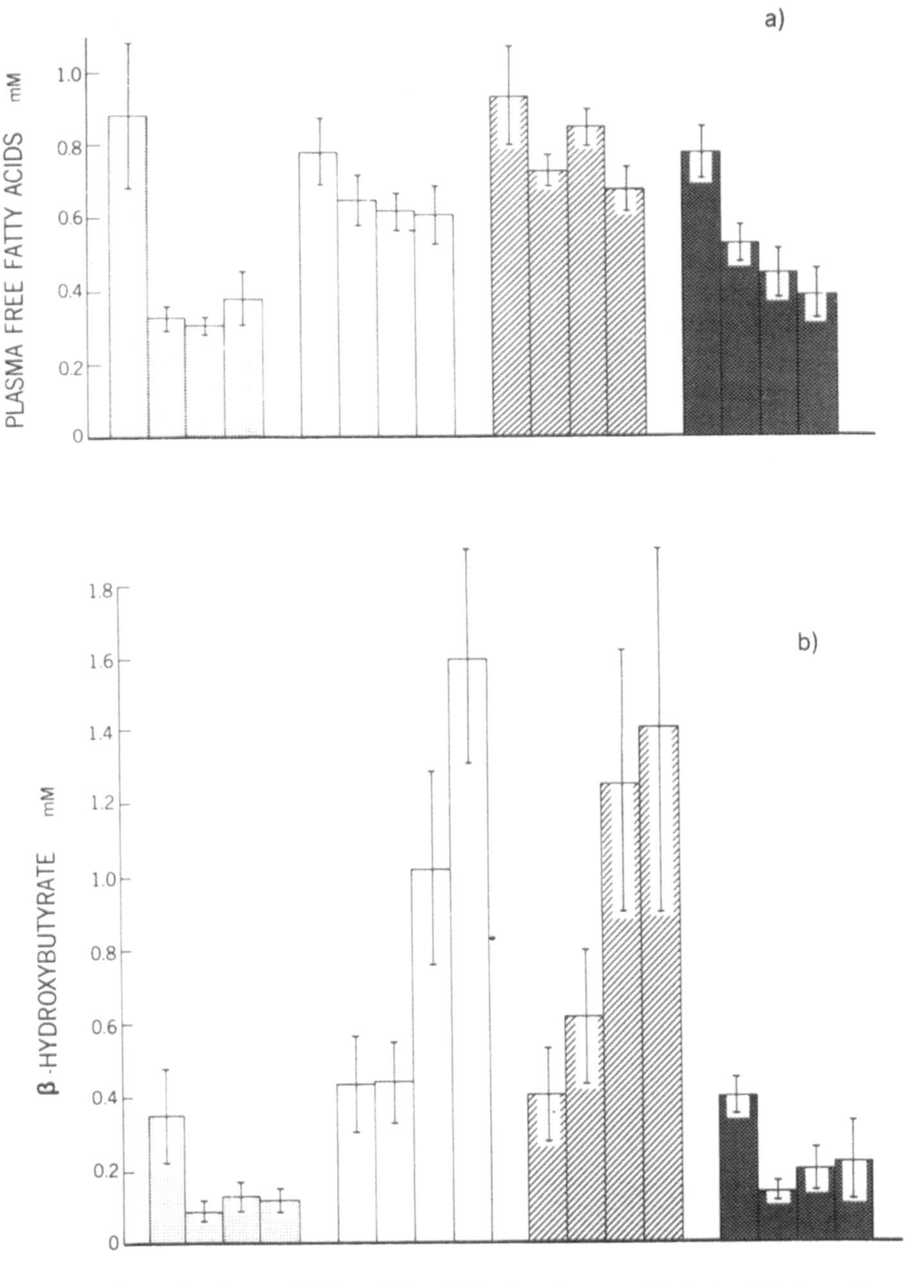

Figure 2. Plasma free fatty acid (a) and blood β-hydroxybutyrate (b) during infusions of glucose, protein, protein plus lipid and protein plus glucose after operation (0) and on the first, second and third post-operative days. Values are mean ± S.E.M.

depended exclusively on glucose as the main source of calories (4). In contrast the technique developed by Wretlind (5) and used widely in Europe included lipid as a major source of calories. In view of animal studies suggesting a special role for carbohydrate in sparing nitrogen (1) it became crucial to determine the relative efficacy of glucose and lipid in promoting nitrogen retention.

DISCUSSION OF SPECIFIC CONSIDERATIONS

Role of amino acids

To determine the role of amino acids in promoting nitrogen retention Greenberg et al. (6) designed a study in which patients were randomly allocated to groups receiving glucose alone (G) (550 kcals per day), amino acids alone (P) (1 g/kg/day), amino acids infused in the above dosage together with either 550 kcals/day of glucose (PG) or lipid (PL) (Intralipid[R], Pharmacia, Montreal, Canada).

Hence there were two groups receiving glucose, G and PG and two without glucose P and PL. The results of substrate profile and nitrogen balance are given in Figs. 1, 2 and Table 1. The substrate profile showed that the two groups receiving glucose (G and PG) had significantly higher pyruvate ($P < 0.05$) and lactate ($P < 0.05$) levels than the groups not receiving glucose (P and PL). In contrast the groups not receiving glucose, P and PL, had higher levels of plasma free fatty acids ($P < 0.005$) and ketones ($P < 0.001$). The results of these studies have already been published (6) in detail and the interested reader is referred to this paper (6). Consistent with this substrate profile the plasma insulin levels ($P < 0.05$) were significantly higher in patients receiving glucose, in contrast glucagon levels were higher in P and

Table 1. Cumulative nitrogen input and balance*

System	Input	Balance	P values**
Glucose (7)***	0.0 ± 0.0	− 45.1 ± 5.05	–
Protein (7)	41.8 ± 2.41	− 20.4 ± 3.45	< 0.001 (vs glucose)
Protein + lipid (7)	38.5 ± 2.03	− 17.3 ± 4.61	< 0.001 (vs glucose) > 0.3 (vs protein)
Protein + glucose (8)	39.6 ± 2.59	− 20.8 ± 3.97	< 0.001 (vs glucose) > 0.95 (vs protein) > 0.70 (vs protein + lipid)

* g of nitrogen/3 days (mean ± SEM).
** For the comparisons indicated.
*** Figures in parentheses denote no. of observations.

PL. Hence the glucose infused groups had higher insulin levels and a glucose induced substrate profile. In contrast P and PL had a profile with high free fatty acids and ketones, with low insulin levels. This profile is believed by Blackburn to be most conducive to nitrogen retention (3). Despite these very different substrate-hormone profiles Greenberg et al. (5) noted that the cumulative nitrogen balance was comparable in the three protein infused groups (P, PL and PG) and significantly greater ($P < 0.001$) than in those receiving glucose alone. In short the source of non-protein calories did not seem to influence nitrogen balance and the substrate hormone profile did not affect the nitrogen retention.

From these studies it appeared that amino acid infusion alone was protein-sparing. To test this hypothesis further we infused patients with two different amounts of amino acids. One group received 1 g/kg and the other 2 g/kg of amino acids only, without added non-protein calories. The results showed that the patients receiving 2 g/kg/day were in mean positive nitrogen balance amounting to + 16.3 g over a 7-day period compared with those receiving 1 g/kg/day who showed a mean negative nitrogen balance of – 26.1 g/kg/day ($P < 0.01$). This finding confirmed that the amount of amino acid infused determined the degree of nitrogen-sparing (in the hypocaloric situation). In contrast to the suggestion that increased fat mobilization may aid nitrogen retention we found that the free fatty acids and ketones were lower in the patients receiving 2 g/kg/day of amino acids and who were in positive nitrogen balance. Hence our studies in patients infused with hypocaloric solutions showed that when non-protein calories do not meet the requirements, the amount of protein infused alone determines the degree of nitrogen retention. Furthermore in order to obtain a positive nitrogen balance under these circumstances about 2 g/kg/day should be infused.

Relation of source of non-protein calories to nitrogen balance

Now turning to the situation where the amount of non-protein calories exceeds the requirements of the patient, we set out to determine if glucose and lipid calories were equally effective in maintaining nitrogen retention. To do this we infused patients with a constant background of amino acids providing 1 g/kg/day with all the other nutrients and trace elements except non-protein calories. With this background the patients were allocated to receive in random order either glucose (glucose system) or lipid (lipid system) amounting to a total of 40 kcals/kg/day of non-protein calories. The infusion was continued for 7 days after which the patient was switched to the alternate source of calories for another 7 days. For example, if the patient

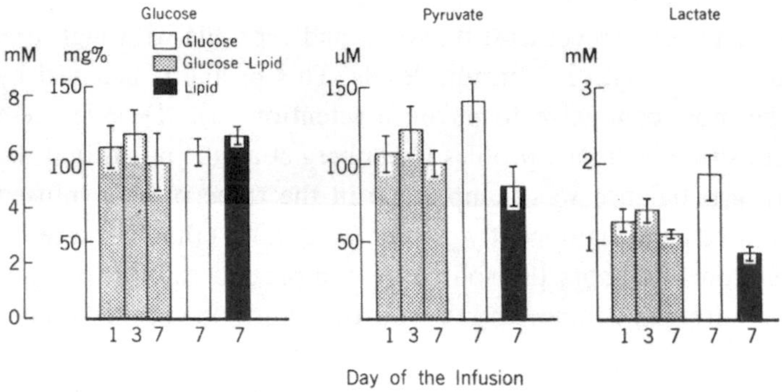

Figure 3

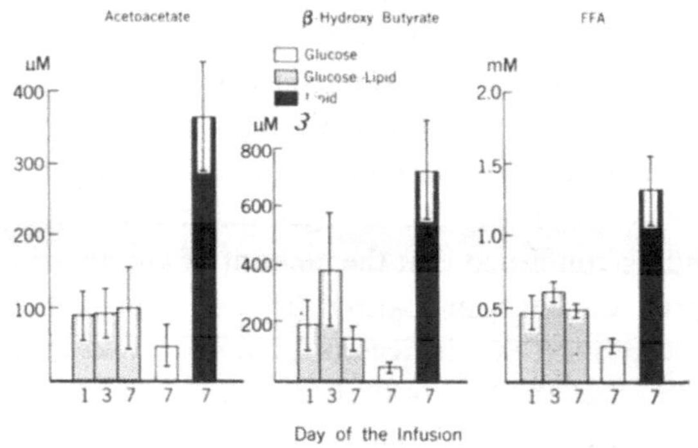

Figure 4

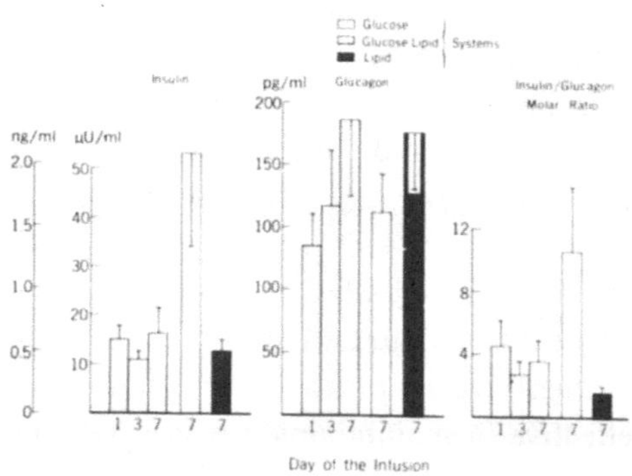

Figure 5

Figures 3, 4, 5. Blood levels of glucose, pyruvate, lactate, acetoacetate, and β-hydroxybutyrate (ketone bodies), plasma free fatty acids (FFA), insulin and glucagon levels during total parenteral nutrition using different ratios of glucose to lipid as non-protein calories. All studies were isocaloric. In the figures the open bars (glucose) represent studies where glucose alone was the source of non-protein calories. The stippled bars represent studies where equal calories of glucose and lipid were infused. The black bars (lipid) represent the system where 83% of the calories were given as lipid.

had received glucose initially for 7 days he was switched to lipid for the next 7 days. The details have already been published and the interested reader is referred to the paper (7). In another study the patients were randomly switched from either glucose or lipid to a mixture containing 50% of calories as glucose and 50% as lipid (50-50 system) (8).

In these studies since the order of infusion did not influence the final substrate-hormone profile we have grouped the results of each system together. The results are shown in Figs. 3, 4 and 5. It is clear from the figure that patients receiving the glucose system had higher pyruvate and lactate levels (Fig. 3) whereas those receiving the lipid system had higher levels of free fatty acids and ketones (acetoacetate and β-hydroxybutyrate) (Fig. 4). The patients receiving the 50-50 system had substrate-hormone profiles intermediate to these two extremes and in the post-prandial range of subjects eating a normal diet (Figs. 3 and 4). Correspondingly insulin levels were high in patients receiving the glucose system and low in those receiving the lipid system with the glucagon levels being in the other order. Hence J/G ratios were high in patients given the glucose system and low in patients receiving the lipid system. It should be noted that when patients received

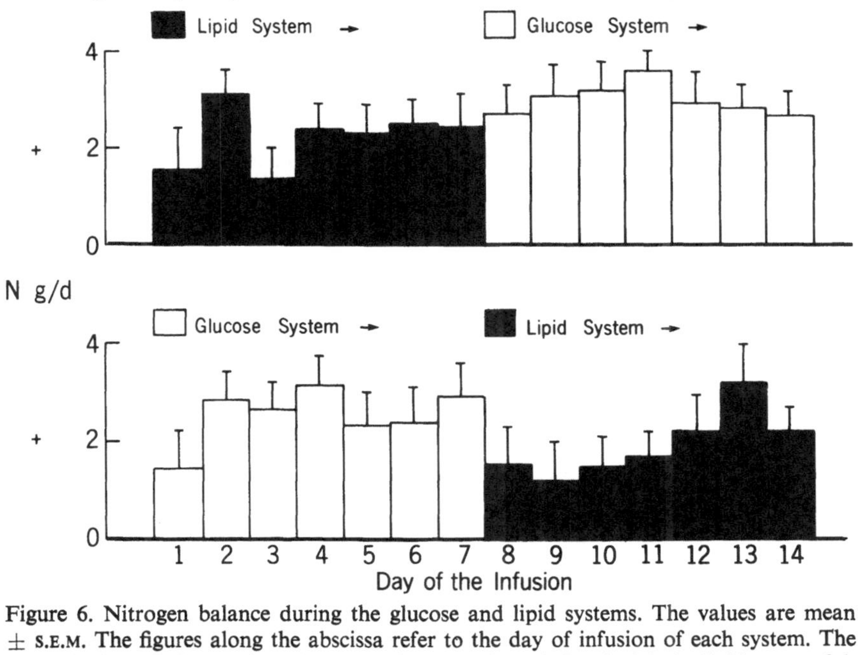

Figure 6. Nitrogen balance during the glucose and lipid systems. The values are mean ± S.E.M. The figures along the abscissa refer to the day of infusion of each system. The upper half of the figure gives the results for 13 patients infused with the lipid system followed by the glucose system. The lower half shows the results for 14 patients infused in the reverse order.

the 50-50 system the insulin levels were in the post-prandial range of orally fed man (Fig. 5).

Despite these very different substrate-hormone profiles and insulin-glucagon ratios the nitrogen balance after equilibrium had been established (days 5, 6 and 7 of the studies) was not significantly different in the two groups (Fig. 6). Furthermore in patients receiving the 50-50 system the same conclusions applied when they were compared with those given the glucose or lipid systems.

Hence it can be concluded that the source of non-protein calories does not influence nitrogen balance. The patient uses the substrate that is given and secretes the appropriate hormone to utilize this substrate. When glucose is given glucose is the main substrate with high pyruvates and lactates. To utilize this substrate a high insulin level is generated. In contrast when lipid is infused there is an increase in lipid-related substrates such as free fatty acids and ketones. Since these substrates do not require high insulin levels for utilization the patients are in positive nitrogen balance despite lower insulin levels noted with this system. The system supplying 50% of calories as glucose and 50% of calories as fat generates equivalent substrates from each source and functions with a moderate circulating insulin level.

What is the significance of these findings? They show that it is possible to obtain equivalent positive nitrogen balance with a variety of combinations of non-protein calories. However there are special features of each of these combinations which make it useful for certain situations. Firstly the system providing 50% of calories as lipid and 50% as glucose provides the most physiological levels of substrate-hormone profile and simulates the normal diet. Recently Myers et al. (9) have shown that even when glucose alone is given as the source of non-protein calories a significant amount of calories is derived from body fat. This finding again suggests that the ideal mixture of non-protein calories is a combination of glucose and lipid. Secondly since the system infusing lipid as the major source of calories requires low insulin levels it is ideal for diabetics who cannot generate high insulin levels or who have insulin resistance. Thirdly a system using a lipid as the major source of calories is isotonic and can be infused through a peripheral vein. This system has allowed us to give TPN peripherally up to 40 days. The interested reader is referred to earlier publications for details (7, 8, 10). Finally because the 50% glucose-50% lipid system generates moderate insulin levels it can be discontinued abruptly without hypoglycemia and is useful for patients receiving TPN at home (11, 12) where they can disconnect themselves at will and go about their normal daily activities unencumbered with pumps and bags.

Relationship of energy and amino acid input to nitrogen balance

The results are seen in Fig. 7. It is clear from this figure that the nitrogen

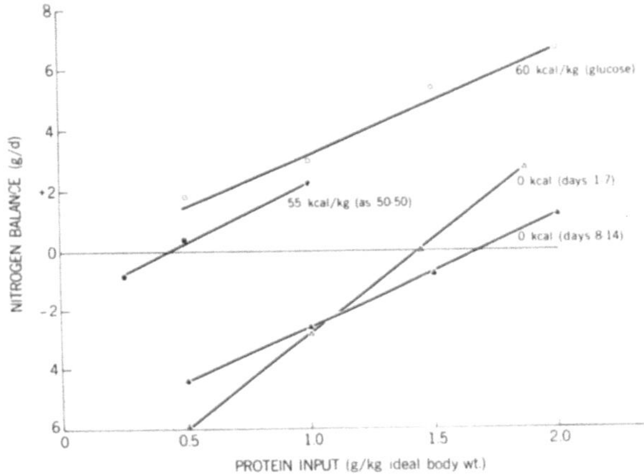

Figure 7. Relationship of the inputs of non-protein calories and of total nitrogen, to nitrogen balance.

retention is related to intake with increasing retention observed as the input is increased from 0.25 g/kg/day to 2 g/kg/day. The addition of non-protein calories shifts the curve to the left so that at each level of amino acid input the retention is greater with added non-protein calories than without. Hence nitrogen balance may be achieved with 1.7 g/kg/day amino acids without added calories and with only 0.4 g/kg/day where added non-protein calories amount to 55 kcals/kg/day. Thus both input of calories and of protein determines the degree of nitrogen retention. Furthermore when the infusion of glucose-lipid non-protein calories at 55 kcals/kg/day is compared with that using only glucose at a level of 60 kcals/kg/day, as in patients studied by Rudman et al. (13), it becomes clear that the results are as would be expected from total calories infused and are independent of the source of non-protein calories, confirming our previous result.

In conclusion we can state that amino acid infusions will spare protein in the hypocaloric state and the amount of protein required to attain nitrogen balance is 1.7 g/kg in the absence of added non-protein calories. When such calories are added there is further protein-sparing depending on the total amount so used. The source of calories does not determine the degree of nitrogen retention but an infusion providing 50% calories as glucose and 50% as lipid appears to be most physiological. Where peripheral TPN is desirable or in diabetics, an infusion using lipid as the major source of calories is useful.

ACKNOWLEDGEMENT

Acknowledgement is kindly made to the editors of the following publications for permission to use material appearing originally therein: the New England Journal of Medicine (Figures 1 and 2, and Table 1), the Proceedings of the Symposium on Fat Emulsion in Parenteral Nutrition, American Medical Association, Chicago (Figures 3, 4 and 5) and the Journal of Clinical Investigation (Figure 6) and the Annals of The Royal College of Physicians and Surgeons of Canada (Figure 7).

We are grateful to the Ontario Ministry of Health for Grant # PR.228 which has allowed us to undertake these studies.

We thank Mrs. J. Chrupala for her expert typing.

REFERENCES

1. Munro, H. N., General aspects of the regulation of protein metabolism by diet and by hormones. In: *Mammalian Protein Metabolism*, vol. I, Chapter 10. Munro, H. N. and Allison, J. B. (eds), Academic Press, New York, 381-481 (1964).
2. Gamble, J. L., Companionship of water and electrolytes in the organization of body fluids. Stanford University Press, Stanford. *Lane Medical Lecture 5*: 71 (1951).
3. Blackburn, G. L., Flatt, J. P. and Clowes, G. H. A., Jr., et al., Nitrogen-sparing therapy during periods of starvation with sepsis or trauma. *Ann. Surg. 177*: 588-594 (1973).
4. Dudrick, S. J. and Ruberg, R. L., Principles and practice of parenteral nutrition. *Gastroenterology 61*: 901-910 (1971).
5. Wretlind, A., Complete intravenous nutrition. *Nutr. Metabol. 14*: Suppl. 1-57 (1972).
6. Greenberg, G. R., Marliss, E. B., Anderson, G. H., Langer, B., Spence, W., Tovee, E. B. and Jeejeebhoy, K. N., Protein-sparing therapy in post-operative patients. Effects of added hypocaloric glucose or lipid. *New Eng. J. Med. 294*: 411-416 (1976).
7. Jeejeebhoy, K. N., Anderson, G. H., Nakhooda, A. F., Greenberg, G. R., Sanderson, I. and Marliss, E. B., Metabolic studies in total parenteral nutrition with lipid in man: comparison with glucose. *J. Clin. Invest. 57*: 125-136 (1976).
8. Jeejeebhoy, K. N., Marliss, E. B., Anderson, G. H., Greenberg, G. R., Kuksis, A. and Breckenridge, C., Lipid in Parenteral Nutrition. Studies of Clinical and Metabolic Features. In: Meng, H. C. and Wilmore, D. W. (eds.), Fat Emulsions in Parenteral Nutrition, *Am. Med. Assoc.*, Chicago, 45-54 (1976).
9. Myers, R. N., Smink, R. D., Skutches, C. L., Paul, P. and Reichard, G. A., Jr., Plasma glucose metabolism during parenteral hyperalimentation. *J. Clin. Invest.* (in press).
10. Zohrab, W. J., McHattie, J. D. and Jeejeebhoy, K. N., Total parenteral alimentation with lipid. *Gastroenterology 64*: 583-592 (1973).
11. Langer, B., McHattie, J. D., Zohrab, W. J. and Jeejeebhoy, K. N., Prolonged survival after complete small bowel resection using intravenous alimentation at home. *J. Surg. Res. 15*: 226-233 (1973).
12. Jeejeebhoy, K. N., Langer, B., Tsallas, G., Chu, R. C., Kuksis, A. and Anderson, G. H., Total parenteral nutrition at home: studies in patients surviving 4 months to 5 years. *Gastroenterology 71*: 943-953 (1976).
13. Rudman, D., Millikan, W. J., Richardson, T. J., Bixler, T. J., Stackhouse, W. J. and McGarrity, W. C. Elemental balances during intravenous hyperalimentation of underweight adult subjects. *J. Clin. Invest. 55*: 94-104 (1975).

Panel discussion

Carbohydrate - versus fat - versus proteincalories

FISCHER: The title of the carbohydrate-/versus fat-/versus protein calories panel is intended to discuss an outstanding issue. This same group of people met in Vail last March and devoted an entire day to this subject. The basic question that the panel wants to discuss is: is a carbohydrate-calorie the same as a fat calorie? If it is not, why not, and if it is, are the two interchangeable?

Dr. Jeejeebhoy will forgive me if I paraphrase his recent presentation you can manipulate the system any way you wish. The only possible advantage is perhaps in the first three or four days: there seems to be some slight advantage, at least numerically and perhaps even not statistically significant to a glucose substrate load as opposed to a lipid substrate load. As the study periods get longer, you get to the point where the two systems are equivalent. Dr. Wilmore showed us some data yesterday, which has perhaps a slightly different message in it. Perhaps you would like to begin the discussion?

WILMORE: Although it is well known that fat and carbohydrate calories exert equal effects and nitrogen retention in normal man, there is some question whether these two differing non-protein calorie sources effect protein metabolism in a similar manner in the stressed patient.

We evaluated varying doses of carbohydrate and fat in thermally injured patients receiving a constant infusion of 11.7 g/nitrogen/m^2 per day. Increasing the carbohydrate dose improved nitrogen retention and hence enhanced nitrogen balance. Increasing the dose of intravenous fat did not exert a comparable effect (Table 1).

This finding is not unique. Dr. Halmagyi and Professor Heller studied stressed patients and presented their findings at this symposium. Fat calories did not exert the same nitrogen retention as was achieved with carbohydrate energy.

The influence of carbohydrate calories on nitrogen balance was just described by Shaffer, Coleman and Dubois (1, 2) at the turn of this century.

Table 1. Nitrogen excretion during each study period

From Long, J. M., Wilmore, D. W., Mason, A. D., Jr. and Pruitt, B. A., Jr., Effect of carbohydrate and fat intake on nitrogen excretion during total intravenous feeding. *Ann. Surg.* April, 1977.

		Nitrogen intake: 11.7 g/m²/day			
		Carbohydrate intake (kcal/m²/day)			
		110	350	875	1450
Fat intake (kcal/m²/day)	0	12.0*	9.3	8.0	7.0
	575	—	—	7.2	5.4
	1100	11.6	9.5	8.0	6.7

* Mean urea nitrogen excretion (g/m²/day) on third day of each infusion period.

Studies in patients with typhoid fever demonstrated that nitrogen balance could be improved with the addition of protein or carbohydrate to the diet, but not fat. These studies served as the basis for utilizing high carbohydrate high protein diets in critically ill patients.

1. Shaffer, P. A. and Coleman, W. Protein metabolism in typhoid fever. *Arch. Int. Med. 4*: 538-600 (1909).
2. Coleman, W. and Dubois, E. F., Calorimetric observations on the metabolism of typhoid patients with and without food. *Arch. Int. Med. 15*: 887-938 (1951).

BLACKBURN: An increase in hydroxyproline excretion during starvation and during infusion of glucose-free isotonic crystalline amino acids has been demonstrated (Kaminski, M. et al., J. Parent. Ent. Nutr. 1:3, Oct. 1977). It is also well recognized that glucose and lactate will enhance collagen content in wounds. However there are no observations that would allow one to conclude that more is better. Clearly glucose produces a different collagen content in this study than do glucose-free parenteral feedings but the clinical significance is uncertain.

FISCHER: Professor Munro in his 1951 review based on oral data made the same point about fat and protein sparing. Would you care to comment on your own opinion in this area. We return to the possible differences between these two sets of data in a minute, because there may be some reconciliation possible.

MUNRO: The problem is compounded by two separate phenomena – caloric intake and a specific carbohydrate component which operates an insulin-dependent mechanism for which I showed you a diagram yesterday (see p. 59).

As you will remember, the effect of the carbohydrate administration was an immediate transfer of blood amino acids into muscle and we did find in these rats that the liver actually lost protein during this period (Munro, 1964)*. Similarly, if you give a meal containing protein and you manipulate the carbohydrate either to be taken separately from the meal or with the meal, when both are in the same meal there is an increased nitrogen retention which we think goes into muscle. The mechanism is very limited in capacity. In the rat it lasts about 4 days; in man, it probably lasts rather longer and a

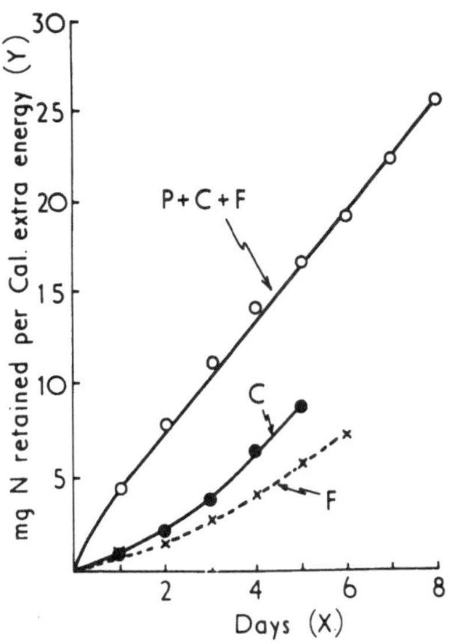

Figure 1. Effect on cumulative N balance energy (700 kcal/day) to the diet of an adult male subject.
C = extra carbohydrate;
F = extra fat;
P+C+F = extra protein + carbohydrate + fat
(From Munro, 1964).

* Munro, H. N., General aspects of the regulation of protein metabolism by diet and by hormones. In: Mammalian Protein Metabolism, Vol. 1, pp. 267-319 (H. N. Munro and J. B. Allison, eds.). Academic Press, New York (1964).

small amount of carbohydrate is sufficient to give you a very considerable response. In other words, 50 g or 100 gr of carbohydrate per day probably operates the mechanism just as well as 400 gr would. This mechanism is not very prolonged, but long enough to confuse brief metabolic studies on post-operative patients, and I think this phenomenon gives rise to a difference between carbohydrates and fat, because the fat does not have this specific effect. The second mechanism depends on caloric intake (Munro, 1964).* Fig. 1 shows some studies I did in 1934, in which I overfed myself with calories on a constant diet to which was added energy either as fat, as carbohydrate or as protein, carbohydrate and fat. The diagram shows cumulative

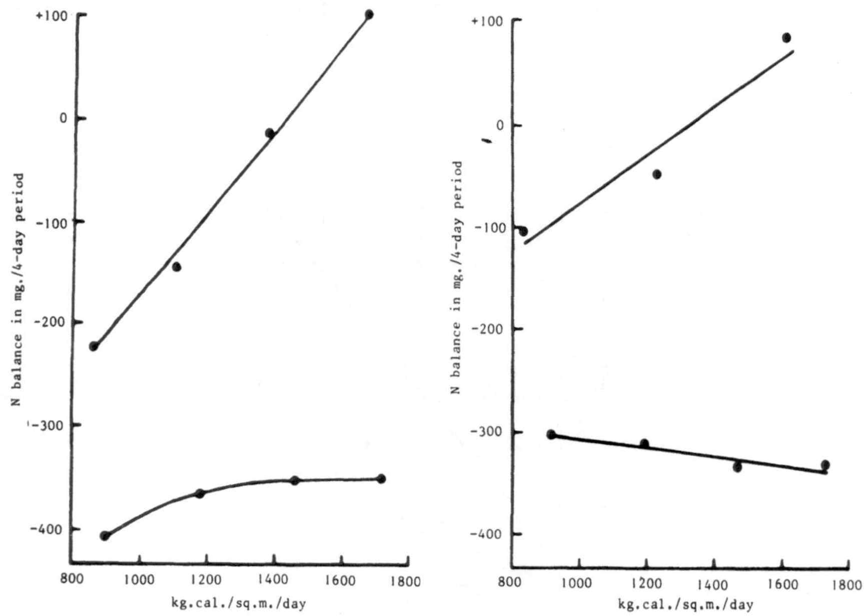

Figure 2a. The effect on nitrogen balance of changes in energy intake produced by alterations in dietary carbohydrate. Upper regression line, protein-containing diet. Lower line (drawn freehand through points), protein-free diet. Each point is the mean result obtained with four rats. (From Munro and Naismith, 1953).
Figure 2b. The effect on nitrogen balance of changes in energy intake produced by alterations in dietary fat. Upper regression line, protein containing diet. Lower regression line, protein-free diet. Each point is the mean result obtained with five rats or four rats (From Munro and Naismith, 1953).

* Munro, H. N. and Naismith, D. J., The influence of energy intake on protein metabolism. *Biochem. J. 54*: 191 (1953).

nitrogen retention continuously rising as over-feeding proceeds. The slope of the line is about 2-3 mg of nitrogen per calorie. Note that the presence of the protein in the supplement gives an extra boost to the slope as well as to the initial start. This is supported by many data in the literature. In general, both carbohydrate and fat given over quite long periods to rats and to human subjects induce retention. The fat takes several days to begin inducing the retention; the carbohydrate has a more rapid effect for the reason I gave you earlier: the specific action. So one tends to get a mixture of two phenomena – one of which is energy and one is for carbohydrate using a specific action associated with muscle protein deposition. Regarding energy, we (Munro and Naismith, 1953)* have shown in the rat that changes in energy content of the diet from addition of carbohydrate or fat can be effective at an

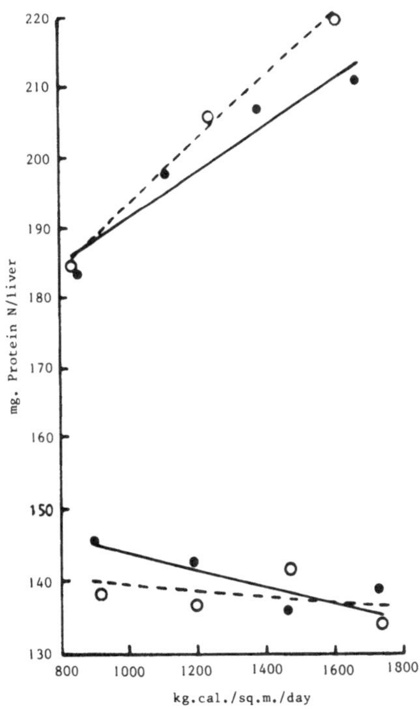

Figure 3. Changes in liver-protein nitrogen produced by variations in energy intake from carbohydrate (∼—∼) or from fat (#—#). The upper two curves represent the regression lines obtained when the diet contained protein. The lower two regression lines were obtained when the diet was free from protein. Each point is the mean result obtained with four or five rats (From Munro and Naismith, 1953).

adequate protein level in changing nitrogen balance, but not at a low protein level.

Notice that on a protein-free diet carbohydrate addition causes a certain amount of nitrogen retention (Fig. 2A) whereas added fat depresses nitrogen balance (Fig. 2B).

Regarding the liver, addition of extra carbohydrate or fat increases liver protein at an adequate level of protein intake but on a protein-free diet this is not so and added carbohydrate even tends to reduce liver protein content perhaps by diverting amino acids into muscle instead of into liver (Fig. 3).

There is evidence that the N retention with extra calories is proportional to the protein content of the diet (Plough and Iber, 1956). At a high protein level, instead of 1 or 2 mg nitrogen per calorie the subjects retained 5 or 6 mg nitrogen per calorie added. This gives rise to the problem that nitrogen balance cannot be defined solely in terms of protein intake but protein and calorie intake combined. This is illustrated on p. 65, showing the effect of caloric level and the effect of protein intake on the relationship to balance which I have just described.

FISCHER: Dr. Jeejeebhoy, in the two studies which you did, the patients had Crohn's disease and were presumably non septic. Perhaps a few of them had fever and abscesses, but most were treated for gut rest, is that correct?

JEEJEEBHOY: I think they did have a degree of sepsis. They came in with inflammatory bowel masses and things like that. But certainly they didn't have raving temperatures. We have carried out about 10 oxygen consumption studies with these patients to date and from these we would say that about 25 percent are hypermetabolic.

FISCHER: Nowhere near?

JEEJEEBHOY: Oh no, nothing like that, no. They were certainly in a completely different ballpark, these patients.

FISCHER: Could that be a possible explanation for the differences between your two studies?

JEEJEEBHOY: I think it is like this. Perhaps I'll go one stage further and say that if you have an energy substrate and you want it to be utilized it has to be mobilized and available in the circulation. In situations of total fasting and the patients Dr. Wilmore talked about – the burns – they had complete mobilisation of fat substrates. They are just so high that in the situation adding more fat, just cannot manipulate the system like we are doing. That is the problem, in other words: under those conditions you cannot see an effect of fat.

FISCHER: There is another group; maybe Dr. Wilmore wants to talk for himself. In that group there was a group of patients, who got carbohydrate sufficient to cover the measured metabolic rate. Are those the data that Jimmy Long and yourself published in 1975? Were they mobilizing fatty acids maximally? There was no change in nitrogen balance, even if they were covered with enough carbohydrate to cover the basic metabolic rate. Did you measure the free fatty acids in that group?

WILMORE: We have measured free fatty acids in our patients and they are suppressed somewhat by these large carbohydrate loads. If insulin is added, more carbohydrate can be administered. However, free fatty acids are still elevated and more important fat mobilization remains accelerated. Addition of up to 1000 calories of fat per meter square body surface area (approximately 1500-2000 fat calories in a usual patient) doesn't exert a major impact on nitrogen balance. However, these patients have normal body composition before injury and fat mobilizing occurs at accelerated rates.

FISCHER: There is another study in which the patients are presumably even in better shape than yours: Brennan's study* in normal volunteers. He was unable to show any effect of a comparable amount of Intralipid over and above the glycerol content. At least on urea-nitrogen excretion if I remember the data correctly, nitrogen balances were not carried out, patients were on a protein-free diet.

JEEJEEBHOY: If I remember correctly, what he tried to do was to fast these patients and of course, once you fast a patient then you are giving him a fat substrate. So whatever effect you have got, it has been achieved by maximum mobilization of fat.

If you add exogenous fat you cannot do anything further, I think. And of course, the second part Dr. Munro pointed out to us was that the fat-

* Brennan, M. F., Fitz Palsian, G. F. Cohan, R. Metal, Glycerol major contributor to the short term protein-sparing of fat emulsions in normal man. Ann. Surg. 182: 786 (1975).

energy effect is only seen in the presence of added nitrogen. I think this is an important point, and all our studies were done with the added nitrogen.

WILMORE: The impact on the 2 caloric sources is different on a nitrogen-free diet and this needs to be kept in mind as you look at the various studies. So that the first slide that I demonstrated just took a patient that was on a nitrogen-free diet and gave fat and showed no impact and then gave carbohydrate it showed marked retention. And that is why we went into the study where we gave definitive levels of nitrogen to see if that same difference was present at that point in time.

BLACKBURN: I wonder if I can try one more time to resolve the differences because I can see the two points quite well.

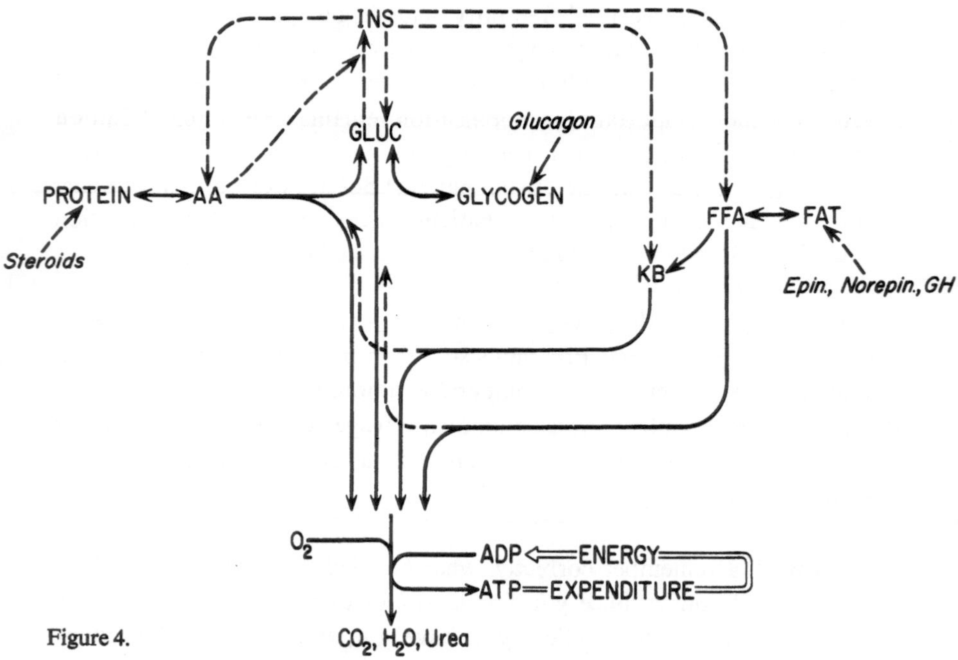

Figure 4.

In figure 4 we tried to integrate these substrates: amino acids, the carbohydrate and the fat. The various hormones that we have mentioned today and their effect is also graphically shown. Insulin has a universal storage effect, whereas there is a localized effect from the steroids on protein, glucagon in the liver on glycogen and catacholamines and growth hormone on the peripheral fat. The common denominator and rate limiting step is at the bottom: the energy requirement. If one is to spare protein, one must minimize the protein contribution to energy expenditure. This occurs by allowing non-protein calories to meet most of the requirements either from the body stores of glycogen or fat or dietary carbohydrate or fat. We can see in figure 5 that the same protein intake during stress and carbohydrate resistance decreases the endogenous sources of non-protein calories both from fat or glucose. Thus carbohydrate intake contributes to hyperglycemia while this glucose contribution to the calorie requirement is not proportionally increased. More of the body protein must be catabolized. Thus the respiratory quotient shifts and the first order of survival for each cell is to meet its energy requirement. In figure 6 there were 4 patients in the study that I have shown you, who did not keto-adapt. They therefore lost some of 400-500 of the calories that would normally come from 100 g of ketones. This loss of energy substrate had the effect on the same amount of protein intake to cause its oxidation and production urea N resulting in a nitrogen balance similar to those receiving 5% dextrose. The sepsis group did not

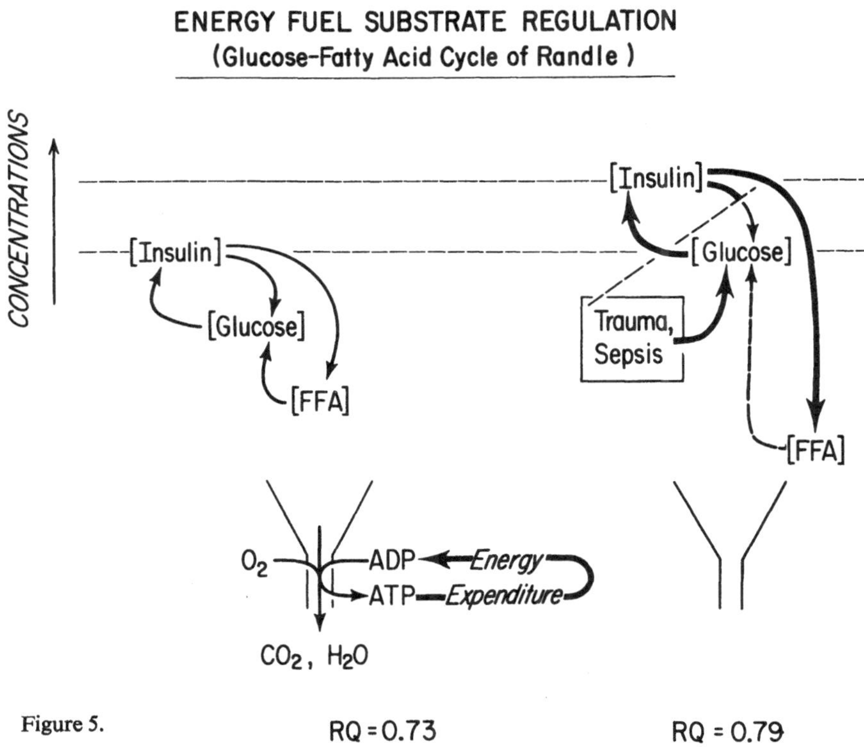

Figure 5.

keto-adapt, had no ketonuria and the nitrogen loss approaches the nitrogen loss that was shown in the glucose group. So, again we would believe that there is a relationship between nitrogen and calories and the dietary nitrogen will influence nitrogen balance if it does not have to be consumed for calories. Clearly when there are no ketones and the debt of calories cannot be made up by either glucose availability or the free fatty acids, the nitrogen balance decreases. This is owing to an increase in urea N production and excretion. Fig. 7. Again the potassium balance was the same way. Those patients could not develop positive potassium balance, and therefore body cell mass remained negative, similar to that of the dextrose group. Fig. 8. The difference is that, as Dr. Wilmore has pointed out, hypermetabolic patients keto-adapt poorly. They are maximally energy expending, usual for the major burn group. This is strikingly different from infection, Crohn disease, routine surgery or surgical injury group. Energy fuel utilization is going to be in-

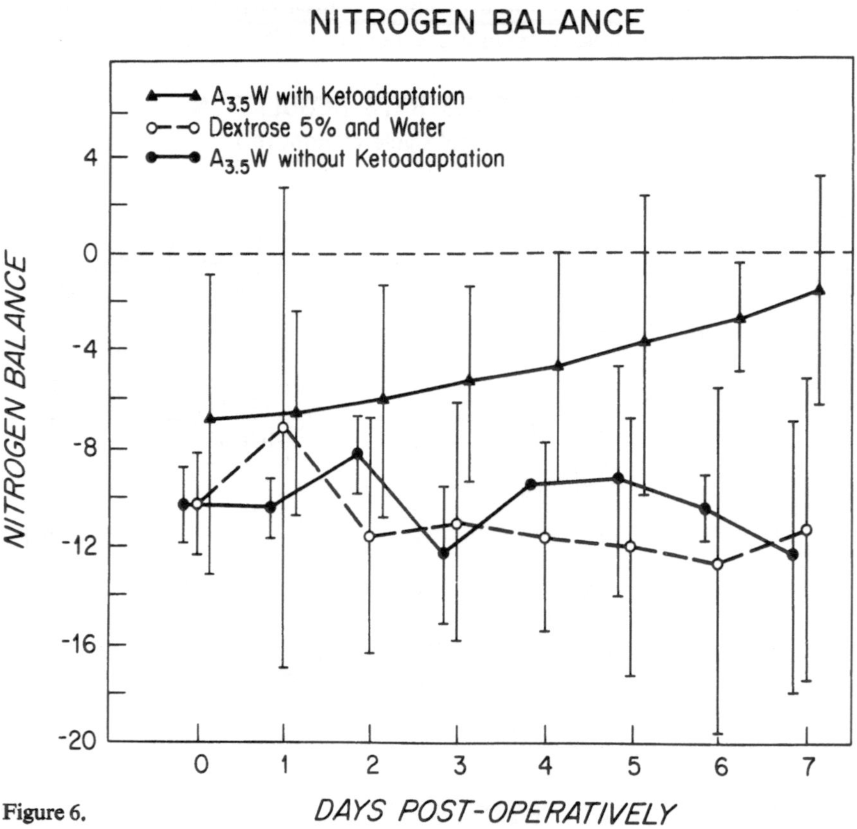

Figure 6.

fluenced by the non-protein calories available and certainly if this requirement is not going to be contributed to by ketone-bodies and there is no carbohydrate in the system, there is more protein broken down and oxidized (Fig. 9). This matrix is drawn from the work of Dr. Wilmore, Dudrick, Duke, Gump, Kinney, Winters and ourselves and many people trying to integrate the degrees of malnutrition with the degrees of hypermetabolism. Dr. Wilmore is working in that left lower matrix-square, whereas obviously Dr. Jeejeebhoy's data and much that we are talking about, is not there. It is either in the left upper or middle square, the exact middle, the whole area on the top and certainly not in these severe areas.

I would suggest for a consideration of each set of data that the first criterion is to decide which category of patients is being reported. Then using

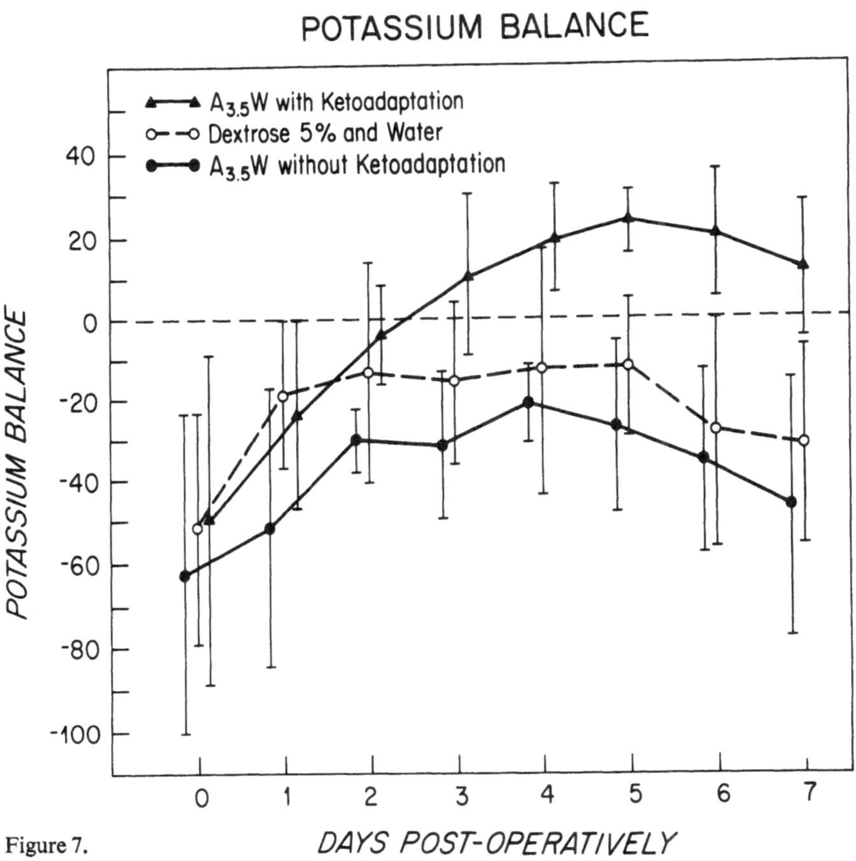

Figure 7.

that model we showed you, you can pick your system and help to predict what sort of results you are going to have.

I do not believe that Dr. Wilmore's criteria for efficacy can continue to be based on nitrogen balance and in the next slide (Fig. 10) we think that you must define to make sure that the improved nitrogen balance is a function of the viscera, whether it is leucocytic activities, bone marrow erythrocytosis, acute phase proteins synthesis albumin and transferrin that reflect criteria of efficacy. If the improved nitrogen balance reflects these changes, then that is strong evidence in support of the technique reported. These data are not available in adequate volume to the best of my knowledge from any of our laboratories and many of us are looking at this issue now.

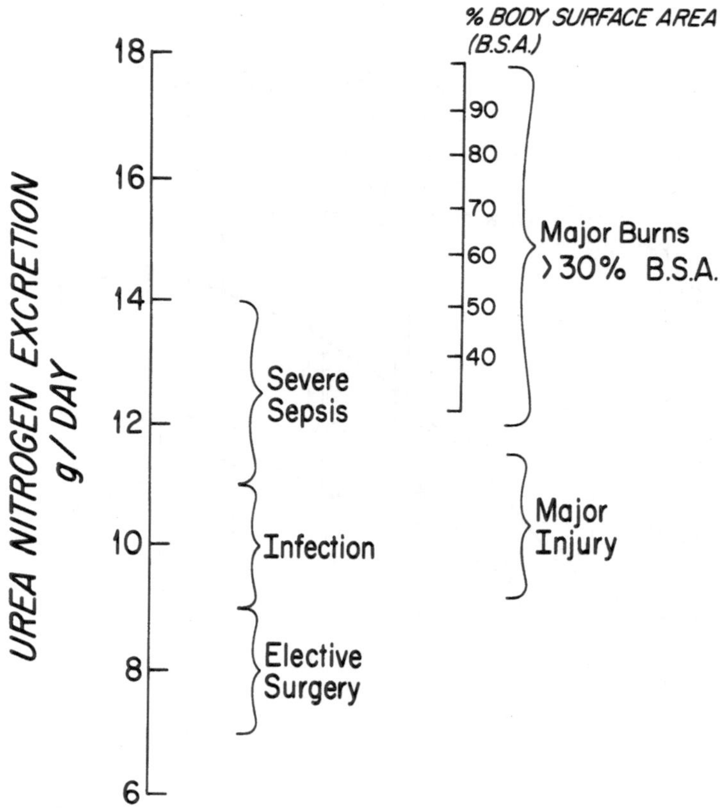

Figure 8.

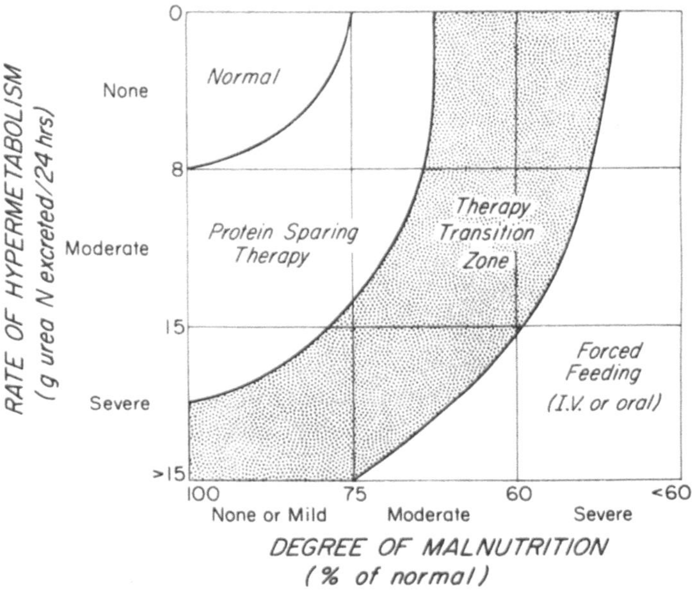

Figure 9.

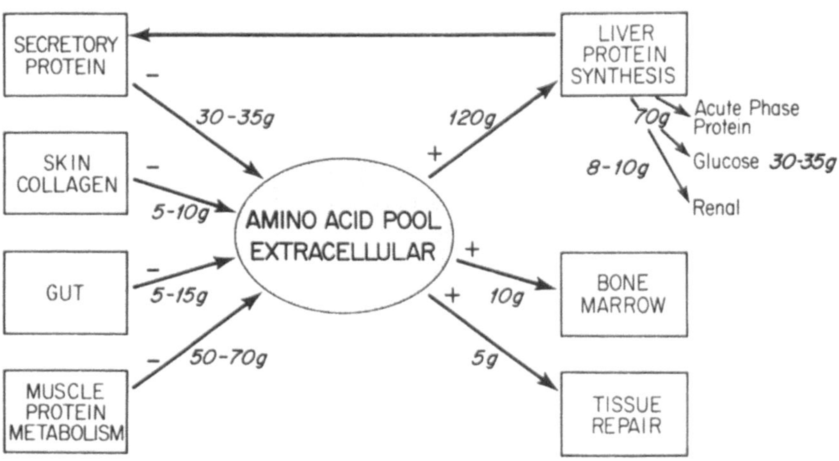

Figure 10

FISCHER: I personally would take issue with the last statement, certainly people die from the lack of lean body mass too – we usually call it death from pneumonia – it generally means they cannot breathe enough to clear their own secretions – they get pneumonia and they die. So that the positive nitrogen balance itself is a perfectly reasonable thing, independent of where it goes.

BLACKBURN: You mean that all your positive nitrogen balance hyper-alimented patients survive?

FISCHER: No, it just means that if you have positive nitrogen balance, it is a perfectly valid thing that you don't have to limit it just by visceral protein. You just watch these patients – they can't walk, they can't talk, they can't breathe?

AARIMA MARKKU – FINLAND: I have a comment on what Prof. Blackburn said that the various forms of therapy do not influence the healing of the wound. I would like to show you a slide (Fig. 11) on which you see the effect of a glucose infusion versus amino acids infusion on the collagen production of the fibroblast in the wound. We see that there are two kinds of patients – it concerns patients with resection of the stomach and aorto-femoral reconstruction and they were divided into 2 groups. One group received only

	RESECTED		A-F RECONSTR.		mean of all patients
	patient	production of collagen	patient	production of collagen	
GLUCOSE	1 2 3 mean	5 3 9 5.7	7 8 9 mean	6 8 7 7.0	6.3
AMINO ACIDS	4 5 6 mean	1 4 2 2.3	10 11 12 mean	2 6 6 4.7	3.5

Figure 11.

glucose from the beginning of the operation for 5 days on. And another group received only amino acids from the beginning of the operation again 5 days on. The collagen production was measured by cell stick method, and here on the right we see a summary of the results. We see that those patients who received only glucose had a much better production of the collagen than those who received only amino acids. These patients had their sodium balance measured too and there was a difference like that described earlier.

I would like to comment that we do not know if the hyperglycemia which so constantly occurs in the course of trauma, has any beneficial effects or if it is only a lapsis of the nature or a phenomenon without any importance. But we could maybe discuss that the hyperglycemia in the course of trauma means that the dead spaces that remain are concentrated in the dead spaces, there is more glucose which serves on the one hand as an energy source to the various forms of cells, for example in the wound, and on the other hand, it serves as a source of lactate which in turn could be of importance in stimulating the growth of capillaries.

FISCHER: Any comments from the floor?

NUBEE – LEIDEN – THE NETHERLANDS: I should like to ask Dr. Blackburn. You have shown your graph with a nitrogen balance with dextrose alone and physiological saline. Both groups had the same nitrogen intake you said. But in an article a few years ago, you reported 2 groups of patients and there was a difference between the groupsl. One group received 90 gr. of amino acids and the other group 70. And in my opinion, that could explain the difference yon found in nitrogen balances. Are these results new results or are they same as a few years ago?

BLACKBURN: (Fig. 12), see next page. These studies are all new. These are from the first 7 days postoperatively and the groups that you refer to were patients that were not controlled from outward phenomena, but patients who were on I.V.'s for some time. I will point out that if you read that article (Blackburn et al. Am. J. Surg. 125: 447, 1973) in which I gave 70 g of amino acids plus glucose compared to the amino acid group alone, there is no statistical difference. Only when comparing glucose alone versus amino acids was there a statistical difference.

A. C. DOUWES – AMSTERDAM: I'd like to comment on the paper of Dr. Blackburn. He states that in periods of hypercatabolism during stress, it is better

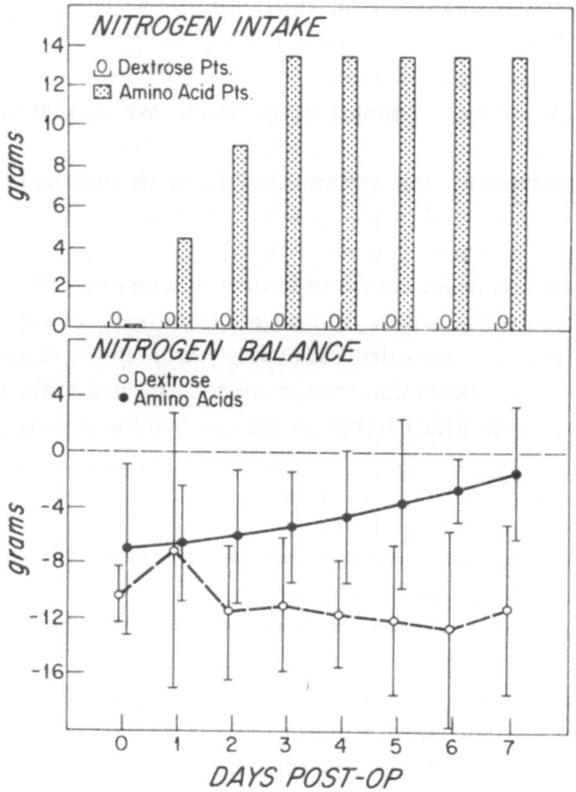

Figure 12.

to provide aminoacids only. The problem is that in my opinion he did not probe by metabolic and hormonal parameters, that his patients were really stressed. If they were not, they were just starving. In that situation one can supply any energy substrate just as Dr. Jeejeebhoy indicated, and it will be tolerated and utilized well. Much evidence exists for a difference in hormonal profile during catabolism from stress and catabolism from starvation. It is generally known that during catabolism from operative stress, the blood insuline-response is depressed by epinephrine and therefore, the blood sugar is high, especially in those patients which receive glucose infusions. It is also known that lipoprotein lipase-activity during stress is decreased so that Intralipid is not well tolerated. Aminoacids are the only substrates, that can be metabolized in the state of stress.

Starving patients will profit more by providing them any sort of intra-

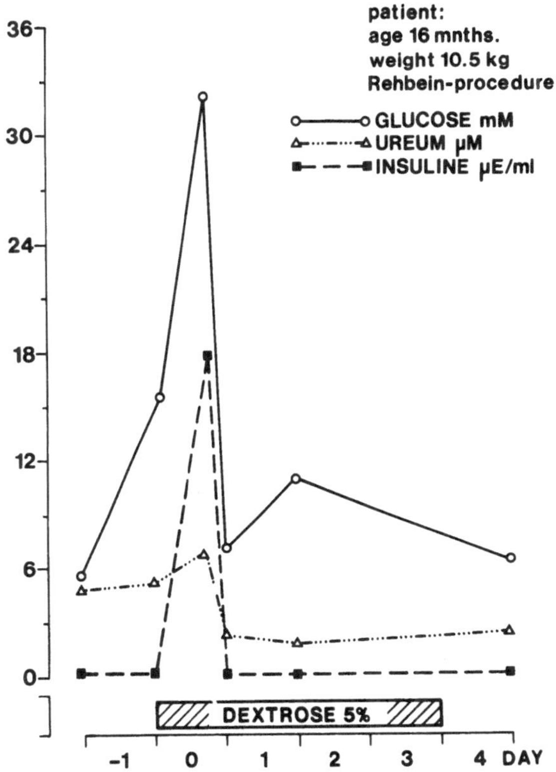

Figure 13. Measurements in venous blood. Patient is operated on day zero.

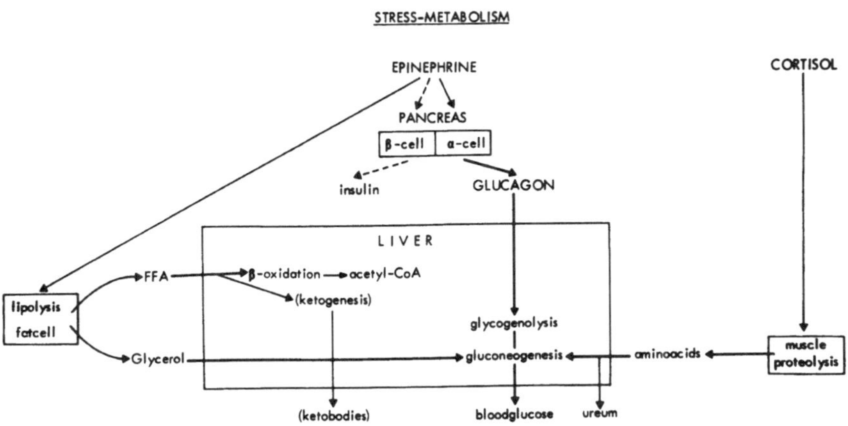

Figure 14. Proposed simplified scheme for the interaction of hormones and fuel substrate during stress. ——→ stimulation - - - - -→ inhibition.

venous feeding you have. So it is important to know whether the patient is in stress or not.

Fig. 13: I have a slide with me concerning postoperative patients. We investigated 5 children. They were all operated upon for Morbus Hirschsprung and we intended to find parameters which could define the presence of stress. All patients received 5% dextrose i.v. during and after operation and were followed for about 5 days. On the first slide you see the bloodsugar rising to 32 mmols one hour after the end of surgery. The first point is basal; the next after anaesthesia; the next one hour after operation and this point next morning. The insulin response of 18 units to the hyperglycemia is very low. The urea curve in the blood goes up at the time of surgery, then goes down below preoperative values next morning and subsequent days. These features were found in all 5 patients. We concluded that none of them was in stress one day after surgery.

In the urine, one can find an increased urea nitrogen excretion during day zero and on the first postoperative day. On day 2 however, the urea-nitrogen total nitrogen ratio of the urine is only 24%. This too means that the patient was not in stress anymore. He was just starving.

Fig. 14: On the next slide, you see an outline of stress metabolism composed from literature data. You see that in stress metabolism epinephrine depresses the insulin response and simultaneously stimulates glucagon output. This results in an increased glycolysis and gluconeogenesis from amino-acids and glycerol and abnormally high bloodsugars. Lipolysis is directly enhanced by epinephrine, providing free fatty acids and glycerol to the liver. What I want to underline is that there is a definite difference between the effects of catabolism from stress and catabolism from starvation. These differences do have important effects on the utilisation of parenteral feedings. I think this might explain some of the differences between the figures of Dr. Jeejeebhoy and Dr. Blackburn.

FISCHER: If I may just amplify the question with your permission, there are now 3 studies that I am aware of and there may be more. Your patients: following gastrectomy, cholecystectomy, moderate degree of operative trauma, given glucose and amino-acids versus amino-acids alone. Dr. Wilmore's in severely burned patients in the 19-24 g of negative nitrogen balance range, and a third study as yet unpublished, but to be presented at the Surgical Tripartite Meeting the week after next from Peter Brigham Hospital by Bruce Wolfe et al. In that study, very much as you did, the amount of glucose that was provided was a little different: the same amount of protein in normal volunteers. The amounts of glucose were 150 and 600 g. Dr. Jeejeebhoy's study did not show any advantage to adding glucose to amino-acids. Dr. Wilmore's study seemed to show some advantage to adding glucose to amino-acids in proportion to the amounts added and Wolfe's study done in Dr. Moore's lab seemed to show a fractionally better nitrogen balance with 150 g of glucose and naturally with 600 g of glucose, there was a considerable improvement in nitrogen balance. I think basically, this is the area you tried to define.

BLACKBURN: First, to characterize our patients, we are talking about stress within the moderate category. There was not complete inhibition of ketone bodies. The protein-sparing effect from fat mobilization was not maximized, but the non-protein calories from body fat were in significant amounts.

I should point out that in designing parenteral therapy we should consider both risk benefits and cost benefits of therapy. This study of which I speak of includes patients in a condition in between those in the controlled starvation study of Wolfe and those maximally stressed patients that Wilmore reports on. The common practice in hospitals today is to ignore the nutritional requirements of postoperative patients with adequate nutritional reserves; those patients are treated for long periods (7-10 days) on dextrose. It does not seem wise to continue therapy that leads to substantial iatrogenic malnutrition, a condition prevalent in hospitals. Our goal is to point out the consequences of the prolonged use of hypocaloric infusions using glucose alone; we advocate the substitution of a nutrient that everybody seems to agree is quintessential – amino acids – in standard fluid and electrolyte therapy. When one adds 5% glucose, it represents an additional cost, produces hyperosmolality and vein intolerance with no demonstrated benefit. If one delays this form of nutritional support and allows nosocomial malnutrition you will have to go on intravenous hyperalimentation. Peripheral amino acid therapy will in no way replace hyperalimentation nor is it a treatment for malnutrition. Its purpose is to minimize the starved state, a condition that occurs too frequently in every hospital I've ever been in.

FISCHER: Professor Lee wants to say something.

LEE: Well, I am just a little bit bothered you see. We came here yesterday to reassure the audience that one thing they won't do after today is to allow their patients to starve to death in hospital, because they were all agreed that Prof. Dudrick, Fischer, everybody around the table have been showing you slides of how people starve to death in hospital. We all know what it looks like. You don't need a nitrogen balance to recognise a starving patient. You don't need to do any metabolic profiles at all in fact to recognise the emaciated patient. I'll reiterate, if a patient loses more than 30% of his initial body weight in an acute metabolic illness, then his chances of survival are remote.

I am fearful, therefore, because of the recent discussions, that many of you may feel that parenteral nutrition is too dangerous and that you decide not to use it. This is the very reverse of what this Symposium was meant to achieve. Clearly, there are some areas of different opinion with respect to energy substrate utilisation and influence on metabolic profiles. However, these problems should in no way interfere with the normal application of parenteral nutrition to the vast majority of patients who have need of it. If one is going to discuss stress in more detail then one should begin with often the first stage, namely, anaesthesia. Here it has been shown that the metabolic needs are entirely different from the post-trauma and later post-operative periods which we have been discussing, where indeed fat energy may be better utilised than glucose (Ref. Biebuyck, J. F. (1973) Anaesthesiology 39, 188-198). But may I re-iterate for the purposes of this Symposium we are not talking about this particular period. Furthermore, most of us would agree that during the first twenty-four hours after any major trauma or elective procedure, our preoccupation is with circulatory, acid base regulation and oxygenation homeostasis. Only after twenty-four to forty-eight hours do we really become concerned with the real problem of nutrition.

I do not think there is any real argument that there are different groups of patients who can handle either fat or carbohydrate preferentially, irrespective of time duration effects. There are those patients who cannot keto-adapt in the early stages (Smith, R., Fuller, D. J., Wedge, J. H., Williamson, D. H. and Alberti, K. G. M. M. (1975) Lancet 1, 1-3). Then other patients, such as those described by Dr. Wilmore, become fully keto acid-adapted and maybe it is unreasonable to expect they could use fat energy substrate to greater advantage. Again, reference has been made to normal controls, but I would stress we are not dealing with normals and I cannot see the relevance of making comparisons between the metabolic requirements of normal volunteers (Brennan, M. F., Fitzpatrick, G. F. Cohen, K. H. and Moore, F. D. (1975) Ann. Surg. 182, 386-393.) and the types of patients we are dealing with. A sick patient is an entirely different proposition. I would also like to stress that confusion must not be made between the metabolism of long term adapted starvation situations with a type of acute starvation problems described in our patients. I agree entirely with Dr. Blackburn that amino acids are certainly better than the old formula of a drop of water and a dash of salt, which curiously some of my peers used to think extremely valuable nutritionally!

I think, therefore, we are to a large degree agreed about our parenteral nutrition approaches according to the degrees of catabolism met with in different groups of patients. A fair idea of the catabolic rate can be gained by measuring the 24-hour urinary urea excretion and using either Blackburn's or my approach for converting into nitrogen equivalents. In the moderately catabolic group once the first thirty-six hours of resuscitation has been completed, there is general agreement that one proceeds to provide nitrogen as amino acids and appropriate quantities of energy divided 50/50 between fat and glucose calories, such as Jeejeebhoy and myself would recommend, or greater emphasis on glucose with or without insulin, if you are a Blackburn disciple. The indisputable facts about parenteral nutrition in such patients is that you do correct the metabolic abnormalities, correct the deficiencies and improve the survivorship of your patients. This is what the whole Symposium is about.

It is an entirely different matter when one considers some of the implications of liverslice work, which no doubt does have bearing on the greater metabolic problems. But this should not prevent us from applying what is known *now* to the improved management of our patients. There can be no excuse for allowing patients to starve to death, for the appropriate ways of treating them are available and can be applied with a fair degree of clinical acumen only in the absence of large laboratory back-ups. Obviously, it is nicer if you have good laboratory back-up services but if you don't, then assess your patient on a day by day basis and with the simple measurement of urinary urea nitrogen production, one can have a fair assessment of degree of catabolism one is coping with and treat accordingly. Therefore, I plead let's think about the nutritional requirements of our patients if they are seen to be in need, let's treat them and where parenteral nutrition is indicated, let's use it because it does work, it can be extraordinarily safe, though one would not minimise that complications can occur if one is not careful.

SHIZGAL – MONTREAL: With your permission I would like to show a few slides. During the past several years we have investigated many of the areas which the panel has been discussing this morning. In order to avoid the problems normally associated with nitrogen balance we have employed a multiple isotope dilution technique to quantitate the various components of

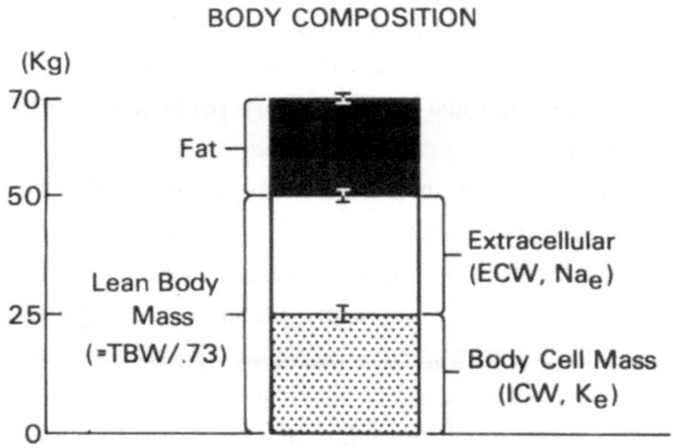

Figure 15.

body composition (Fig. 15). The total body water volume is obtained by measuring the volume of distribution of tritiated water. The lean body mass is then calculated by assuming that it is equal to total body water divided by 0.73. Body fat is subsequently calculated as the difference between body weight and the lean body mass. The lean body mass is divided into two major components; the body cell mass and the extracellular mass. The body cell mass is the most important component of body composition, at least from our view point, as it is the total mass of living, functioning, oxygen consuming cells in the body. The size of the body cell mass is estimated by measuring either the intracellular water volume or the total exchangeable potassium. Both of the latter parameters are linearly related to the size of the body cell mass. The extracellular supporting component of body composition can also be estimated by measuring either the extracellular water volume or total exchangeable sodium.

I would now like to show you body composition data which supports the protein sparing hypothesis first proposed by Dr. Blackburn. Two groups, of 19 patients each, were studied. The first group received all of their intravenous fluids and electrolytes as a 5% glucose solution. The patients in the second group received all their intravenous water and electrolytes as a 5% casein hydrolysate (Amigen) solution. Thus, isocaloric infusions were administered to both groups. All of the patients, in both groups, underwent either a gastrectomy or colon resection, i.e., an elective operation of moderate severity. To assess the effects of the two intravenous solutions administered, body composition measurements were performed preoperatively and on the fifth post-operative day. The following results were obtained (Fig. 16).

Change in body composition

	Glucose	Amigen
Body weight (kg)	-2.6 ± 0.6*	-2.0 ± 0.5*
Body fat (kg)	-1.9 ± 0.9*	-3.7 ± 0.6*
Lean body mass (kg)	-0.8 ± 0.6	$+1.8 \pm 0.7$*

* $p < .05$

Figure 16.

In both groups there was a decrease in body weight, which was statistically significant, and of similar magnitude. However, in the two groups, changes in different components of body composition were responsible for the weight changes observed. In the patients who received glucose, body weight decreased by 2.6 kg secondary to a decrease in the lean body mass and body fat. In contrast, in the patients receiving the amino acid solutions following operation, a similar loss of body weight was experienced post-operatively. However, this entire loss of body weight resulted from a loss of body fat. The lean body mass actually increased slightly. However, this increase was not statistically significant. The differences between the two solutions are even more striking if one looks at the changes which occurred in the two major components of the lean body mass (Fig. 17). In the glucose group there was a significant decrease in the exchangeable potassium and intracellular water, both are excellent measures of the body cell mass. In contrast a similar decrease in the body cell mass was not seen following operation in the Amigen group. In fact, there was a slight increase in exchangeable potassium post-operatively. However, this change was not statistically significant.

These changes are summarized on the next slide (Fig. 18). The patients, who received amino acids intravenously following operation, experienced a slight decrease in body weight secondary to a loss of body fat. Both the extracellular mass and the body cell mass remained unchanged. In contrast, in the glucose group, there was a similar decrease in body weight post-operatively. This loss of body weight was secondary to the loss of body fat and a decrease in the lean body mass. The decrease in the lean body mass did not totally reflect the loss of body cell mass since these patients also experienced a significant expansion of the extracellular mass. The concomitant extracellular expansion with a loss of body cell mass, is characteristic of malnutrition and is reflected by the ratio of exchangeable sodium to exchangeable potassium (Fig. 19).

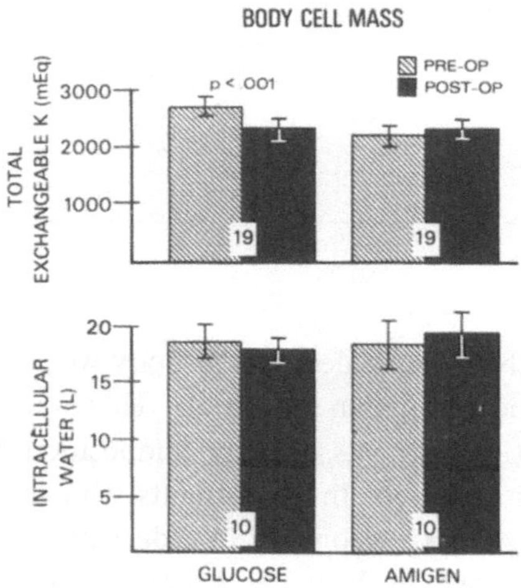

Figure 17.

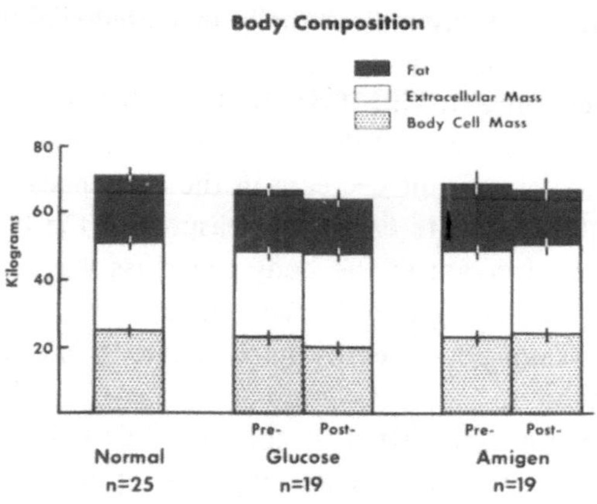

Figure 18.

In our experience, this ratio was an accurate measure of nutritional status. In 25 normal volunteers this ratio was almost unity with a small standard error. A similar ratio was obtained in both patient groups preoperatively. The ratio remained unchanged in the patients receiving amino acids postoperatively. However, this ratio significantly increased in the glucose group. Thus a minor degree of malnutrition occurred in the patients undergoing an elective operation of moderate severity who received intravenous solutions containing glucose. The infusion of protein prevented this from occurring.

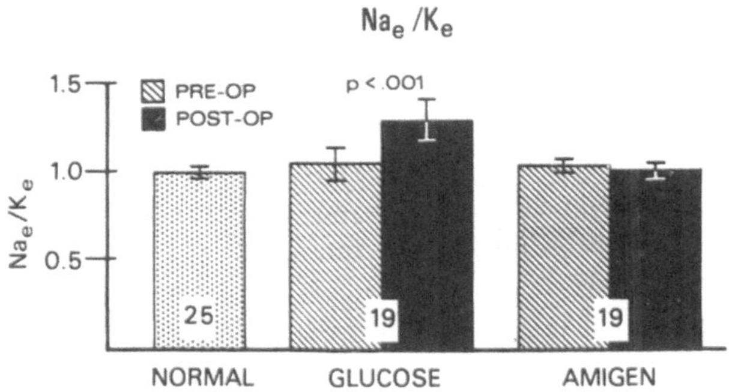

Figure 19.

The next slide (Fig. 20) is for Dr. Lee's benefit. We recently carried out a study to determine the caloric requirements of patients receiving total parenteral nutrition. Body composition measurements were performed prior to, and following a period of total parenteral nutrition. The mean daily change in exchangeable potassium was plotted against the mean kcal/kg infused per day. A statistically significant relationship was obtained with an intercept of 46 kcal/kg/day. This is the same figure which Dr. Lee obtained on the slide which he showed earlier today. This data therefore indicates that in the average patient requiring total parenteral nutrition, nutritional balance is achieved when 46 kcal/kg/day is infused. Furthermore, the infusion of calories in excess of this amount will result in a re-building of a depleted body cell mass.

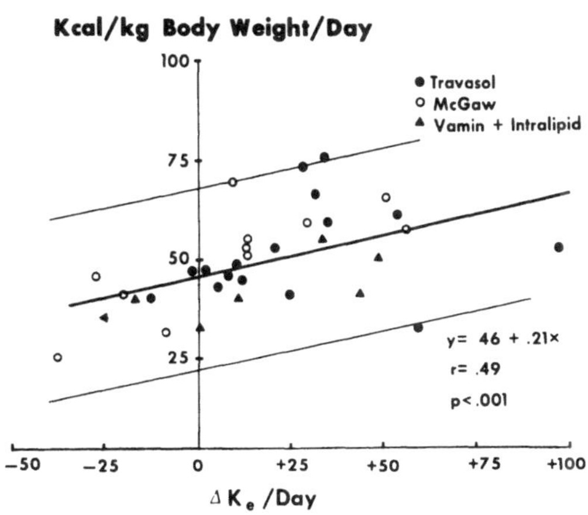

Figure 20.

FISCHER: Are there any other comments about the issues we have discussed, if not we will go on to some questions from the floor. There are two questions of practical nature – surprisingly. They both concern the mixing of fat, amino-acids and carbohydrate. One concerns the storage of mixture in polyvinylchloride bags at 4°C, and the question is: I have heard that the fat particles become greater after 2-3 days. Have you any experience in the stability of fat emulsion presumably under these circumstances?

WRETLIND: Intralipid is quite stable from physical and chemical point of view. It is a general recommendation not to add anything but fat soluble vitamins to Intralipid to prevent any possible interactions. However, it has been shown by Prof. Solassol and Dr. Joyeux in Montpellier, that Intralipid is stable enough to be mixed with the regular infusion solutions for intravenous nutrition containing aminoacids, glucose and all other nutrients (*Solassol and Joyeux*, Ann. Anesth. Franç. Spécial II, pp. 75-86, 1974). Such mixtures have been stored for several months. The changes of the particle size and of other parameters investigated have been negligible. The reason why we don't recommend this type of mixing is that it has to be handled by experts in order to prevent any interactions and bacteriological contaminations. Each single container of the mixture has to be investigated from bacteriological point of view because the mixture can not be heat-sterilized.

FISCHER: Another question along the same line is: apparently the questioner, who has not identified himself – suggests that there is a difference in the site of entry between your system and Prof. Lee's system, which I think is caused by the schematic presentation you gave. They both enter at the same site?

WRETLIND: Yes, about the same.

FISCHER: Next question concerns trace elements. What trace elements must be added to TPN, what is their dosage, can you expect deficiency states in the absence of trace elements in TPN. What are they and after what time do they appear?

JEEJEEBHOY: I think in objective terms, a part of this remains poorly explored. I will not say unexplored, but poorly explored and several groups, including ourselves, are involved in this. The answer to the first is, yes, trace elements are necessary. And to answer your second question, do you meet deficiency – of course you do. Zinc deficiency is known to produce a specific form of skin rash which is very characteristic, and has been corrected specifically by giving zinc. Copper deficiency produces neutropenia and anemia.

Chromium deficiency which we have observed after very long periods of TPN in patients produces diabetes and neuropathy. The other elements like manganese and cobalt and many others are unexplored. I may add that there is also the opposite situation that we noticed in patients with liver disease, the inability to excrete manganese and in fact their blood manganese levels may rise in some cases to unacceptable levels. This is particularly true if you use a solution like Amigen, which is pretty high in manganese. Thus one may see both sides of the story in certain situations.

WILMORE: I think again that you have to characterize the type of patients you are talking about. Dr. Jeejeebhoy has excellent data on a series of very long-term patients that he has carefully followed over a long-term period.

In practical terms, phosphorus and zinc are two of the more common deficiencies that are seen. We have not had the fat emulsion in the U.S. for some time and so people have talked about essential fatty acid deficiencies, which is another trace nutrient deficiency, but in terms of phosphate and zinc, those are the common things which we see in our acutely ill and injured patients.

WRETLIND: I should like to speak in favour of a complete intravenous feeding as an alternative to an adequate oral food intake. It seems not to be any reason to give a patient an incomplete or unbalanced parenteral nutrition and just wait until deficiency symptoms occur. It might be correct as Dr. Wilmore said that in general you don't see any deficiency symptoms in patients on parenteral nutrition. The reason is that such symptoms appear only after the patient has been a few weeks on parenteral nutrition. But, then, you will have a patient, who needs to be repleted with the missing nutrient. In some situations it might be difficult both to reach the correct diagnosis and to make the repletion. It is always much easier to prevent the deficiencies than to cure them. From a practical point of view, there is nowadays no problem to supply all essential nutrients intravenously. The use of an incomplete parenteral nutrition will result in deficiency symptoms, which may be called iatrogenic malnutrition and which only prove well-known nutritional facts, of no use for the patients.

LEE: Could I just make a comment. I entirely agree with what Dr. Wilmore has said about zinc and phosphorus deficiencies probably being the most common ones that we meet. I would just like to comment on the changing scene with respect to potential hypophosphataemia as seen in the United Kingdom. Hitherto, because casein hydrolysates were used which happens to contain over half a gram of phosphate per liter (though never admitted on the labels) phosphate provision was made unwittingly. Now, with the more refined crystalline aminoacid solutions available in the United Kingdom and, of course, in many other parts of Europe, which do not contain inorganic phosphate, hypophosphataemia is beginning to occur even when Intralipid is used as part energy substrate. This is an interesting observation for hitherto it has been assumed that all the Intralipid phospholipid phosphorus was available for metabolic utilisation. However, our recent studies (Tovey, S. J., Benton, K. G. F., and Lee, H. A. (1977) Postgraduate Med. Journal 53, June Issue) cast some doubt on the bioavailability of phospholipid phosphorus. Furthermore, our studies suggest that the daily recommended allowances of phosphorus for the type of catabolic patients we are referring to, have been set too low and we recommend that 0.5 to 0.75 mmols of phosphorus per kg body weight per day, be added to intravenous regimens preferably as some form of inorganic phosphate solution (in the U.K. Boots Neutral Phosphate Solution).

JEEJEEBHOY: In our TPN mixture, we have used the following combination – 3 mg zinc and 1.6 of copper, 2 of manganese and 2 micrograms of chromium, plus selenium and iodine (Iron is given intramuscularly). These amounts were gleaned from known or published data concerning absorption of the amounts available in a diet. In other words, these were ballpark figures which we derived from summarizing the work of Sandstead (Ref: Sandstead, H. H., Burk, R. F., Booth, G. H., Jr. and Darby, W. J. Current concepts of trace minerals. Clinical considerations. Med. Clin. North Amer. *54*: 1509-1531 (1970), Underwood (Ref: Underwood, E. J. Trace elements in human and animal nutrition. Acad. Press, N.Y. and London, (1971) and several other workers in such dietary studies. Thus we gave amounts based on what normal diets should contain and the percentage absorption. Obviously, there are many errors in this kind of computation.

Table: We have looked at the results of 6 patients in whom the TPN had been given for at least 1 year and in some instances up to 5 years at the time of measurement, and you can see they have normal levels of zinc, normal levels of copper, slightly increased levels of manganese and slightly

Table Circulating levels of trace elements*

Patient no.	Plasma		Blood	
	Zn	Cu	Mn	Cr
	μg/dl		ng/ml	
1	110.9	155.5	19.1	3.38
3	105.6	155.5	19.1	
5	105.6	164.4	28.5	1.84
6	105.0	192.5	35.7	3.84
11	100.3	129.6	20.3	2.76
12	192.5	92.5	29.7	1.84
Mean ± SEM	120.0 ± 14.5	148.3 ± 13.9	25.4 ± 2.8	2.73 ± 0.40
Normal range	70–127	69–145	3.0–13.8	4.9–9.5

* September to October 1975

decreased levels of chromium. I will not go into it as it is a subject by itself, but it will appear in the American Journal of Clinical Nutrition *30*: 531-538 (1977). Basically this patient requires ± 20 micrograms of chromium per day. But I may say that the chromium deficiency was only seen after 3 years on total parenteral nutrition. There is one other factor that needs to be explored. Beisel's group (Diabetes *24*: 350-353 (1975) showed that there is a septic-induced chromium deficiency in patients who had been given sandfly fever experimentally. There was glucose intolerance with low concentrations of chromium in blood and a poor response to administered chromium in these patients. The suggestion was that in the septic state chromium may be of great importance. Now that is something which has to be looked at more carefully. This is as far as we have gone.

I'd also like to point out one other thing. We have recently manipulated the zinc levels in the TPN system and I can tell you that the blood zinc levels have no reflection whatever on the zinc balance and looking at literature, I believe this is true. So, you cannot diagnose zinc deficiency purely on plasma concentrations and in fact when the levels go low, the patient is very seriously sick. This has not been explored for copper and other elements so we dont's really know how general this may be.

FISCHER: Another question: which kind of nutritional support will the panel advise for critically ill renal transplant recipients, with septic complications, whether pulmonary or abscesses; are they correlated with a depressed immunologic state or are they result of their former renal insufficiency or a result of prednisone and azathopirine therapy.

LEE: Our Transplant Unit, which has now been operating for five years, has a patient survival rate of 88% which is the best recorded as far as I know of. As far as our regular haemodialysis patients go, they are not malnourished, thus when they are transplanted, they are in excellent nutritional status. My view is, if they do become malnourished, then they are not being properly treated. Therefore, to the transplant patients you give more protein as required and dialysis as required. Of course, you must give them adequate calories and often dialysis time can be used for the provision of further intravenous nitrogen and energy. There is quite an extensive literature on this topic and I would refer the questioner to two recent issues of Clinical Nephrology (Clinical Nephrology (1975) 3, No. 5, and 3, No. 6) in which the dietary requirements of patients on regular dialysis treatment are discussed in detail.

To continue with your question on the post-transplant patient, we use the pulse therapy system where on days 3, 5 and 7 post transplant, we give 2 gms of methyl prednisolone intravenously as part of their immunosuppressive regimen. Our patients, once transplanted, go on to entirely free diets and less then 5% of our patients actually require any intravenous nutrition. They are not in a bad state, at least in our Unit. If indeed you do have a problem with gross sepsis or haematoma formation in the persistently oliguric post-transplant patient, then a case can be made for wanting to delay the first haemodialysis by using the regimen offered by Dr. Fischer and Dr. R. Abel as published in the New England Journal of Medicine, 1973. Certainly, in that situation I would not hesitate to put in a subclavian vein catheter and start feeding parenterally completely with either a glucose-insulin regimen, together with Intralipid in the way I described to you earlier, together with amino acids. The actual nitrogen intake here may appear to be a little less than optimum bearing in mind the massive doses of steroids they are on and it works out at the level of something like 0.12 gms nitrogen per kg body weight. This is somewhat surprisingly lower than in our non-renal failure non-transplanted patients. But I really do not see that the post-transplant patient creates a fundamentally different problem to the sort of immunosuppressed patient that Professor Dudrick was talking about yesterday. I have heard this question posed before and it always amazes me that they should be thought of as constituting a different group. Their nutritional requirements, if they are passing urine, are the same as anybody elses. If they are not passing urine and they are oliguric and you are wanting to delay haemodialysis because of some bleeding problem, then use a Fischer Regimen as I have just referred to.

FISCHER: I just cannot resist the temptation to say that in fact the data you were referring to Dr. Lee, when referring to Dr. Abel's and my data yesterday, were expressing the amount of nitrogen per bottle, not the amount of nitrogen the patients got on a daily basis and the amount the patients get on daily basis is really quite remarkably similar – about anywhere from 2200-3000 calories in renal failure patients and between 22-26 grams of amino-acids and you go up to 35 gr. So, it is not really very different.

FISCHER: There is another question which has been previously asked: heparin enhances Intralipid clearing. This is a statement from Dr. Gevers in Rotterdam. So does any of you use heparin to be able to infuse more Intralipid without inducing lipemia?

WRETLIND: Heparin has been used in order to increase the elimination rate of Intralipid from the blood stream. This fact does not mean that more Intralipid can be given. The general trend is not to add heparin to Intralipid. I should very much like to know the opinion of my clinical colleague Dr. Harry Lee concerning the use of heparin in connection with the infusions of Intralipid.

LEE: It certainly is not my practice to add heparin to Intralipid, but I cannot see the logic in fact. All you do is clear a little faster, you don't in fact utilize more and again a word of warning, that in the uremic situation this is one example of where the post heparin lipolytic activities are totally inhibited and using heparin is only going to cause hemorrhage. You won't cause better lipid utilization. To start doing that, you are adding more things to your lipid bottle. I personally – it's the one thing I say quite clearly to my nursing staff, and junior staff "Thou shalt not add anything to the lipid emulsion in case of cracking it up", and I think that is a safety precaution that should be adhered to and I see no rationale for using heparin. That is a personal view.

FISCHER: The second element of the question: do any of you use heparin to prevent thrombosis of the vein in which the catheter is placed? If you do, what is your dose and if you don't, why not?

BLACKBURN: We add heparin to hyperalimentation solutions given in a central venous catheter because our most dreaded complication is subclavian vein thrombosis. Thrombosis is one problem that discourages our colleagues who do not appreciate that the risk of hyperalimentation is justified. I am not sure of the effects of heparin. In the peripheral vein I use an activated form of steroid such as hydrocortisone in subclinical doses of 5 mg/liter when administering parenteral solutions of 750 mOsm. This has been shown to decrease the inflammation and represents a hardware technique that can keep peripheral veins going when you have a hypertonic solution.

WILMORE: Realistically, a number of critically ill patients receive subclinical doses of heparin. So I have never considered it to prevent subclavian thrombosis, as I look at the patient population that I cared for in the past year.

LEE: At the International Heparin Meeting in London in July, 1975, it was shown by the International Collaborative Study (Kakkar, V. V. and Corrigan, T. P. (1976) in Heparin-Chemistry and Clinical Usage Eds. Kakkar, V. V. and Thomas, D. P. p. 229-245, Academic Press Ltd. London) that using subcutaneous heparin, 5000 units b.d. per day post-operatively or the immediate seven days post myocardial infarction, dramatically reduced the incidence of pulmonary emboli. The results were drawn from large numbers of patients. Professor Bonnar (Bonnar, J. (1976) ibid p. 247-260) showed a similar beneficial effect of subcutaneous heparin during the last trimester of pregnancy, where in the U.K. it has been shown that pulmonary emboli is still an important cause of maternal death. I would entirely agree that subcutaneous heparin can do no harm, in fact it has been shown to do good, is a perfectly safe dose to use and what is more important, does not require special monitoring.

FISCHER: Just a word of caution – I don't really know whether heparin added to the bottle really stays in that form or is inactivated. Dick Giovannoni and John Webb of our pharmacy have done a number of studies on what happens to materials added to a bottle of hypertonic glucose and aminoacids (things like digoxin, antibiotics etc.). They were broken down in a very short period of time, so whether or not heparin really stays unchanged in the bottle I do not know.

One gentleman I was talking with yesterday, did say that by adding heparin to the bottle they had dramatically decreased their incidence of subclavian thrombosis. That may be well so.

PARTICIPANT: That was me. It was not the subclavian vein thrombosis, but clotting of the catheter.

FISCHER: I think clotting of the catheter is not much of a problem, I think what we are really concerned with is subclavian vein thrombosis. It may very well be that you need a different type of material other than p.v.c. which is less reactive.

FISCHER: One additional question: does anyone here give total parenteral nutrition to new-borns, in the umbilical vein or artery and how long do they do so?

I personally have seen 2 cases of aortic thrombosis secondary to administration of hypertonic dextrose solution into the umbilical artery and I think it is a practice which should be condemned.

DUDRICK: I think that is in the umbilical artery and I think the same can be said of the umbilical vein. The incidence of late omphalitis with all of its disastrous complications like bleeding varices etc. could probably be rather high, don't you think so?

JANSSEN, *Belgium*: Are amino-acids metabolized in a different way when they are given intravenously instead of given orally?

MUNRO: One would think that they would be, but in fact the Swedish group (Fürst et al., 1970)* did a study about 7-8 years ago. Volunteers were given intravenous mixtures and also by mouth. At first, the oral nitrogen balance was less favourable than the intravenous; the reason for that was that the oral dose was given so quickly that the liver responded by making urea. When they slowed down the drip to the same rate as the intravenous drip, then there was no difference between the balance by the two routes. So the answer would be that the body compensates even if you do not give it via the portal vein.

FISCHER: There appears to be an increase in splanchnic blood flow in Dr. Heberg's studies with certain aminoacids given by vein. What the significance of this is, I don't know, but maybe someone else does.

WILMORE: Increased oxygen consumption occurs in the liver and is associated with the specific dynamic effect of aminoacids. This is a very nice tech-

* Fürst, P., Jonsson, A., Josephson, B. and Vinnars, E., Distribution in muscle and liver vein protein of ^{15}N administered as ammonium acetate to man. *J. Appl. Physiol. 29*: 307 (1970).

nique for increasing visceral heat production and increasing splanchnic blood flow.

FISCHER: Dr. Blackburn suggests that we should say something about the different catheter materials. There are silastic catheters available and there is a vicral type of catheter available in the U.S. I would say that our experience with that as far as thrombosis concerns, even in people who have previously thrombosed one subclavian vein, has been very good. The problem is the catheter is very difficult to fix in place, it kinks easily and you have to use a wire suture to do so which apparently many people do not like or really don't know about, so that has been a problem with catheters falling out. The study in dogs which are certainly different from patients as far as their clotting systems are concerned, leave no doubt that silastic or teflon or some type of non-reactive material are superior to p.v.c. I think the problem is engineering, of getting the catheter that has all the desirable characteristics that you want: short bevel, easy placement, radio-opaque, easy to fix, doesn't fall out, doesn't kink, drive the nurses crazy. This is a large number of characteristics to achieve with a small thing.

LEE: There was a very nice paper published earlier this year (Dinley, R. J. (1976) Current Med. Research and Opinion 3, 607-617) which I recommend you read, reviewing the incidence of phlebothrombosis as opposed to the septic complications with i.v. catheters. A much higher incidence was found with p.v.c. catheters than with the teflon type. Furthermore the important question of plasticizers in p.v.c. (di-2-ethylhexyphthalate) was also reviewed and may have some bearing on the production of phlebothrombosis. Another important point brought out in this paper was something that both Dr. Fischer and Miss Colley referred to earlier, was that one should never use the feeding line for giving other than parenteral nutrients, whenever possible. It has been clearly shown that the incidence of phlebothrombosis rises rapidly when blood is passed through a feeding catheter. This is a very important practical point to bear in mind.

Silastic based and furthermore there is an important question of plasticizers with a thallic component which seems to be very much involved in producing the phlebothrombosis and the other point to find in his paper was something Dr. Fischer mentioned yesterday and I know Miss Colley too has never used your feeding line for other things like plasma or blood. Because certainly you would find a rapidly increased incidence of phlebothrombosis when blood has been passed through that feeding catheter. So, it is a very important point to bear in mind.

JEEJEEBHOY: We have in our long-term TPN patients, 3 deaths and in those patients who have survived on this between 1 and 3 years, we have looked at the catheter at post-mortem and this is a patient who died of intercurrent pneumonia and this catheter had been in place for 3 years and this is the superior vena cava dissection specimen. You can see that the silastic catheter in this particular system seems to be quite non-reactive and we have confirmed this in 2 other patients although not for as long as this. So that there may be some virtue in using the silastic catheter.

FISCHER: I can confirm that, that is an observation that a number of people have made.

BLACKBURN: I have had one thrombosis on a silastic catheter. Dr. Broviac included it in his series. Interesting in that case, we subsequently used the stilette contained in a black silicone rubber catheter (Vicra USA) and drove it through the thrombosis to continue the hyperalimentation. In that patient, we kept the silicone catheter in for 1 year before returning to surgery. I am sure there will be an increasing role for the silicone rubber catheters to play even for short-term use. Another thing is that it is now possible to bind heparin to polyethyline and in other catheter material. This is encouraging to us in our effort to prevent thrombosis.

Index

TPN = Total Parenteral Nutrition.